Chronic Obstructive Pulmonary Disease

COPD

Chronic Obstructive Pulmonary Disease

COPD

Amit Kumar Verma
MBBS, MD (Pulmonary Medicine), MAMS

Associate Professor
Division of TB and Chest
Department of Medicine
University College of Medical Sciences
(University of Delhi)
Delhi

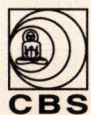

CBS

CBS Publishers & Distributors Pvt Ltd

New Delhi • Bengaluru • Chennai • Kochi • Kolkata • Mumbai
Bhopal • Bhubaneswar • Hyderabad • Jharkhand • Nagpur • Patna • Pune • Uttarakhand • Dhaka (Bangladesh)

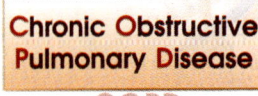

Chronic Obstructive Pulmonary Disease
COPD

ISBN: 978-93-87964-84-6

Copyright © Author and Publisher

First Edition: 2019

Published by Satish Kumar Jain and Produced by Varun Jain for

CBS Publishers & Distributors Pvt Ltd

4819/XI Prahlad Street, 24 Ansari Road, Daryaganj, New Delhi 110 002, India.
Ph: 23289259, 23266861, 23266867   Fax: 011-23243014   Website: www.cbspd.com
e-mail: delhi@cbspd.com; cbspubs@airtelmail.in.

Corporate Office: 204 FIE, Industrial Area, Patparganj, Delhi 110 092
Ph: 4934 4934   Fax: 4934 4935   e-mail: publishing@cbspd.com; publicity@cbspd.com

Branches

- **Bengaluru:** Seema House 2975, 17th Cross, K.R. Road,
  Banasankari 2nd Stage, Bengaluru 560 070, Karnataka
  Ph: +91-80-26771678/79   Fax: +91-80-26771680   e-mail: bangalore@cbspd.com
- **Chennai:** 7, Subbaraya Street, Shenoy Nagar, Chennai 600 030, Tamil Nadu
  Ph: +91-44-26680620, 26681266   Fax: +91-44-42032115   e-mail: chennai@cbspd.com
- **Kochi:** 42/1325, 1326, Power House Road, Opp. KSEB Power House
  Ernakulam 682 018, Kochi, Kerala
  Ph: +91-484-4059061-65   Fax: +91-484-4059065   e-mail: kochi@cbspd.com
- **Kolkata:** 6/B, Ground Floor, Rameswar Shaw Road, Kolkata-700 014, West Bengal
  Ph: +91-33-22891126, 22891127, 22891128   e-mail: kolkata@cbspd.com
- **Mumbai:** 83-C, Dr E Moses Road, Worli, Mumbai-400018, Maharashtra
  Ph: +91-22-24902340/41   Fax: +91-22-24902342   e-mail: mumbai@cbspd.com

Representatives

• Bhopal	0-8319310552	• Bhubaneswar	0-9911037372	• Hyderabad	0-9885175004	• Jharkhand	0-9811541605
• Nagpur	0-9021734563	• Patna	0-9334159340	• Pune	0-9623451994	• Uttarakhand	0-9716462459
• Dhaka (Bangladesh)	01912-003485						

Printed at Goyal Offset Printers, GT Karnal Road, Industrial Area, Delhi, India

to

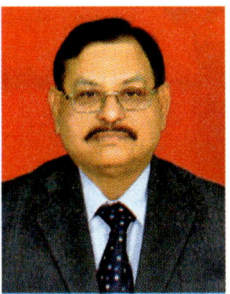

Prof (Dr) Sudhir Chaudhari
my mentor and guide

गुरुर ब्रह्म गुरुर विष्णु, गुरुर देवो महेश्वरः
गुरुः साक्षातपरम ब्रह्म तस्मै श्री गुरुवे नमः

Contributors

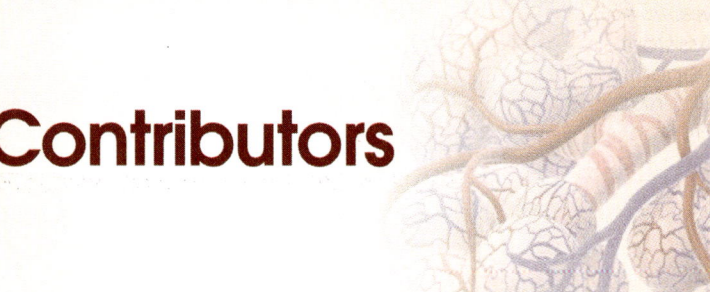

Adesh Kumar
MBBS, MD (Respiratory Medicine)
Professor
Department of Respiratory Medicine
UP University of Medical Sciences , Saifai
Etawah
Uttar Pradesh

Aditya Kumar Gautam
MBBS, MD (Respiratory Medicine)
Assistant Professor
Department of Respiratory Medicine
UP University of Medical Sciences, Saifai
Etawah, Uttar Pradesh

Ajay Kumar Verma
MBBS, MD (Respiratory Medicine)
Associate Professor
Respiratory Medicine
King George's Medical University
Lucknow
Uttar Pradesh

Amir Maroof Khan
MBBS, MD (Community Medicine)
Associate Professor
Department of Community Medicine
University College of Medical Sciences
Delhi

Amit Kumar Verma
MBBS, MD (Respiratory Medicine), MAMS
Associate Professor
Division of TB and Chest
Department of Medicine
University College of Medical Sciences
Delhi

Anand Kumar
MBBS, MD (Respiratory Medicine)
Associate Professor and Head
GSVM Medical College
Kanpur
Uttar Pradesh

Anubhuti Singh
MBBS
Department of Respiratory Medicine
King George's Medical University
Lucknow
Uttar Pradesh

Apoorva Tomar
MBBS
Postgraduate Student
Department of Medicine
University College of Medical Sciences
Delhi

Arpita Singh
MBBS, MD (Pharmacology)
Assistant Professor
Department of Pharmacology
Government Medical College
Kannauj
Uttar Pradesh

Arun Sampath
MD (Respiratory Medicine)
Senior Consultant
Miot Hospital
Chennai
Tamil Nadu

Ashish Kumar Gupta
MBBS, MD (Respiratory Medicine)
Assistant Professor
Department of Respiratory Medicine
UP University of Medical Sciences
Etawah
Uttar Pradesh

Ashok Kumar Singh
MBBS, MD (Respiratory Medicine)
Professor
Department of TB and Chest
Lady Hardinge Medical College
Delhi

Harender Singh
MBBS, MD (Respiratory Medicine)
Junior Resident
Department of Respiratory Medicine
UP University of Medical Sciences
Etawah, Uttar Pradesh

Hemant Kumar Aggarwal
MD (Respiratory Medicine)
Assistant Professor
Department of Pulmonary Medicine
Institute of Liver and Biliary Sciences
Delhi

Jasmeet Kaur
Assistant Dietician
Department of Dietics
Guru Teg Bahadur Hospital
Delhi

Kamlesh Sethi
Senior Dietician
Department of Dietics
Guru Teg Bahadur Hospital
Delhi

Mayank Agarwal
MBBS
Junior Resident
Department of Physiology
King George's Medical University
Lucknow, Uttar Pradesh

Nishtha Singh
MBBS
Subharti Medical College
Meerut
Uttar Pradesh

Prashant Yadav
MBBS, MD (Respiratory Medicine)
Senior Resident
Department of Respiratory Medicine
UP University of Medical Sciences
Etawah
Uttar Pradesh

Priyanka Gogoi
MBBS, MD (Pathology)
Associate Professor
Department of Pathology
University College of Medical Sciences
Delhi

Riddhi Jaiswal
MBBS, MD (Pathology)
Department of Pathology
King George's Medical University
Lucknow
Uttar Pradesh

Shiva Narang
MBBS, MD (General Medicine)
Associate Professor
Department of Medicine
University College of Medical Sciences
Delhi

Shraddha Singh
MBBS, MD (Physiology)
Professor
Department of Physiology
King George's Medical University
Lucknow, Uttar Pradesh

VG Prabhu Ramnath
MBBS, DNB, DTCD, FCCP
Consultant Pulmonologist
Sri Gokulam Hospital
Salem, Tamil Nadu

Foreword

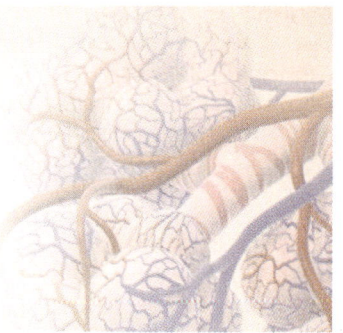

I am delighted to write the Foreword to this book. As a teacher in the field of respiratory medicine, I felt that COPD in itself is not a single disease, rather it is a group of diseases. Hence, better we refer it as chronic obstructive pulmonary syndrome in place of chronic obstructive pulmonary disease, to highlight the nature of this disease affecting many organ systems of the body.

To help in achieving excellence in management of patients with COPD, this book beautifully deals with all the aspects right from epidemiology, physiology and pathology to recent advances in management.

This book will be a great help to postgraduate students, teachers and practitioners in the field of pulmonary medicine. The contributors have full knowledge of subject and hence very efficiently dealt with respective topics and details.

Indian literature is lacking in various aspects of COPD and this book enthusiastically fills this gap. A few things which attracted me of this book are use of language which is easily understandable by Indian practitioners, chapters on physiotherapy and yoga, nutrition, discharge and prevention of COPD patient. These chapters are hard to find in other available books on COPD.

Dr Amit Kumar Verma is an excellent teacher and clinician. He has thoroughly evaluated the subject and hence given the best efforts in bringing forth the recent updates on COPD through this book.

Rajendra Prasad

MD, DTCD, FAMS, FCCP (USA), FRCP (GLASG), WHO Fellow (Japan)
FNCCP (India), FICS, FCAI, FIAB, FIMSA, FCCS, DSC (Hon. Causa)
Certificate in Respiratology (Japan), Certificate in Thoracic Oncology (Mumbai)
Dr BC Roy National Awardee
Director, Medical Education, and
Head, Department of Pulmonary Medicine
Era's Lucknow Medical College and Hospital, Lucknow
former Director, Vallabhai Patel Chest Institute, Delhi
former Director, UP Rural Institute of Medical Science and Research, Saifai
former Professor and Head, Department of Pulmonary Medicine, KGMU, Lucknow

Preface

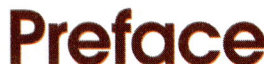

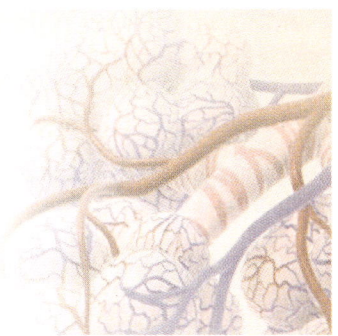

COPD is one of the commonest diseases presenting in any physician's clinic. In spite of this, its understanding and management varies. When a physician is willing to gain knowledge about COPD, he has to refer to the books on respiratory medicine, journal articles, and available guidelines. But all these provide knowledge which is in piecemeal and scattered. On the top of that, most of the literature is written in the Western context, which many a times found difficult to be followed by the Indian physicians. Hence, there was need of a book which will give wholesome knowledge on COPD while keeping in mind the socioeconomic scenario in India.

This book aims to cover all topics related to COPD, right from physiology and pathology to the recent advances. The special interest is in management of COPD, which takes the lion's share of the book. While going through this book one may find that there is repetition of certain facts as each chapter is written by different authors, and while editing this book it is maintained so that readers get insight to see the same thing from different angles and at last there is no doubt in mind.

Let me mention a few facts in the epidemiology chapter, here data is presented as 'thousands/lakhs/crore' against the 'million/billion/trillion' format. This enables our readers to put no efforts to understand the facts.

In the chapter on physiology I have tried to give details of various processes which occur in patients with COPD, and in pathology, the inflammation in COPD is discussed in detail including oxidative stress.

When students want to read about comorbidities in COPD, again data is very much scattered. Although I have tried to explain comorbidities but it may not be complete. The main stress point for this chapter is that the readers must be able to suspect these illnesses in patients of COPD and should be able to provide timely management of comorbidities at least at the first level of contact with healthcare system.

I have also given in-depth knowledge of physiotherapy, yoga and nutrition in COPD. It is expected that after going through these chapters physicians will be able to know about how to prescribe them in COPD patients.

In the chapter on prevention, along with smoking cessation, I have given stress to vaccination for exacerbation prevention and special mention of Pradhan Mantri Ujjwala Yojana (PMUY) is made so that a doctor can easily guide his poor patients as to how to get the benefit of PMUY and make their life smoke-free.

In the chapter on recent advances and future, special attention is being made to upcoming molecules, with detailed description about them and their place in current clinical practice.

At last I hope that this book will help the physician manage COPD better and will be able to create a new hope in the life of patients.

Amit Kumar Verma

Acknowledgements

First of all thanks to Lord Hanuman for choosing me to write this book **Chronic Obstructive Pulmonary Disease.**

I acknowledge my teachers and seniors at my alma mater KGMU, Lucknow, and GSVM Medical College, Kanpur, from where I learnt basic and advanced skills in the field of medical sciences. I specially thank my mentor Prof Sudhir Chaudhari for grooming me in the field of respiratory medicine.

I would like to express my gratitude to the contributors spread over the entire country, who have shared their knowledge and put tremendous efforts by contributing their chapters. I also appreciate their patience and kind-heartedness to incorporate my comments in the chapters.

I acknowledge Mr SK Jain (CMD) and Mr Varun Jain (Director), CBS Publishers & Distributors Pvt. Ltd, and Mr YN Arjuna (Senior Vice President—Publishing, Editorial and Publicity) along with his entire team who entrusted me on writing this book and also thank them for decent and aesthetic formatting of this book, and Mr Sunil Dutt (Promotion and Development Manager).

I would like to thank Dr Rajneesh Awasthi, Professor and Head, Department of Medicine, and senior faculty members and my colleagues of the UCMS, Delhi, for creating a conducive environment so that this book could be conceived.

I also want to thank my family, who supported and encouraged me in spite of all the time it took me away from them.

Last, I pray to God for his love, blessings and enable me to write this book and more worthy for his world.

Amit Kumar Verma

Contents

Contributors   vi

Foreword by Rajendra Prasad   viii

Preface   ix

Abbreviations   xv

Section I: Basics of COPD

1. **Epidemiology**   3
   Amir Maroof Khan

2. **Physiology**   13
   Shraddha Singh, Mayank Agarwal, Nishtha Singh, Ajay Verma

3. **Pathology**   31
   Riddhi Jaiswal, Priyanka Gogoi

4. **Diagnosis**   48
   Anand Kumar, Shraddha Singh, Amit Kumar Verma

5. **Comorbidities**   67
   Ashok Kumar Singh, Amit Kumar Verma

Section II: Management of COPD

6. **Stable COPD**   79
   Arun Sampath, Amit Kumar Verma

7. **Acute Exacerbation of COPD**   106
   Arun Sampath, Amit Kumar Verma

8. **Comorbidities** 119
   Ashok Kumar Singh, Amit Kumar Verma

9. **Discharge** 125
   Ajay Kumar Verma, Anubhuti Singh, Arpita Singh

10. **Guidelines and their Deficiencies** 132
    Adesh Kumar, Aditya Kumar Gautam, Ashish Kumar Gupta,
    Prashant Yadav, Harender Singh

11. **Nutrition** 147
    Kamlesh Sethi, Jasmeet Kaur

12. **Physiotherapy and Yoga** 165
    VG Prabhu Ramnath

13. **Prevention** 177
    Shiva Narang, Apoorva Tomar, Amit Kumar Verma

14. **Recent Advances and Future** 198
    Hemant Kumar Aggarwal, Amit Kumar Verma

Index 217

Abbreviations

AAT Alpha antitrypsin

ABG Arterial blood gases

ACE Angiotensin converting enzyme

ACOS Asthma COPD overlap syndrome

ACV Assist control ventilation

AECOPD Acute exacerbation of chronic obstructive pulmonary diseases

AVAPS Average volume around pressure support

BOLD Burden of obstructive lung disease

C-ANCA C-type antineutrophilic cytoplasmic antibodies

CAT COPD assessment test

CAT Score COPD assessment score

COTPA ACM Cigarette and other tobacco products prohibition of advertisement and regulation of trade and consume

CPAP Constant positive airway pressure

CVA Cardiovascular accident

DALY Disability adjusted life years

DLCO Diffusion capacity of carbon monoxide in lung

DPI Dry powder inhaler

ECLIPSE Evaluation of COPD longitudinally to identify predictive surrogate endpoints

FEV_1 Forced expiratory volume in one second

FFM Fat free mass

FVC Forced vital capacity

GARD Global alliance against chronic respiratory diseases

GERD Gastro esophageal reflux disease

GOLD Global initiative for chronic obstructive lung diseases

IAP Indoor air pollution

ICMR Indian Council of Medical Research

ICS Indian Chest Society

ICS Inhaled corticosteroids

IMV Invasive mechanical ventilation

INSEARCH Indian Study on Epidemiology of Asthma Respiratory Symptoms and Chronic Bronchitis

LAMA Long acting muscarinic antagonist

LTOT Long term oxygen therapy

LVRS Lung volume reduction surgery

mMRC Modified Medical Research Council

MVV Maximum voluntary ventilation

NCCP National College of Chest Physician

NCD Non-communicable diseases

NCMH National Commission of Macro-economics and Health

NIPPV Non-invasive positive pressure ventilation

OSAS Obstructive sleep apnoea syndrome

PAL Practical approach to lung health

PCM Pressure control mode

PEEP Peak end expiratory volume

pMDI Pressurized meter dose inhaler

PMUY Pradhan Mantri Ujjwala Yojana

PSV Pressure support ventilation

REE Respiratory energy expenditure

SI Smoking index

SAMA Short acting muscarinic antagonist

SpO$_2$ Oxygen saturation by pulse oximeter

TDEE Total daily energy expenditure

TPM Total particulate matter

USPSTF United States Preventive Services Task Force

VC Vital capacity

VCV Volume control mode

VSV Volume support ventilation

WHO World Health Organization

WHO FCTC World Health Organization framework convention on tobacco control

Section I
Basics of COPD

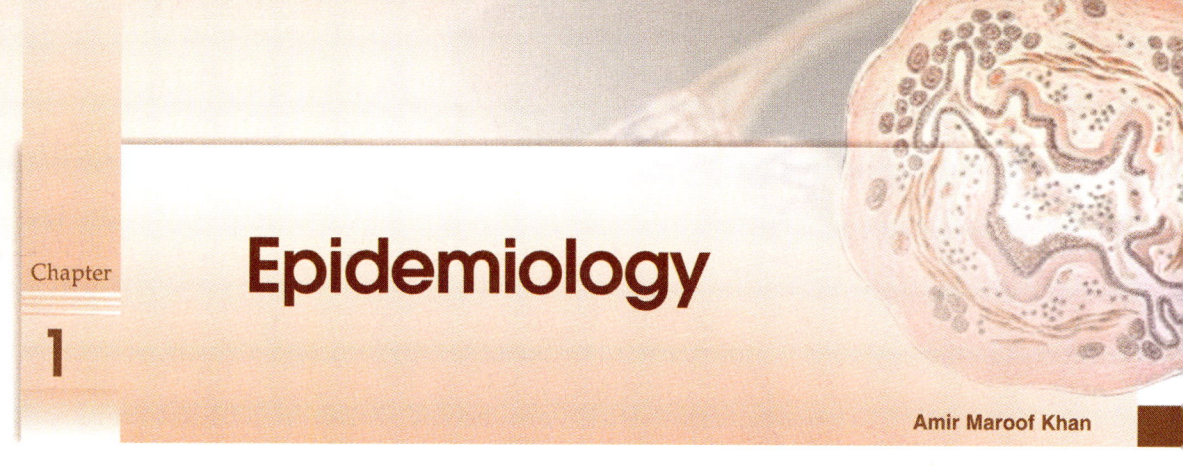

Amir Maroof Khan

Epidemiology

INTRODUCTION

Chronic obstructive pulmonary disease (COPD) is an underdiagnosed, progressive, incurable lung disease. Its prevalence is on the increase globally as well as in India. There it has overtaken tuberculosis and pneumonia, with respect to the number of deaths caused. The mortality in India by COPD is expected to rise from 9 lakhs to 16 lakhs between 2005 and 2030. There is a lack of consistent data from the Indian settings. Indian Study on Epidemiology of Asthma, Respiratory symptoms and Chronic Bronchitis (INSEARCH) studies have attempted to provide multicentric data for COPD in the recent years.

COPD is incurable but preventable disease and the progression of the disease can also be slowed. Smoking is the main cause of the disease. Indoor air pollution is responsible for the majority of COPD cases and other respiratory illnesses occurring among women and children worldwide. Even though traditionally COPD has been seen in the context of smoking only, non-smoker's COPD is now a recognized entity which also needs more attention and research.

The World Health Organization has been proactive in developing guidelines and advocating the control and prevention of this disease. The response from the policymakers at the national level seems to be lacklustre when seen in context of the huge burden of the disease. A multisectoral approach is needed to control this disease of growing public health importance.

DEFINITION

As per the Global Initiative for Chronic Obstructive Lung Disease (GOLD) 2016 COPD is a common, preventable and treatable disease that is characterized by persistent respiratory symptoms and airflow limitation that is due to airway and / or alveolar abnormalities usually caused by significant exposure to noxious particles or gases.

The terms 'chronic bronchitis' and 'emphysema' which were till recently very commonly used as independent diagnosis are now included under the term Chronic Obstructive Pulmonary Disease (COPD).

Persistent reduction in the airflow is the characteristic feature of this lung disease. COPD is an umbrella term which is used to describe chronic lung disease that causes obstruction in lung airflow. The abnormal inflammatory response of the lung to noxious particles and gases leads to this condition. It develops gradually and usually manifest after 40 years of age. The triads of symptoms of COPD are:

1. Breathlessness

2. Chronic cough and

3. Sputum production.[1]

As the disease progresses the simple daily activities become nearly impossible. Patients complaining of breathlessness on exertion at first and later affecting their daily routine activities. This is also associated with episodic exacerbations of these symptoms which may last from a few days to a few weeks. Usually routine medical care is needed but during severe exacerbations, hospitalization may be required. COPD is preventable but not curable. Treatment can help slow the disease progression but cannot stop and it gradually worsens over time.

The term 'chronic bronchitis' is defined as presence of cough and sputum production for at least three months in each of two consecutive years in a patient and all other causes of chronic cough have been excluded. This is a relevant and useful clinical and epidemiological definition. However, it may not be associated with airflow limitation which is the essential feature of COPD.

A low peak flow detected by spirometry as a confirmatory test for COPD. But it is not specific to COPD. Patients with symptoms of cough, sputum production should be subjected to spirometry but if spirometry is not available, then other available tools of diagnosis should be used. The clinical signs and symptoms may help in making a diagnosis of this condition. The presence of established risk factors further strengthens the suspicion of COPD.[2]

GLOBAL BURDEN OF COPD

Respiratory diseases including asthma and COPD are the fourth leading causes of non-communicable disease (NCD) deaths. 90% of deaths from COPD occurred in low and middle income countries (WHO 2004). NCD deaths are projected to rise to five crore and twenty lakhs by 2030; NCDs will lead to five times as many deaths and three times as many DALYs (disability adjusted life years—are the years of life lost to disability and to premature deaths) as communicable diseases. Thirty lakh deaths have been attributed to COPD in 2015 globally, or in other words, it kills one person every 10 seconds around the world. In 2004, 6.4 crore had COPD and 5% of all deaths were attributed to COPD. A fifth leading cause of death in 2002, COPD is poised to become the third leading cause of death by 2030 worldwide.

Data from middle and low income countries regarding COPD is hardly available even though they are bearing the maximum burden of the disease. With indoor air pollution exposure to women in low income countries and increased tobacco use among women of high income countries, the prevalence of COPD is nearly equal in men and women at the global level.[3]

Different survey methodologies and variable definitions used for COPD render epidemiological data from different countries not fit to be compared. Mostly, due to the difficulty in data collection regarding COPD, the burden is underestimated. In 2001, the estimated prevalence of COPD was 1013 per one lakh, higher in males (1206 per lakh) than females (810 per lakh). This data is for all age groups, thus underestimating the burden as its prevalence is higher among the higher age groups than the younger age groups. Regionwise, Western Pacific has the highest prevalence of COPD (1675 per lakh population) and the lowest prevalence was found in Sub-Saharan Africa (179 per lakh population). Currently it is estimated that around 21 crore people suffer from COPD globally. In 1996 the global prevalence of COPD was estimated to be 9.34/1000 males and 7.33/1000 females for all age groups.[4]

Out of the total 27.48 lakh deaths annually due to COPD, India contributed to 5.56 lakh deaths (>20%), whereas China contributed to more than 50% as per the WHO Global Infobase Jan 2011. The age standardized death rate is 64.7 per one lakh due to COPD in India.[5]

The burden of any disease is quantified in terms of a comprehensive indicator known as disability adjusted life year (DALY). World over, 280 lakhs DALYs were lost due to COPD in 2002 with the highest from the Western Pacific region, India contributing to 67.4 lakhs DALY. In terms of DALYs lost COPD was ranked 12th in 1990 but is expected to be 5th in 2020.[6]

INDIAN SCENARIO

In India, NCDs were responsible for 53% of all deaths and 44% of DALYs lost in 2005. Of these 7% of the deaths and 3% of the DALYs lost were because of chronic respiratory diseases.[7] It is crudely estimated that there are 3 crore COPD patients in India.[8]

India contributes to more than one-fifth of the total COPD mortality all over the world. Due to the varying methodologies and definitions used, we get varying results. Furthermore, a lack of spirometry-based data underestimates this disease burden. In 2001 a study reported a COPD prevalence ranging from 2 to 22% in men and 1.2 to 19% in women.[9]

The INSEARCH study 2012[10] reported prevalence of chronic bronchitis as 3.49% (4.29% among men and 2.7% among women). It is estimated that 1.48 crore people suffer from COPD in India. This study was questionnaire based and thus the asymptomatic cases might have been missed resulting in an under-reporting of the disease. Salvi S from Pune found that with post-bronchodilator spirometry in addition to the questionnaire estimated the COPD burden as about twice that detected by questionnaire alone.[11] There is a lack of real time data collection for COPD in India, but the available data show increasing trends of COPD morbidity and mortality from 1990 to 2010.

In 2004–06—ICMR INSEARCH-I showed the prevalence of COPD as 4.1% (5% among men and 3.2% among women).[12]

According to National Commission on Macroeconomics and Health (NCMH) estimates in 2006 there were about 1.7 crore COPD patients in India and will increase to 2.2 crore by 2017.[13]

In year 2005 estimated economic burden of COPD in India is 35000 crore or Rs. 350 billion and by around 2010 it was expected to cross 48000 crores or 480 billion.[13]

WHO compiled morbidity and mortality data and reported in 2004 that COPD and asthma were the leading causes of NCD deaths after road traffic accidents in India and there were around 5.5 crore cases of COPD and asthma combined.[14]

In the last 50 years trends highlight that COPD has overtaken tuberculosis (TB) and pneumonia as a leading cause of death.[15] COPD mortality in India is expected to increase from 9 lakh to 16 lakh.[16]

India has huge population and it has rich diversity and there are variable definitions and resource intensive procedures such as performing spirometry in community-based settings to study COPD prevalence. This makes it difficult to have its burden estimates. However, studies by certain authors in years 2005-6, have reported the COPD prevalence as 5% in Indian popu-lation.[17, 18] The varying age group cut-off used in various such studies is another challenge for inconsistent findings regarding burden of COPD in India.

RISK FACTORS OF COPD

1. **Tobacco use:** Smoking is the primary cause of COPD. Data suggests that there are about 100 crore smokers globally and 600,000 crore cigarettes are smoked.[19] In

India, 70,000 crore bidis (rolled dried leaves filled with tobacco) are annually consumed. Smoking is estimated to cause 42% cases of chronic respiratory disease. Prevalence of smoking is the highest in the European region (29%) and the lowest in African region (8%). Men smoked more than women across all regions. Second-hand smoke or passive smoking is also a risk factor for COPD.[20]

In the high and middle income countries tobacco smoke is the biggest risk factor but in low income countries indoor air pollution from biomass fuels for cooking and heating leads to burden of COPD. A large majority of Indians use the non-conventional forms of tobacco (Fig. 1.1) such as hookah single or multi-stemed instrument for smoking tobacco where smoke is passed through water before inhalation), bidi (rolled dried leaves filled with tobacco) and chillum (a straight conical pipe usually made of clay and used for smoking). There is a common misconception among Indians that hookah is not harmful as the smoke passes through water before it is inhaled by the smoker. But studies have shown that it is also hazardous to health.[21, 22] In a multi-centric study (INSEARCH-I, 2004–06) it was found that smokers of all types, i.e. cigarettes, bidis, or hookah, had three times more risk to develop COPD when compared to non-smokers. It was also reported that among the smokers the bidi smokers had a higher risk (8.2%) of COPD than cigarette smokers (5.9%).[12] Around one-fifth of the Indian urban males and less than one percent of the Indian females smoke.

Dose response relationship has been found to exist with respect to smoking and COPD. A recent systematic review and meta-analysis showed that as compared to the non-smokers, the risk of developing COPD is higher among ex-smokers (2.35 times), ever smokers (2.89 times) and current smokers (3.51 times). The risk of developing COPD increased with pack years and duration of smoking.[23]

2. **Indoor air pollution (IAP):** This is a major risk factor for women developing COPD and mainly affects the poor and vulnerable section of the community. Around three crore Indian households use solid fuels (wood, crop wastes, charcoal and dung) in open fires and leaky stoves for cooking and heating homes.

Around one-third of premature deaths from COPD in adults in low and middle income countries are due to exposure to household air pollution. Women exposed to IAP are two times more likely to suffer from COPD than women who use cleaner

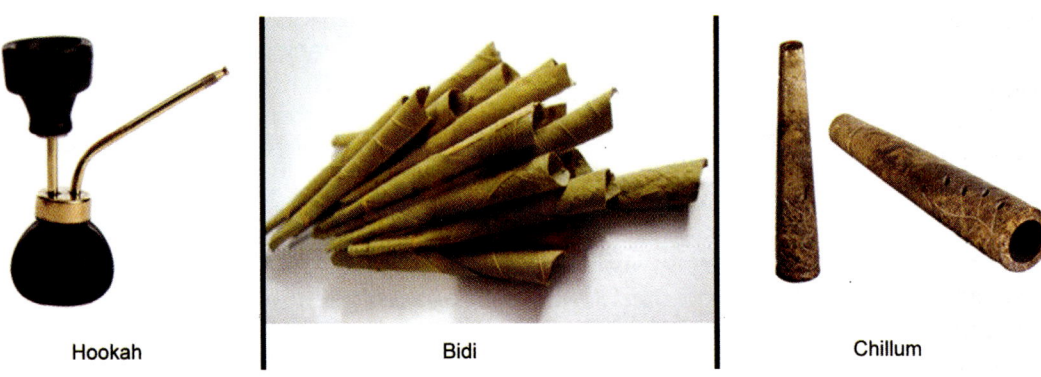

Hookah   Bidi   Chillum

Fig. 1.1: Non-conventional forms of tobacco use

fuels. In poorly ventilated houses, the indoor smoke may be 100 times higher than the acceptable limits.

Around 43 lakh people in a year die due to the illness attributable to IAP. 22% of these deaths are from COPD.[24] Of these, 20 lakh women and children die each year. Exposure to biomass fuels like animal dung, crop residues and woods is widely prevalent in India. 70% of the homes use biomass fuels for cooking (90% in rural and 32% in urban) for cooking and heating.[25, 26]

Mosquito coil emissions are another source of indoor pollution in many houses. The particulate matter emanating from one mosquito coil in one night is equivalent to inhaling 100 cigarettes. As mosquito coils are commonly used in India as a mosquito repellent, the burden of this risk factor might also be high.[27]

3. **Non-smoker's COPD:** Traditionally COPD has been thought of to be primarily related to smoking but facts show some interesting data. A study among 12000 slum dwellers in Pune showed that the prevalence of COPD was 6.5% and 69% of them were non-smokers. This factor other than smoking cannot be neglected while considering controlling and preventing COPD.

4. **Post-TB COPD:** This is defined as post-bronchodilator FEV_1/FVC less than 0.7. Healed TB has a higher prevalence of COPD as diagnosed by spirometry. Some experts argue whether this will be labelled as COPD or not, as it is a structural abnormality resulting from TB sequel. However, with the awareness about non-smoker's COPD, its acceptance is increasing.

5. **Others:** The other risk factors are outdoor air pollution exposure to occupational dusts and chemicals, and frequent lower respiratory tract infections in childhood.

COPD MANAGEMENT GOALS[28]

WHO has recommended four components for effective disease management: (1) Assess and monitor disease; (2) reduce risk factors; (3) manage stable COPD; (4) manage exacerbations.

The goals of effective COPD management are to:

- Prevent disease progression
- Improve exercise tolerance
- Prevent and treat complications
- Prevent and treat exacerbations
- Reduce deaths due to COPD

Component 1: Assess and Monitor Disease

- Early diagnosis and management forms the mainstay of managing the disease, once it happens. Screening may help and high risk groups can give high yield when screened. COPD may be symptomatic or asymptomatic. The diagnosis of this is made by the presence of risk factors in history taking and on investigation, airflow limitation which is not fully reversible. Screening for COPD can be done either with the help of question-naires such as COPD-6, respiratory health screening questionnaire and other or also by using spirometry but the US Preventive Services Task Force (USPSTF) states that there is no direct evidence to quantify the benefits and harms of COPD screening with questionnaires or hand-held spirometry, nor is there evidence to estimate the treatment benefits in screen-detected populations.

- For the diagnosis and assessment of COPD, spirometry is the gold standard as it is the most reproducible, standardized, and objective way of measuring airflow limitation.

- Airflow limitation which is not fully reversible is confirmed when the FEV_1/FVC <70% and a postbronchodilator FEV_1 <80%.

Component 2: Reduce Risk Factors

- Identification of risk factors is the most cost effective way of controlling and preventing COPD. As this is a progressive disease, even with treatment, the ideal management strategy should focus on reduction of risk factors. Reduction of total personal exposure to tobacco smoke, occupational dusts and chemicals, and indoor and outdoor air pollutants are important goals to prevent the onset and progression of COPD.

Component 3: Manage Stable COPD

- The severity of the disease should be assessed first and foremost. Based on the level of severity, a stepladder approach should be followed where more intensive management is reserved for more severe cases.

- Nonpharmacological interventions such as exercise training programs have shown improvement in all patients of COPD as the tolerance to exercise has increased and the relief from symptoms such as shortness of breath and dyspnoea is reduced. The long-term administration of oxygen (>15 h per day) to patients with chronic respiratory failure has been shown to increase survival.

- For further details on management of COPD, please refer to Chapter 6.

Component 4: Manage Exacerbations

- In more than half of the cases of COPD exacerbations, the cause is infection of the tracheobronchial tree and air pollution. However, in around one-third of the cases, the cause cannot be found out.

- Inhaled bronchodilators (particularly inhaled β_2-agonists or anticholinergics), theophylline, and systemic, preferably oral, gluco-corticosteroids are the mainstay and effective treatments for acute exacerbations of COPD.

- Patients experiencing COPD exacerbations with clinical signs of airway infection (e.g. increased volume and change of colour of sputum, or fever) may benefit from antibiotic treatment.

- More intensive treatment involves non-invasive positive pressure ventilation (NIPPV) in acute exacerbations. It improves blood gases and pH, reduces in-hospital mortality, decreases the need for invasive mechanical ventilation and intubation, and decreases the length of hospital stay.

- For further details on management of COPD, please refer to Chapter 7.

WHO'S RESPONSE TO CONTROLLING COPD[29]

WHO is the global coordinating agency with regard to controlling COPD at the global level. The main role of WHO is to raise public awareness, to increase awareness among health professionals. Coordinate global surveillance and develop and implement an optimal strategy for prevention. There are three large-scale initiatives taken up by WHO to control COPD are given below.

Global Alliance against Chronic Respiratory Diseases (GARD)

WHO leads the Global Alliance against Chronic Respiratory Diseases (GARD), which is a voluntary alliance of national and international organizations, institutions and agencies from a range of countries working towards a common goal of improving global lung health. Its vision is a world where all people breathe freely. GARD promotes an integrated approach that capitalizes upon synergies of chronic respiratory diseases with other chronic diseases. GARD focuses specifically on the needs of low and middle income countries and vulnerable populations. The Global Initiative for Chronic Obstructive Pulmonary Disease (GOLD) is part of GARD.

WHO Framework Convention on Tobacco Control (WHO FCTC)

The WHO Framework Convention on Tobacco Control (WHO FCTC) was developed in response to the globalization of the tobacco epidemic, with the aim to protect crores of people from devastating impact of tobacco consumption and exposure to tobacco smoke. It is the first global health treaty negotiated under the auspices of the World Health Organization, and has been ratified by more than 140 countries.

Programme on Indoor Air Pollution

WHO, as the global public health agency, collects and evaluates the evidence for the impact of household energy on health and for the effectiveness of interventions in reducing the health burden on children, women and other vulnerable groups. Cooking and heating with solid fuels on open fires or traditional stoves results in high levels of indoor air pollution. Indoor smoke contains a range of health-damaging pollutants, such as small particles and carbon monoxide, and particulate pollution levels may be 20 times higher than accepted guideline values.

As the problem of indoor air pollution mainly affects the low and middle income countries, WHO through this programme provides support to the developing countries. This is based on capacity building, training, research and evidence for policymakers.

PRACTICAL APPROACH TO LUNG (PAL) HEALTH[30]

Objectives

- To improve the quality of respiratory case management for the individual patient.
- To improve the efficiency and cost-effectiveness of respiratory care within health systems.

Focus of PAL

- Tuberculosis (TB)
- Acute respiratory infections (ARIs), with a focus on pneumonia
- Asthma
- Chronic obstructive pulmonary disease (COPD)

Components

- Standardization of health service delivery through the development and implementation of clinical practice guidelines.
- Coordination among different levels of healthcare as well as between TB control programmes and the organization and management of general health services.

STEPS TAKEN BY GOVERNMENT OF INDIA TO PREVENT AND CONTROL COPD

National Health Mission: COPD is included in the list of non-communicable diseases. However, it is not one of the priority areas as a public health problem by the Government of India. More advocacy is needed so that political will is generated to tackle this health issue. There is no national health programme on COPD by the Government of India.

Some steps taken by the government indirectly play role in keeping lungs healthy, thus preventing COPD also. For example, the cigarette and other tobacco products, prohibition of advertisement and regulation of trade and commerce (COTPA Act) attempts to reduce tobacco use and also prohibits smoking in public places.

Another good example is the Pradhan Mantri Ujjwala Yojana (PMUY) (Fig. 1.2) which aims to safeguard the health of women and children by providing them with a clean cooking fuel—LPG, so that they do not have to compromise their health in smoky kitchens or wander in unsafe areas collecting firewood.[31]

SUMMARY

Chronic obstructive pulmonary disease is a disease of growing public health importance. With increasing pollution levels and smoking levels it is bound to increase. It is a progressive and incurable disease. At the global level the World Health Organization is making efforts to control the disease by supporting the various countries. Even though the burden of COPD has overtaken the burden of pneumonia and tuberculosis in India, the government has only recently started taking some initiatives regarding control of this problem and much more needs to be done in this field. There is a need for more national level, multisectoral initiatives to prevent and control COPD in India.

KEY POINTS

1. COPD is a progressive lung disease with irreversible airflow obstruction.

2. It may be symptomatic or asymptomatic. Spirometry is the mainstay of diagnosis.

3. COPD is incurable, but its progression can be slowed.

4. COPD is preventable.

5. Globally it is the fourth most common cause of deaths among NCDs and kills one person in every ten seconds.

6. In India, COPD has overtaken TB and pneumonia with respect to the number of deaths caused.

7. Smoking, indoor air pollution, exposure to certain chemicals and vapours are the predisposing factors.

8. Non-smoker's COPD should also be suspected when making a diagnosis, as it is a recognized entity now.

9. Practical Approach to Lung (PAL) Health has been recommended by WHO to improve the quality of respiratory case management for the individual patient.

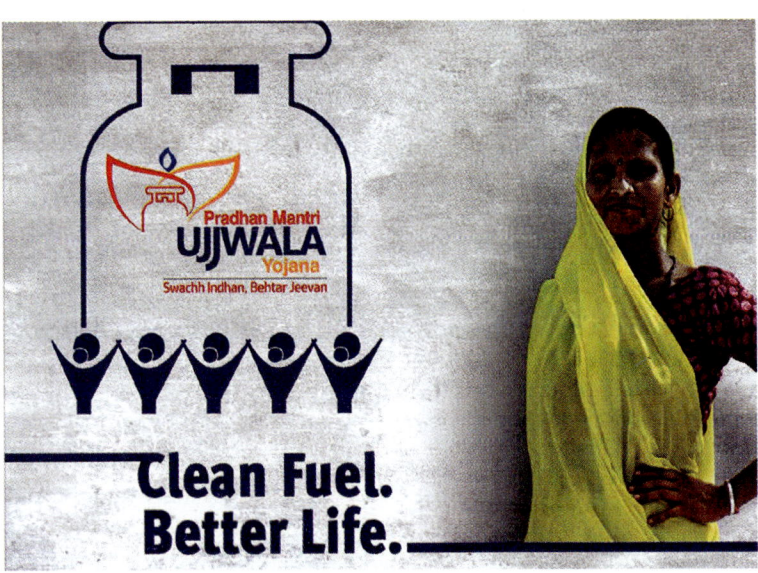

Fig. 1.2: Pradhan Mantri Ujjwala Yojana logo

REFERENCES

1. World Health Organization; COPD: Definition. Chronic Respiratory Diseases.[Internet]. Geneva: World Health Organization; 2017 p. 1. Available from: http://www.who.int/respiratory/copd/definition/en/ Accessed on: February 3 2017.

2. World Health Organization. Diagnosis of COPD. Chronic Respiratory Diseases. [Internet]. Geneva: World Health Organization; 2017 p. 1. Available from: http://www.who.int/respiratory/copd/definition/en/ Accessed on: February 3 2017.

3. World Health Organization. Burden of COPD. Chronic Respiratory Diseases. [Internet]. Geneva: World Health Organization; 2017 p. 1. Available from: http://www.who.int/respiratory/copd/burden/en/ Accessed on: February 3 2017.

4. Murray CJ, Lopez AD. Evidence-based health policy—lessons from the Global Burden of Disease Study. Science. 1996; 274: 740–743.

5. Lopez AD, Shibuya K, Rao C, Mathers CD, Hansell AL, Held LS, *et al.* Chronic obstructive airway disease: Current burden and future projections. Eur Resp J 2006; 27: 397–412.

6. Shibuya K, Mathers CD, Lopez AD. Chronic Obstructive Pulmonary Disease (COPD): consistent estimates of incidence, prevalence and mortality by WHO region. Global Programme on Evidence for Health Policy, World Health Organisation, 2001.

7. ICMR-MRC Workshop. Building Indo-UK Collaboration in chronic diseases; 2009. p. 16.

8. Salvi S, Agarwal A. India needs a national COPD prevention and Control program. J Assoc Physicians India 2012; 60 Suppl: 5–7.

9. Jindal SK, Aggarwal AN, Gupta D. A review of the population studies from India to estimate national burden of chronic obstructive pulmonary disease and its association with smoking. Indian J Chest Dis Allied Sci 2001; 43:139–47.

10. Jindal SK, Aggarwal AN, Gupta D, Agarwal R, Kumar R, aur T, *et al.* Indian study on epidemiology of asthma, respiratory symptoms and chronic bronchitis in adults (INSEARCH). Int J Tuberc Lung Dis 2012; 16:1270–7.

11. Salvi S, Juvekar S, Londhe J, Brashier B, Madas S, Barnes PJ. Prevalence of COPD in a rural population in India. Eur Respir J 2011; 2954.

12. Jindal SK, Aggarwal AN, Chaudhry K, et al. A Multicentric Study on Epidemiology of Chronic Obstructive Pulmonary Disease and its Relationship with Tobacco Smoking and Environmental Tobacco Smoke Exposure. Indian J Chest Dis Allied Sci. 2006; 48:23–29.

13. Murthy KJR, Sastry JG. Economic burden of chronic obstructive pulmonary disease: NCMH Background Papers-Burden of Disease in India, 2005.

14. Nongkynrih B, Patro BK, Pandav CS. Current status of communicable and non-communicable diseases in India. J Assoc Physicians India. 2004; 52: 118–123.

15. Ramanakumar AV, Aparajita C. Respiratory Disease Burden in Rural India: A review from Multiple Data Sources. Int J Epidemiol. 2005; 2:2.

16. Mathers CD, Loncar D. Updated projections of global mortality and burden of disease, 2002–2030: Data sources, methods and results. Evidence and Information for Policy Working Paper Evidence and Information for Policy World Health Organization October 2005.

17. Murthy KJR, Sastry JG. Economic burden of chronic obstructive pulmonary disease. National Commission on Macroeconomics and Health Background Papers—Burden of Disease in India. National Commission on Macroeconomics and Health, Government of India, 2005.

18. Jindal SK. *Emergence of chronic obstructive pulmonary disease as an epidemic in India*. Indian J Med Res 2006; 124: 619–30.

19. Shafey O, et al. The tobacco atlas, 3rd ed. Atlanta, GA, American Cancer Society, 2009.

20. Global estimate of the burden of disease from second-hand smoke. Geneva, World Health Organization, 2010.

21. Koul PA, Hajni MR, Sheikh MA, Khan UH, Shah A, Khan Y, *et al.* Hookah smoking and lung cancer in the Kashmir valley of the Indian subcontinent. Asian Pac J Cancer Prev 2011; 12:519–24.

22. Singh S, Soumya M, Saini A, Mittal V, Singh UV, Singh V. Breath carbon monoxide levels in different forms of smoking. Indian J Chest Dis Allied Sci 2011; 53: 25-8.

23. Forey BA, Thornton AJ, Lee PN. Systematic review with meta-analysis of the epidemiological evidence relating smoking to COPD, chronic bronchitis and emphysema.

BMC Pulm Med. 2011 Jun 14; 11:36. Available from: https://bmcpulmmed.biomedcentral.com/articles/10.1186/1471-2466-11-36 Accessed on: Feb 15 2017.

24. World Health Organization. Household air pollution and health. Fact Sheet number 292. [Internet] World Health Organization. Available from: http://www.who.int/mediacentre/factsheets/fs292/en/ Accessed on: Feb 3 2017.

25. Prasad R, Singh A, Garg R, Giridhar GB. Biomass fuel and respiratory disease in India. Biosci Trends 2012:6: 219–28.

26. International Institute of Population Sciences (IIPS) and Macro International. 2007. National Family Health Survey (NFHS-3, 2005-2006.: India: Volume II, Mumbai: IIPS 2007).

27. Liu W, Zhang J, Hashim JH, Jalaludin J, Hashim Z, Goldstein BD. Mosquito coil emissions and health implications. Environ Health Perspect 2003; 111: 1454–60.

28. World Health Organization. COPD Management. World Health Organization. Available at: http://www.who.int/respiratory/copd/management/en/Last accessed on February 3 2017

29. World Health Organization. WHO's role and activities: COPD. Chronic respiratory diseases. [Internet]. Geneva, World Health Organization. Available from: http://www.who.int/respiratory/copd/activities/en/ Accessed on February 3 2017

30. World Health Organization. Practical Approach to Lung Health. [Internet]. Geneva: World Health Organization. Available from: http://www.who.int/tb/health_systems/pal/background/en/index2.html Accessed on: February 3 2017

31. PradhanmantriUjjwalaYojana. Ministry of Petroleum and Natural Gas.Government of India. Available from: http://www.pmujjwalayojana.com/about.html Accessed on: Feb 15 2017.

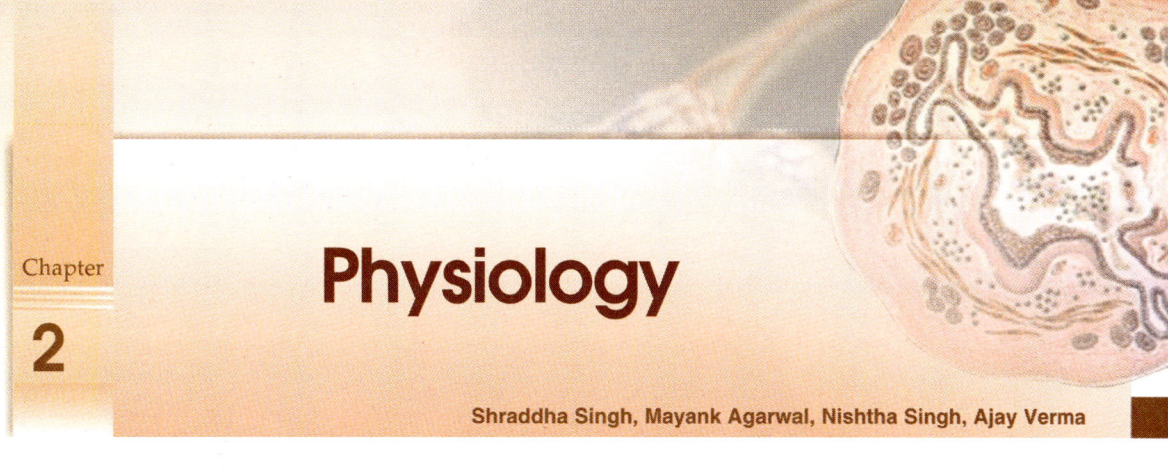

Physiology

Shraddha Singh, Mayank Agarwal, Nishtha Singh, Ajay Verma

INTRODUCTION

Chronic obstructive pulmonary disease (COPD) is an umbrella term covering any long-term, irreversible damage to the lungs that interferes with breathing, specifically with getting air out of the lungs. The term 'COPD' is split into four parts, which implies:

1. Chronic means, "always present" (as opposed to acute, which refers to a short-term condition that disappears after treatment)
2. Obstructive means, "blocking"
3. Pulmonary refers to the lungs, including the airways and tissues that allow your body to pull in oxygen and push out carbon dioxide and other gases
4. Disease is a condition that harms a specific bodily function and/or your overall health

So chronic obstructive pulmonary disease is a condition in which a person has trouble getting the air out of the lungs because the airways are continually blocked.

Many previous definitions of COPD have emphasised the terms "emphysema", and "chronic bronchitis", which are not included in the definition used in GOLD (Global Initiative for Obstructive Lung Diseases) reports. Emphysema is permanent enlargement of the airspaces, distal to the terminal bronchioles, accompanied by destruction of their walls without obvious fibrosis (Fig. 2.1). Emphysema is a pathological term that is often (but incorrectly) used clinically and describes only one of several structural abnormalities present in patients with COPD. Chronic bronchitis (Fig. 2.1) is the presence of chronic productive cough on most of the days for three months in two consecutive years, in a patient in whom other causes of a productive cough have been excluded. Chronic bronchitis remains a clinically and epidemiologically useful term but is present in only a minority of subjects.

The fact of these definitions is that emphysema is a pathological definition while chronic bronchitis is a clinical definition and both of them do not cover the primary abnormality in disease, i.e., inflammation. Hence the GOLD comes in picture. The current definition as suggested by the global strategy for the diagnosis, management, and prevention of chronic obstructive pulmonary disease-2016 report by GOLD, is as follows: "Chronic Obstructive Pulmonary Disease (COPD) is a common, preventable and treatable disease that is characterized by persistent respiratory symptoms and airflow limitation that is due to airway and/or alveolar abnormalities usually caused by significant exposure to noxious particles or gases".

Inhalation of cigarette smoke or other harmful particles, such as smoke from

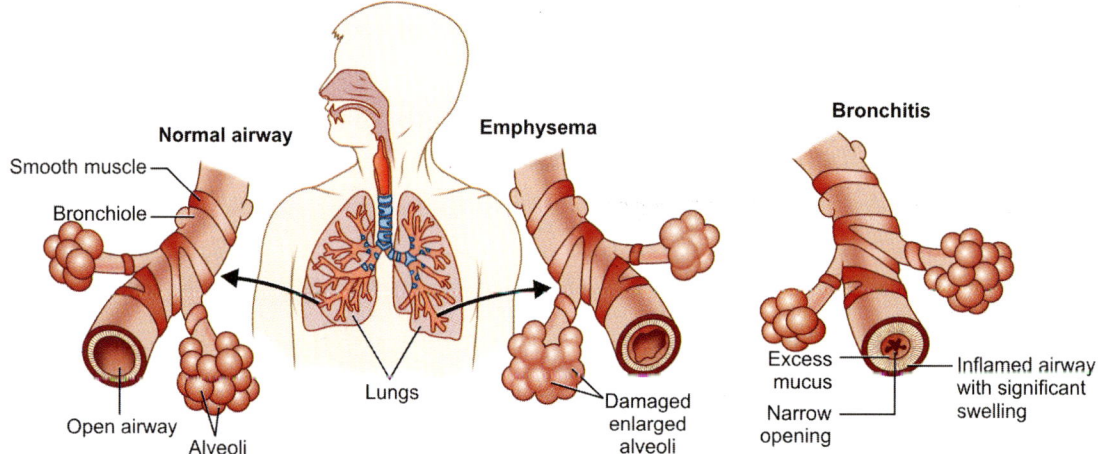

Fig. 2.1: Emphysema harms the tiny air sacs in lungs, eventually destroying them, while chronic bronchitis inflames and narrows airways

biomass fuels, causes lung inflammation. Lung inflammation is a normal response that appears to be modified in patients who develop COPD. This chronic inflammatory response may induce parenchymal tissue destruction (resulting in emphysema), and disruption of normal repair and defence mechanisms (resulting in small airway fibrosis). These pathological changes lead to gas trapping and progressive airflow limitation. This definition provides a better understanding of a complex process by combining the natural history of the condition, the predominant physiological abnormality and the pathological processes involved. It is worth noting that although many guidelines use lung function as the primary defining parameter in severity classification, only GOLD uses symptoms as well (Figs 2.2 and 2.3).

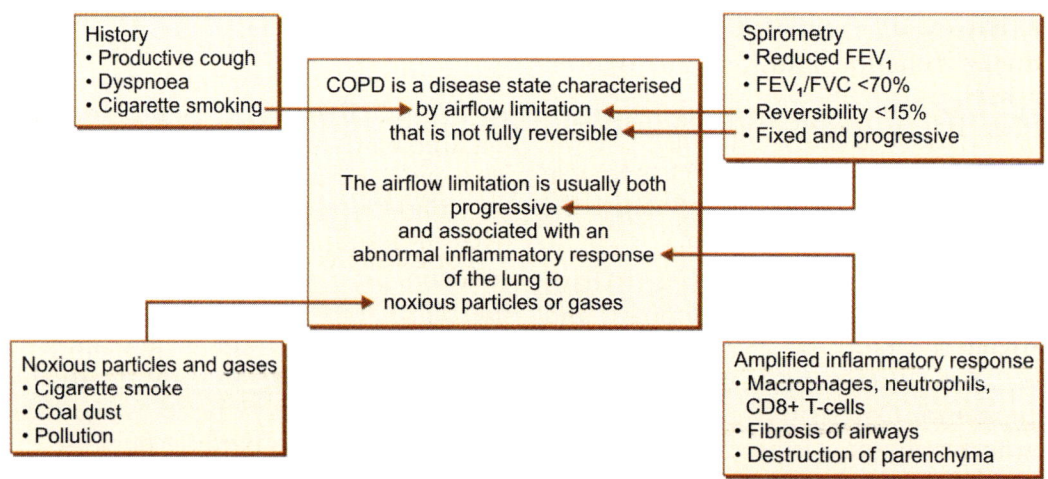

Fig. 2.2: Definition of COPD

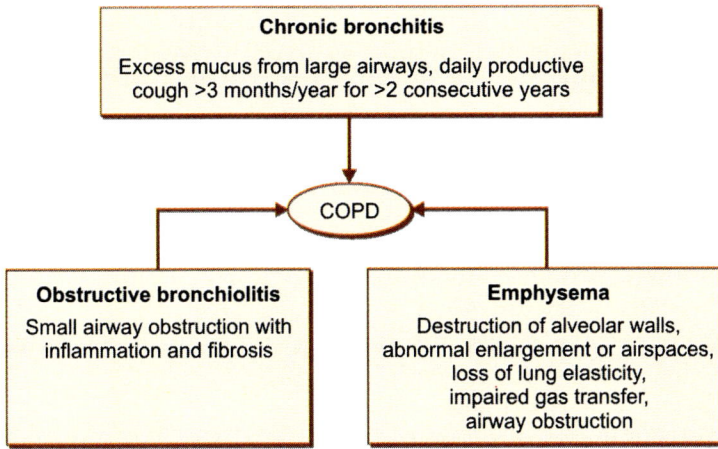

Fig. 2.3: COPD is a multicomponent disease

RISK FACTORS

Risk factors for COPD come under three main headings—behavioural, demographical, and medical history or genetic factors.

Behavioural Risk Factors

Risky behaviours are activities that expose the lungs to harmful gases, fumes, and dust—things that over the course of many years can cause permanent damage to lungs. Some of these behaviours are matters of personal choice, like smoking while some are not, like exposure to noxious elements is virtually inevitable in mine or construction workers; during factory work, especially leather, rubber, and plastics work; textiles, such as cotton workers and weavers; in processing and manufacturing of food products; spray painting or welding.

Smoking

Smoking is the number one risk factor. The correlation between smoking and COPD is exceptionally strong. Doctors and researchers use the term total pack years or smoking index (SI) to quantify the dose of smoking.

Pack years: Pack years equals the number of cigarettes or packs smoked in a day, multiplied by the number of years of smoking.

For example:

1. If there are 20 cigarettes in a pack and 50 cigarettes per day had been smoked for ten years, then:

    Pack years= Number of cigarettes smoked in a day/20 × number of years

2. If five cigarettes a day had been smoked, or a quarter-pack, for ten years, that is only 2.5 pack years (0.25 × 10 = 2.5).

Smoking index (SI): It is defined as average numbers of cigarette smoked per day multiplied by duration in number of years.

SI = Number of cigarettes smoked in a day × number of years.

For example:

1. If a person has smoked five cigarettes per day and total duration of smoking is one year, then:

    SI = 5 × 1= 5

2. If another person has smoked 15 cigarettes per day for three years, then:

    SI = 15 × 3 = 45

Hence we can see that smoking index obviates the need for calculation of the number of cigarettes in a pack.

Table 2.1 shows salient features of pack year and smoking index.

Non-smoker persons may be at risk of COPD if they have around smokers a lot. Second-hand smoke (e.g. environmental tobacco smoke) can damage the lungs just as much as active smoking can. Indeed, some research indicates that second-hand smoke is more dangerous to lungs because there is no filter to block out any of the harmful gases.

Tobacco smoking increases the risk of COPD by 2–3 times. Not all, but around 50% of smokers develop COPD in their lifetime. There are more than 4000 chemicals found in cigarette smoke, of which more than 50 chemicals are known for their carcinogenic activity and cause heart diseases and respiratory diseases like COPD and asthma. However, the major culprit which causes damage to the lungs is the tar present in a cigarette. 70% of smokers in India smoke bidi as it is cheap and easily available as compared to cigarette or hookah. Nicotine content in a bidi is one-fourth of that in a cigarette, but it contains three to five times the amount of tar compared to a cigarette.

Although the causal relationship between cigarette smoking and the development of COPD has been proved, there is considerable variability in response to smoking. Pipe and cigar smokers have a higher risk of developing COPD than people who have never smoked, but the risk is not as high as it is for current and former cigarette smokers. The difference may be in how an individual smokes: Pulling smoke deep into the lungs, as done while smoking cigarettes, is more damaging to lungs than holding the smoke in the mouth or the upper part of the lungs, as most pipe and cigar smokers do. Smoking marijuana alone has not been linked to COPD, but it has been shown to increase

Table 2.1: Salient features of pack year and smoking index

Pack year	Smoking index
Pack years equals the number of cigarettes or packs smoked in a day, multiplied by the number of years of smoking	It is defined as average numbers of cigarette smoked per day multiplied by duration in number of years
Pack years = Number of cigarettes smoked in a day/20 × number of years	SI = number of cigarettes smoked in a day × number of years.
If a person has smoked 20 cigarettes per day for three years, then Pack years = 20/20 × 3= 3	If a person has smoked 20 cigarettes per day for three years, then SI = 20 × 3 = 60
We need to calculate number of cigarettes in a pack	Obviates the need for calculation of the number of cigarettes in a pack
May not be useful in bidi smokers	This is important to Indian setting where number of cigarettes/bidi in a pack is not fixed
No such classification exists	Classification of severity of the disease by smoking index Mild SI = 0–100 Moderate SI = 101–300 Severe SI >301

both the risk and symptoms of COPD in people who are current cigarette smokers.

The nicotine in cigarette smoke gets pulled into the tiny air sacs lining the lungs, where it passes into the bloodstream. Once there, it travels almost immediately to the brain, where it triggers a chain of neurochemical and hormonal responses:

i. Adrenaline level rises. The higher adrenaline levels prompt the release of glucose into the bloodstream.

ii. The neurotransmitter acetylcholine (which controls, among other things, the energy level, heart rate, and the pattern of breathing) is released in multiple areas of the brain.

iii. The high levels of acetylcholine prompt the release of dopamine (one of the brain's most powerful "feel good" chemicals) and endorphins (the brain's natural pain-killers, which like synthetic painkillers, can induce feelings of euphoria).

All these activities also spark the release of a neurotransmitter called glutamate, which plays a role in learning and memory. When someone smokes, glutamate helps his brain to connect the cigarette smoking with the good feelings he get from it. It creates a memory loop that tells the brain how to get those good feelings again—a loop that is strengthened every time a cigarette is smoked.

Most smokers cannot smoke just one cigarette a day because nicotine does not remain in the body for long duration. In fact, an average cigarette has between 8 and 20 mg of nicotine, but the body will only absorb about 1 mg during the smoke. The rest of it is broken down and washed out of the body by liver, kidneys, and bladder. The multiple dosing effect also builds up the tolerance for nicotine; that is why people who started out as teenagers sneaking a cigarette or two a week, ends up being pack-a-day smokers as adults.

Bidi smoking: Bidi is made by rolling a dried, rectangular piece of temburni leaf (*Diospyros melanoxylon*) with 0.15–0.25 g of sun-dried, flaked tobacco into a conical shape and securing the roll with a thread. Bidis are smaller in size and weight when compared to standard size cigarettes. Hence smoking index (SI) is not particularly comparable in these two kinds of smokers, i.e. bidi and cigarettes. Different brands of cigarette and bidi smokers show a little difference in total

particulate matters (TPM) and mean nicotine levels. For example, mean TPM of a regular size cigarette without filter is 21.16–21.94 mg and mean nicotine 1.04–1.21 mg as compared to 23.03–30.03 mg TPM and 1.72–2.05 mg of nicotine in a regular size bidi.

Since cumulative exposure to chemical constituents among these two types of smoking does not differ very much, hence we need not define SI for cigarette and bidi separately. For all practical purposes, we can equate the cigarette and bidi smoking.

Occupational Hazards

Occupational hazards have been linked to many lung diseases, including COPD. Workers who are exposed to so-called "nuisance dust" (dust that the US Occupational Safety and Health Administration defines as containing less than 1 percent silica and that, therefore, is not harmful to the lungs) are almost one and a half times more likely to suffer impaired lung function, and those who are exposed to high levels of dust are more than three and a half times more likely to develop symptoms of asthma or COPD. The link between COPD and people who work underground—like coal or hard-rock miners, tunnel workers, and so on—is well-established. Workers in these occupations tend to breathe in dust from minerals like silica and quartz. This dust can settle deep in the lungs and cause inflammation and scarring.

Working with metal creates tiny particles of metal dust that can be inhaled. Welding adds to the risk because there is exposure not only to metal dust but also to gases emitted by the welding machinery and gases that are created when metal heats up. Some research shows that prolonged exposure to welding fumes have much the same effect as smoking, even among people who have never smoked. Prolonged exposure to welding fumes has been linked to bronchitis.

Occupations that cause exposure to dust from biological sources also can increase the risk for COPD. Plant fibres, pollen, bacteria, and endotoxins (toxic substances that are released when bacteria die) all can cause irritation, inflammation, and scarring in the airways and air sacs. Farmers, grain handlers, sawmill workers, and cotton workers all are exposed to higher-than-average levels of organic or biological dust. So are bakers, hairdressers, and nurses.

The quality of the air inspired also affects the risk of developing COPD, and it does not just apply to the air outdoors. The air in the home, office, car—anywhere, can be laden with particles, gases, and fumes that can irritate the lungs and make breathing more difficult. Prolonged exposure can, in turn, lead to scarring, narrowing of the airways, and deformation or destruction of the air sacs. Mould and mildew are prime irritants and can pose problems indoors and out. Fumes from painting, household cleaners, and even cooking oils can hurt the lungs. Heating fuel, especially wood and kerosene can give off smoke, fumes, and tiny particles that can irritate the lungs.

Demographical Risk Factors

Researchers have linked demographic factors to the risk of developing COPD, although the reasons for these links are not always clear.

A. **Gender:** For years, it was assumed that men and women had roughly the same risk, but recent research indicates that merely being female puts you at higher risk for COPD. This could be so for a number of behavioural, genetic, and environmental reasons. Women seem to be more susceptible to the harmful effects of smoking, possibly because their lungs and airways are smaller than men's, so they get a bigger jolt per puff of the toxic elements in cigarette smoke. Genetic factors may also make women more susceptible. Women's immune systems may respond differently than men's to the assault of cigarette smoke. This may be true of environmental factors, too; women's lungs may be more sensitive to dust, ozone, and other airborne irritants. This seems to be particularly true of biological dust.

B. **Age:** COPD is pretty uncommon in people younger than 40, thus age is a factor in this disease. COPD is the result of years of exposure to smoke, industrial pollutants, and other irritants that cause repeated damage to the lungs, suppressing the body's ability to defend itself and promoting scar tissue that interferes with lung function. This continual irritation to the ageing lungs makes COPD more common in people who are 40 or older.

C. **Socioeconomic status:** Worldwide, COPD is more common among low-income patients than among those with higher incomes. This could be because low-income patients are more likely to be smokers than higher-earning individuals. There also could be an environmental explanation: Poor people tend to be exposed to more environmental hazards than wealthier people. The use of wood or oil for heating, for example, tends to be more prevalent among low-income households; mould and mildew are more common in older, poorly maintained housing; and low-income neighbourhoods tend to have higher concentrations of airborne pollutants and dust particles. Low-income patients also may delay seeking medical care, either because they have a little or no health insurance coverage and a little, if any, means to pay for treatment themselves, or because they lack access to qualified medical care because of transportation issues, inability to take time off from work, or other obstacles. The delay in diagnosis and treatment means the disease progresses further and the symptoms are more debilitating and harder to treat.

Hereditary Risk Factors

Genetics, family's medical history, and own medical history all can influence the overall risk of developing COPD.

A. **Genetic factor:** There is one well-documented genetic risk: A deficiency of a protein called alpha-1 antitrypsin (AAT), which is produced by the liver and plays a crucial role in protecting your lungs. Without this protein, emphysema is virtually a certainty; symptoms usually show up when patients are in their 30s or very early 40s. AAT-deficient people who smoke almost always have symptoms of lung disease—COPD or another disease—at an earlier age than either non-smokers with AAT deficiency or smokers who do not have this condition.

B. **Medical history:** There is some debate about whether a family history of COPD automatically increases the risk of developing it. Some studies have shown a strong correlation; others have not. Factors from the childhood, lifestyle as an adult, even what happened in the womb can influence the COPD risk.

Childhood lung diseases like severe respiratory infections can cause permanent scarring in the lungs. When this scarring occurs, it interferes with the normal growth and development of the lungs. Childhood asthma also may affect the lung function as an adult.

Airway hyper-responsiveness means that the lungs become supersensitive to irritants that other people can tolerate without symptoms. Both asthma and airway hyper-responsiveness are considered risk factors for COPD.

Childhood chronic exposures to second-hand smoke, noxious fumes, car exhaust, mould and mildew as a child can lead to reduced lung function and lung disease, including COPD, as an adult. These childhood exposures also can lead to airway hyper-responsiveness. Maternal smoking during and after pregnancy is associated with reduced infant, childhood and adult ventilatory function, days, weeks and years after birth, respectively.

If lungs did not develop properly or wholly in the womb, the maximum lung function would be reduced, and that increases the risk for COPD. Low birth weight and childhood exposures also can affect lung growth and development, which in turn may increase the risk for COPD.

PHYSIOLOGICAL CHANGES IN COPD (Fig. 2.4)

Exposure to tobacco smoke leads to initiation of series of inflammatory reactions involving small as well as large airways and can impair host defence systems. In predisposed person, this leads to pathophysiological changes that we have come to recognise as chronic bronchitis and emphysema. To name these are **mucous hypersecretion and ciliary dysfunction, airflow limitation** and hyperinflation, gas exchange abnormalities, ventricular muscle dysfunction, cardiovascular disturbances, pulmonary hypertension, reduced exercise capacity and systemic effects. The biochemical and physiological changes caused by either cigarette or bidi are similar.

Mucous hypersecretion and ciliary dysfunction. Mucous hypersecretion results in a chronic productive cough. This is characteristic of chronic bronchitis, but not necessarily associated with airflow limitation, while not all patients with COPD have symptomatic mucous hypersecretion. Mucous hypersecretion due to an increased

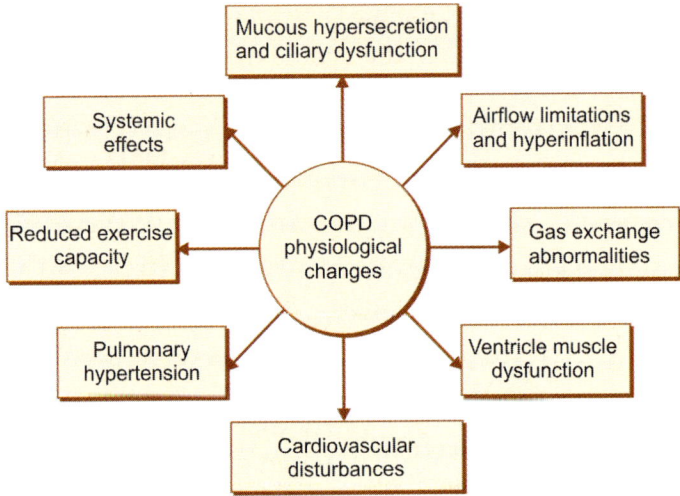

Fig. 2.4: Physiological changes in COPD

number of goblet cells and increased the size of bronchial submucosal glands in response to chronic irritation caused by noxious particles and gases. Ciliary dysfunction is due to squamous-metaplasia of epithelial cells and results in dysfunction of the muco-ciliary escalator and difficulty in expectorating.

Airflow limitation and hyperinflation/air trapping. Chronic airflow limitation is the physiological hallmark of COPD. The main site of airflow limitation occurs in the small conducting airways that are <2 mm in diameter. This is because of inflammation, narrowing (airway remodelling) and inflammatory exudates in the small airways. Other factors contributing to airflow limitation include loss of lung elastic recoil (due to the destruction of alveolar walls) and destruction of alveolar support (from alveolar attachments).

The airway obstruction progressively traps air during expiration, resulting in hyperinflation of the lungs at rest and dynamic hyperinflation during exercise. Hyperinflation reduces the inspiratory capacity and, therefore, the functional

residual capacity during exercise. These features result in the breathlessness and impaired exercise capacity typical of COPD.

Gas exchange abnormalities. Gas exchange abnormalities occur in advanced disease and are characterised by arterial hypoxaemia with or without hypercapnia. An abnormal distribution of ventilation/perfusion ratios—due to the anatomic alterations described in COPD—is the main mechanism accounting for abnormal gas exchange. The extent of impairment of diffusing capacity for carbon monoxide is the best physiological correlate to the severity of emphysema.

Ventricular muscle dysfunction: The number of factor leads to ventricular muscle dysfunction in COPD. A major factor is the consequence of lung hyperinflation, which alters the geometry of the thorax and decreases the resting length of the diaphragm, thus placing the diaphragm in a suboptimal contractile position that limits its force generation capacity. It ultimately leads to the inspiratory muscles at a mechanical disadvantage. Severe lung hyperinflation increases intrathoracic pressure that results in reduced preload due to decreased venous return and left ventricle volume. Thus, left ventricle stroke volume decreases and, consequently a reduced cardiac output. Other factors leading to ventricular muscle dysfunction are nutritional alterations, a sustained inflammatory response that affects the contractile apparatus, tissue hypoxia and loss of muscle mass. These factors further affect other skeletal muscles, which further contributes to exercise limitation.

Cardiovascular disturbances: These are common in COPD and may represent a complication of COPD itself or may be triggered by the common risk factor, i.e. smoking. It has also been proposed that lung inflammation may directly affect athero-genesis by driving systemic inflammation.

Pulmonary hypertension: Pulmonary hypertension develops late in the course of COPD at the time of severe gas exchange abnormalities and independently worsens its prognosis. Contributing factors include pulmonary arterial vasoconstriction (due to hypoxia), endothelial dysfunction, remo-delling of the pulmonary arteries (smooth muscle hypertrophy and hyperplasia) and destruction of the pulmonary capillary bed. The development of structural changes in the pulmonary arterioles results in persistent pulmonary hypertension and right ventri-cular hypertrophy/enlargement and dys-function.

Reduced exercise capacity: It may result from the lack of physical activity and can be an independent factor in exercise limitation. Physical activity is conventionally defined as any bodily movement produced by skeletal muscles that result in energy expenditure. Exercise constitutes a subtype of physical activity that is planned, structured, repe-titive and purposeful. Fortunately, reduced exercise capacity responds favourably to a pulmonary rehabilitation programme.

Systemic effects. COPD is associated with several extra-pulmonary effects like:

- Cachexia
- Skeletal muscle wasting
- Increased risk of cardiovascular disease
- Normochromic normocytic anaemia
- Osteoporosis
- Depression
- Secondary polycythaemia

The systemic inflammation and skeletal muscle wasting contribute to limiting the exercise capacity of patients and worsens prognosis, irrespective of the degree of airflow obstruction. There is an increased risk of cardiovascular disease in individuals with COPD and, if present, it is associated with a systemic inflammatory response and vascular dysfunction.

PATHOLOGY, PATHOGENESIS AND PATHOPHYSIOLOGY OF EXACERBATIONS

Exacerbations are often associated with increased neutrophilic inflammation in the airways, and in some mild exacerbations, the presence of increased numbers of eosino-phils. Some exacerbations are infectious in origin (either bacterial or viral), while other potential mechanisms include air pollution and changes in ambient temperature. Viruses and bacteria may activate transcription factors such as NF-κB and the MAP kinases, leading to the release of inflammatory cytokines. In mild exacerbations, the degree of airflow limitation is often unchanged or only slightly increased. Severe exacerbations are associated with worsening of pulmonary gas exchange due to increased ventilation/perfusion inequality and subsequent res-piratory muscle fatigue. The worsening ventilation/perfusion relationship results from bronchoconstriction, airway inflam-mation, mucous hypersecretion and oedema. These reduce ventilation and cause hypoxic vasoconstriction of pulmonary arterioles, which results in impairment of perfusion. Alveolar hypoventilation and respiratory muscle fatigue can contribute to hypoxaemia, hypercapnia and respiratory acidosis which may lead to severe respiratory failure and death. Additionally, hypoxia and respiratory acidosis can induce pulmonary vasoconstriction, which increases the load on the right ventricle, and together with renal hormonal changes, can result in peripheral oedema.

SPIROMETRY

Instruments and Measurements

Different spirometers are available in the markets but all of them work on two basic principles

A. Volume displacing spirometers

B. Flow sensing spirometers

Volume displacing spirometers assess the change in volume with each effort over the time period and calculate flow with the graph while flow sensing spirometers measure the flow and its change over time and calculate the volume accordingly using the formula, volume = flow × time. Volume displacing spirometers are either water seal type (Fig. 2.5), rolling seal type, bellows or

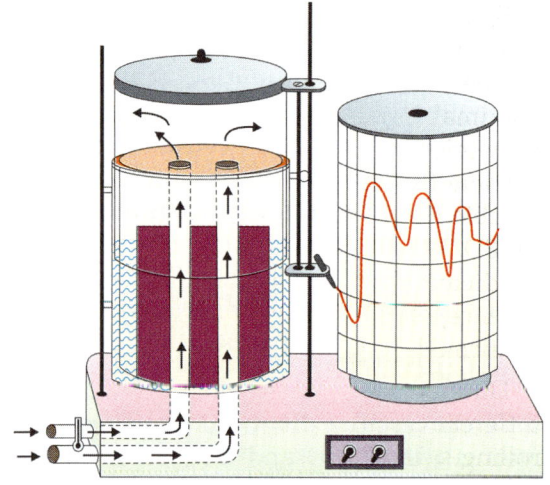

Fig. 2.5: A water seal type of volume displacing spirograph. Change in volume of barrel will draw a graphical pattern on adjacent drum

diaphragm type. Flow sensing spirometers are pneumotachograph, thermister heated wire anemometer, turbine propeller device (Fig. 2.6) or ultrasonic device. Each type has its own advantages and disadvantages. Although volume displacing spirometers are considered to be the ideal one but they are bulky and cannot be carried. Flow sensor devices are portable and are more in use all over the world because of smaller size and good sensitivity and specificity.

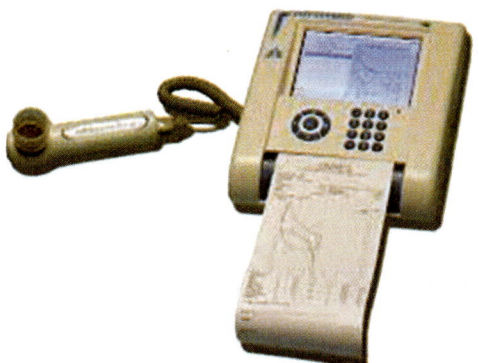
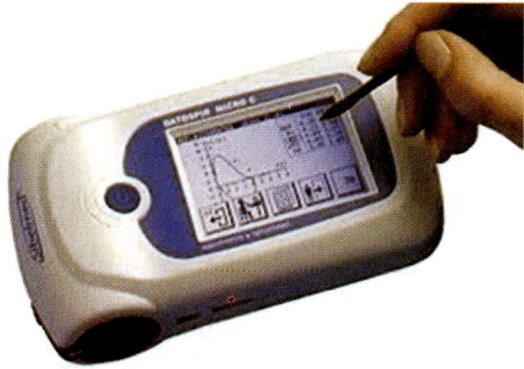

Fig. 2.6: Hand held turbine flow sensing spirometer

Spirometry is a method of assessing lung function by measuring the volume of air that can be expelled from the lungs following a maximal inspiration. The indices derived from this forced expiratory manoeuvre have become the most accurate, repeatable and reliable way of confirming the diagnosis of COPD. When these values are compared to predicted normal values, the presence (or absence) of COPD—and its severity—can be confirmed.

Different types of spirometer are used in different clinical settings. Large bellows or rolling-seal spirometers are not portable and are used mainly in lung function laboratories. They require regular calibration but provide very accurate measurements. Desktop spirometers are compact, portable, quick, and easy to use. They usually have a real-time visual display and provide a paper printout. Some require calibration and others can be checked for accuracy with a 3 litres syringe; any changes need to be made by the manufacturer. They need a little maintenance other than cleaning. Desktop spirometers maintain accuracy over the years and are ideal for use in primary care. Small, inexpensive hand-held spirometers provide a digital record of forced expiratory manoeuvres but not a printout. These devices are useful for simple screening and are still accurate for diagnosis if a desktop spirometer is unavailable. Many spirometers provide two forms of traces. One is a plot of the volume of air exhaled versus time, while the other is a plot of flow versus volume of air exhaled (Fig. 2.7). The latter is called a flow/volume trace and is helpful in identifying airflow obstruction.

How to Perform Spirometry

American Thoracic Society (ATS) has gone at lengths to standardise spirometry. "Standardisation of spirometer" guidelines are freely available to all on ATS website. The excerpts are as follows: Spirometry should be undertaken when the patient is clinically stable. Ideally, short-acting bronchodilators should be withheld for the previous 6 hours, long-acting bronchodilators for 12 hours and sustained release theophylline for 24 hours. When performing spirometry for the first time, most patients (once comfortably seated) need clear, concise and unhurried instruction by a skilled and experienced operator. The following practical points need to be followed:

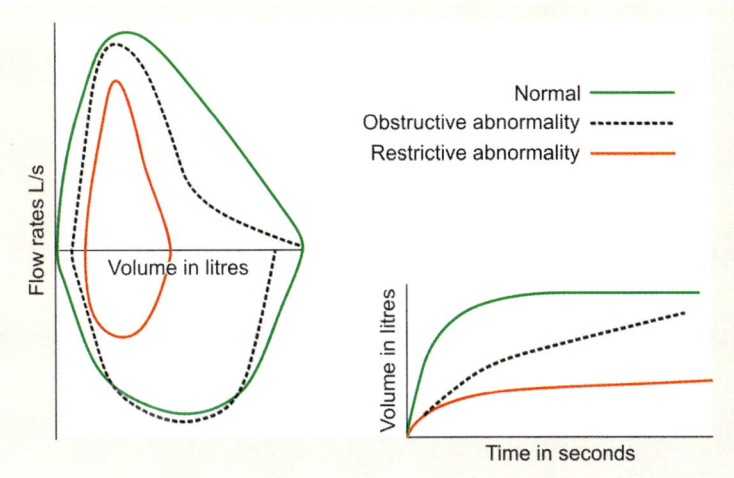

Fig. 2.7: Graphic display of flow volume loop and volume *versus* time spirogram

- Record the patient's age, height, gender and ethnicity; enter the data into the spirometer or computer, add correction factor if required.
- Document when bronchodilator was last used.
- Attach a sterilised, preferably disposable, one-way mouthpiece to the spirometer.
- The use of a nose clip is optional.
- Ask patients to breathe in fully until the 'lungs feel full'.
- Ask patients to hold their breath long enough to seal their lips tightly around the mouthpiece.
- Ask patients to 'blast' air out as forcibly and as fast as possible until there is no more air left to expel; the operator should encourage the patient to keep blowing during this phase.
- Observe the patient carefully during the manoeuvre.
- Check that an adequate flow/volume curve or trace has been achieved; with electronic spirometers, the leak of a small volume of air into the mouthpiece while sealing the lips may register as an attempt.
- Ask the patient to repeat the manoeuvre at least three times until three acceptable and reproducible traces are obtained (with a maximum of eight efforts).
- The best two traces should be within 100 ml or 5% of each other.
- Record the highest FEV_1 and FVC obtained.

Contraindications to Spirometry

There are a few absolute contraindications to performing spirometry, but it should probably not be pursued in any of the following circumstances:

- Recent (in the last month) myocardial infarct, uncontrolled hypertension or stroke.
- Moderate or large volume haemoptysis of unknown origin.
- Known or suspected pneumonia and tuberculosis.
- Recent or current pneumothorax.
- Recent thoracic, abdominal or eye surgery.
- Pregnancy beyond 28 weeks of gestation

Accuracy and Quality of Traces

The most common cause for a poor quality traces is suboptimal patient performance (sometimes due to inadequate explanation by the operator). It is, therefore, important to observe the patient throughout the manoeuvre and provide advice on how to improve technique. Common problems and pitfalls include the following:

- Inadequate or incomplete inhalation (to total lung capacity).
- Lack of 'blast effort' during exhalation.
- Incomplete emptying of lungs to residual volume (common in COPD where it can take up to 15 seconds).
- An additional breath inwards during the expiratory manoeuvre.
- Lips not tight around the mouthpiece (leaks underestimate FEV_1 and FVC).
- A slow start to the expiratory manoeuvre (doing so underestimates FEV_1).
- Exhaling to some extent through the nose.
- Coughing.
- Poor posture (e.g. leaning excessively forward or backwards).

Equipment Maintenance and Calibration

To provide accurate and repeatable results, spirometers must be regularly cleaned and maintained according to the manufacturer's instructions. Calibration should be performed on a regular basis and the frequency of doing so depends on the individual spirometer.

Infection Control

Precautions are necessary to minimise any cross-infection between patients via the spirometer and its mouthpiece. The use of barrier filters and disposable mouthpieces significantly reduces the risk of infection and helps protect equipment from exhaled secretions. A new filter must be used for each patient.

Training

Training is a key issue in successfully performing spirometry and interpreting results. Those involved in doing so should attend an accredited course to gain a full basic training. Regular updates of ability and knowledge on the interpretation of results are also desirable. Training sessions are frequently conducted by various academic bodies in India including Indian Chest Society and National College of Chest Physician.

Spirometric Indices

The standard manoeuvre is a maximal forced exhalation (with the greatest effort possible) after a maximum deep inspiration (to total lung capacity). Several indices can be derived from this manoeuvre. The important indices are as follows:

- FVC—the total volume of air in litres that can be forcibly exhaled in after a maximal inspiration. FVC value of more than or equal to 80% of predicted FVC is considered normal.
- FEV_1—the volume of air that can be exhaled in the first second while performing maximal forceful expiration. It normally represents ~80% of the FVC. The FEV_1 value of more than or equal to 80% of predicted FEV_1 is considered normal.

- FEV_1/FVC. The FEV_1 and FVC are measured in litres, and the ratio of FEV_1 to FVC is expressed as a decimal; it can also be expressed as a percentage of the predicted values for that individual. Predicted values are calculated from normal individuals and vary with gender, height, age and ethnicity. Normally, the FEV_1/FVC ratio is greater than 0.7.
- Forced expiratory volume in 6 seconds (FEV_6) measures the volume of air that can be forcibly exhaled in 6 seconds. It approximates the FVC, and in healthy individuals, the FEV_6 and FVC are identical. Using FEV_6 instead of FVC may be helpful in patients with more severe airflow obstruction who can take up to 15 seconds to fully exhale.
- Slow vital capacity (SVC)—this parameter is obtained when the patient inhales to total lung capacity and exhales more slowly. SVC usually equals the FVC in normal subjects. SVC is usually larger than the FVC in obstructive lung disorders because the airways tend to collapse and close prematurely due to the increased positive intrathoracic pressure caused by a forceful expiration. This increased pressure leads to air trapping. International guidelines in the future may suggest that the FEV_1/slow VC is the preferred ratio by which to identify airflow obstruction.
- The instantaneous forced expiratory flow (FEF), (Fig. 2.8a), represents the flow of the exhaled air in L/s measured at 25, 50, and 75% of the FVC. Forced mid-expiratory flow (FEF_{25-75}), (Fig. 2.8b), this is the flow of air forcibly exhaled between 25% and 75% of the FVC manoeuvre; this value may be reflective of airflow obstruction in smaller airways.
- Peak expiratory flow (PEF) is usually obtained from flow–volume curve data. It is the maximum expiratory flow achieved

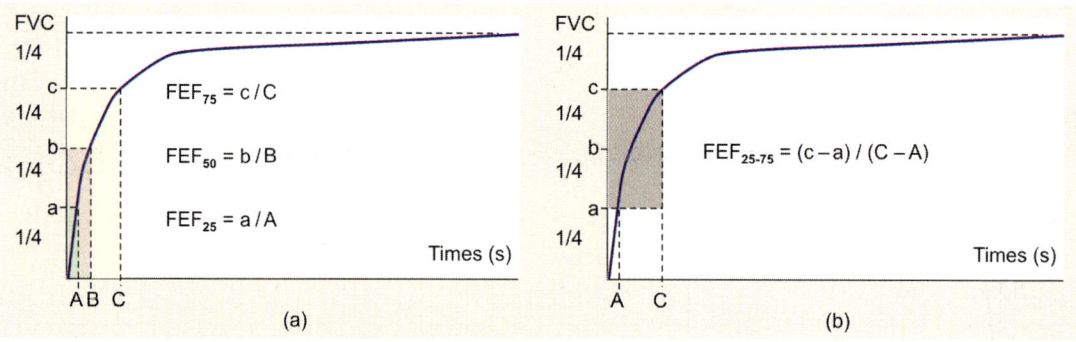

Fig. 2.8: (a) Forced expiratory flow; and (b) Forced mid-expiratory flow

from a maximum forceful expiration done without hesitation from the point of maximal lung inflation. It is expressed in L/s. When PEF is recorded using a patient-administered portable PEF meter, it is often expressed in L/min. PEF drops with a poor initial effort and in obstructive and, to a lesser extent, restrictive disorders.

SPIROMETRIC CURVES

The volume–time curve (spirogram): It is simply the FVC plotted as a volume in litres against time in seconds; both the FVC and FEV_1 can be determined from the curve (Fig. 2.9).

Flow/volume measurement: Most electronic spirometers measure airflow, which allows the flow rate against the volume to be plotted (flow/volume curve shown in Fig. 2.10).

Flow/volume interpretation is a helpful addition to interpreting lung function results and provides a quick and simple check as to whether airflow obstruction is present. It may also identify early stages of airflow obstruction and provide additional help when faced with the interpretation of a mixed pattern of obstruction and restriction.

- A normal trace will have a rapid rise to maximal expiratory flow followed by an almost linear uniform decline in flow until all the air is exhaled.

- In airflow obstruction, a concave dip in the second part of the curve is found, which becomes more marked with increasing obstruction (Fig. 2.11a).

- In more severe COPD where loss of airway elasticity causes airways to collapse during forced exhalation, a characteristic sudden fall in flow occurs after maximal expiratory flow is reached—the so-called steeple curve (Fig. 2.11b).

- In restrictive ventilatory defects, the shape of the flow–volume curve is normal, but a reduction in lung volume—which moves the FVC point to the left compared with the predicted curve—occurs (Fig. 2.11c).

Maximal Voluntary Ventilation (MVV)

The subject is instructed to breathe as hard and fast as possible for 10 to 15 seconds, and the result is extrapolated to 60 seconds. MVV is reported in litres per minute. In a well-performed MVV test in a normal subject, the MVV is approximately forty times of FEV_1 (i.e., $MVV = FEV_1 \times 40$). MVV can be low in – obstructive disease, restrictive disease, neuromuscular disease, heart disease, patients who do not understand/follow the correct procedure, or in a frail patient. Thus, this test is nonspecific, yet it correlates well with a subject's exercise capacity. It is also useful for estimating the subject's ability to

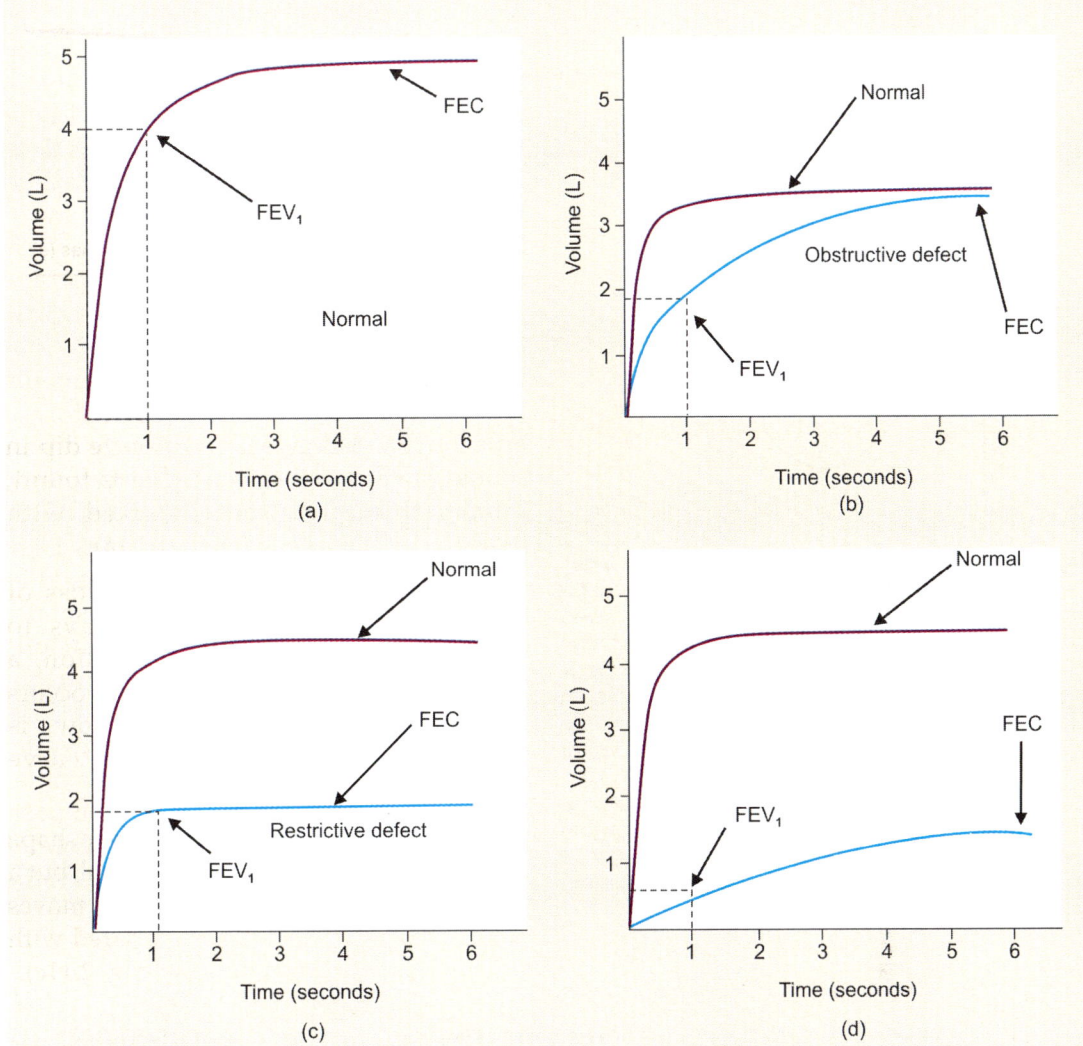

Fig. 2.9: (a) Normal volume/time tracing; (b) An obstructive ventilatory defect; the FEV$_1$ is reduced while FVC is normal; (c) A restrictive ventilatory defect; proportionally reduced FEV$_1$ and FVC; (d) Mixed obstructive and restrictive ventilatory defect; both FEV$_1$ and FVC are disproportionally reduced.

withstand certain types of major operations. An MVV much greater than FEV$_1$ × 40 indicates that the FEV$_1$ test was poorly performed.

Bronchodilator Reversibility Testing

Spirometry before and after treatment with bronchodilators or corticosteroids (rever-sibility testing) is not necessary for suspected COPD, although doing so should be considered when asthma is thought likely or when the response to treatment is surprisingly good. However, asthma can usually be differentiated from COPD on account of the history, examination and baseline spirometry (which is usually normal without an exacerbation). The

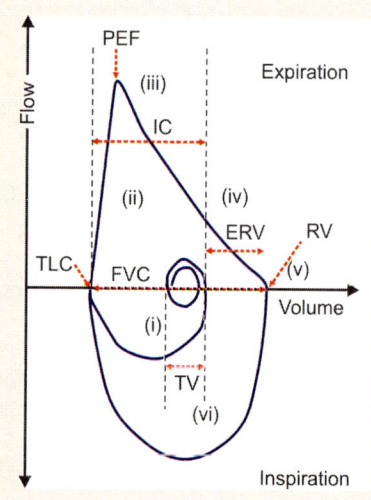

Fig 2.10: Flow/volume curve. A loop of closed whorl represents tidal volume (TV). (i) The curve starts at full inspiration (at the total lung capacity or TLC), followed by maximal and rapid exhalation without hesitation (ii) resulting in a sharp peak (iii) representing peak expiratory flow (PEF). The peak is followed by a smooth downward slope (iv) which curves steeply before reaching the volume axis to the point of zero/near zero below representing residual volume (RV). (v) The inspiratory loop from RV back to TLC should be obtained by rapid and maximal effort. (vi) The width of the curve represents forced vital capacity (FVC). IC, inspiratory capacity; ERV, expiratory reserve volume.

baseline post-bronchodilator spirometry can be done on the first visit if no diagnosis has been made; however, it is best done as a planned procedure. Tests should be performed when patients are free from respiratory infection and are clinically stable. Patients should not have taken—short-acting bronchodilators in the previous six hours, long-acting bronchodilator in the previous twelve hours, or sustained-release theophylline in the previous twenty-four hours. FEV_1 should be measured (minimum twice, within 5% or 150 ml) before a bronchodilator is given. The bronchodilator should preferably be given by metered dose inhaler through a spacer device or by nebuliser to make sure that it has been inhaled. The bronchodilator dose should be selected to be high on the dose/response curve; possible dosage protocols include 400 µg β_2-agonist, or 80–160 µg anticholinergic, or the both of them combined. FEV_1 should be measured again: 15 minutes after a short-acting bronchodilator, or 45 minutes after the combination. An increase in post-bronchodilator FEV_1 that is both greater than 200 ml and 12% above baseline value (pre-bronchodilator FEV_1) is considered

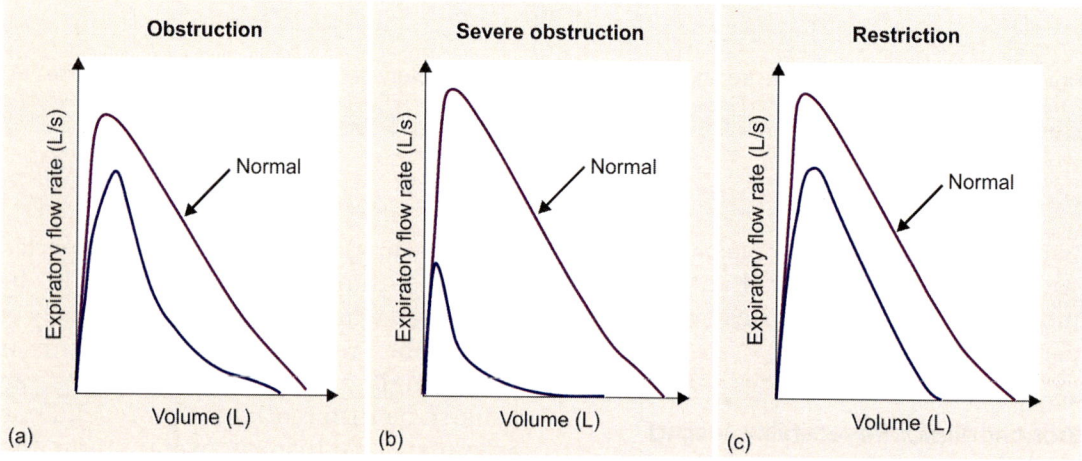

Fig. 2.11: (a) Reduced peak flow, scooped out midcurve; (b) 'Steeple pattern reduced peak flow; rapid fall off; (c) Normal shape, normal peak flow, reduced volume

significant and strongly suggests that asthma is the diagnosis.

SUMMARY

Chronic obstructive pulmonary disease (COPD) is an umbrella term covering any long-term, irreversible damage to the lungs that interferes with breathing, specifically with getting air out of the lungs. Risk factors for COPD can be described under three main headings: Behavioural, demographical, and medical history or genetic factors. In pathophysiological terms, COPD patients can be grouped into three types:

1. Predominantly chronic bronchitis pheno-types,

2. Predominantly emphysematous pheno-type, and

3. A mix of both. In most of the patients, bronchitis and emphysema co-exist, but the percentage of two conditions varies from individual to individual.

Inflammation is present in the lungs, particularly in small airways of all the smokers. Inflammation is a normal protective response to inhaled toxins that is amplified in COPD, which leads to tissue destruction and impairment of defence mechanisms that limit such damage. These, in turn, cause physiological abnormalities such as mucous hypersecretion, ciliary dysfunction, airflow limitation and hyper-inflation, gas exchange abnormalities, pulmonary hypertension and systemic effects. The diagnosis should be considered in any individual >35 years with breath-lessness, chest tightness, wheeze, cough, sputum production and reduced exercise tolerance and who has a history of smoking or other significant risk factors. Spirometry is a method of assessing lung function by measuring the volume of air that can be expelled from the lungs following a maximal inspiration.

BIBLIOGRAPHY

1. Celli BR, Cote CG, Marin JM, Casanova C, Montes de Oca M, Mendez RA, et al. The body-mass index, airflow obstruction, dyspnoea, and exercise capacity index in chronic obstructive pulmonary disease. N Engl J Med. 2004 Mar 4; 350(10): 1005-12.

2. Global strategy for the diagnosis, management, and prevention of chronic obstructive pulmonary disease. Global initiative for chronic obstructive lung disease. 2017 [cited 2017 Jan 1]; Available from: http://goldcopd.org/gold-2017-global-strategy-diagnosis-management-prevention-copd/

3. Hogg JC1, Timens W. The pathology of chronic obstructive pulmonary disease. Annu Rev Pathol. 2009; 4: 435–59.

4. Hu G, Zhou Y, Tian J, Yao W, Li J, Li B, et al. Risk of COPD from exposure to biomass smoke: a meta-analysis. Chest. 2010 Jul; 138(1): 20–31.

5. MacIntyre N, Huang YC. Acute Exacerbations and Respiratory Failure in Chronic Obstructive Pulmonary Disease. Proc Am Thorac Soc. 2008 May 1; 5(4): 530–35.

6. MacNee W, Tuder RM. New paradigms in the pathogenesis of chronic obstructive pulmonary disease I. Proc Am Thorac Soc. 2009 Sep 15; 6(6): 527–31.

7. MacNee W. Pathogenesis of chronic obstructive pulmonary disease. Proc Am Thorac Soc. 2005; 2(4): 258–66.

8. Mannino DM, Watt G, Hole D, Gillis C, Hart A, McConnachie G, et al. The natural history of chronic obstructive pulmonary disease. Eur Resp J. 2006; 27: 627–43.

9. Miller MR, Crapo R, Hankinson J, Brusasco V, Burgos F, Casaburi R, et al. General considerations for lung function testing. Eur Respir J. 2005 Jul; 26(1): 153–61.

10. Miller MR, Hankinson J, Brusasco V, Burgos F, Casaburi R, Coates A, et al. Standardisation of spirometry. Eur Respir J. 2005 Aug; 26(2): 319–38.

11. Pellegrino R, Viegi G, Brusasco V, Crapo RO, Burgos F, Casaburi R, et al. Interpretative strategies for lung function tests. Eur Respir J. 2005 Nov; 26(5): 948–68.

12. Pocket guide to COPD diagnosis, management, and prevention. Global initiative for chronic

obstructive lung disease. 2017 [cited 2017 Jan 1]; Available from: http://goldcopd.org/pocket-guide-copd-diagnosis-management-prevention-2016/

13. Sethi S, Mallia P, Johnston SL. New paradigms in the pathogenesis of chronic obstructive pulmonary disease II. Proc Am Thorac Soc. 2009 Sep 15; 6(6): 532–4.

14. Spirometry for health care providers. Global Initiative for Chronic Obstructive Lung Disease. 2010 [cited 2017 Jan 1]; Available from: http://goldcopd.org/gold-spirometry-guide/

15. Wouters EF. Local and systemic inflammation in chronic obstructive pulmonary disease. Proc Am Thorac Soc. 2005; 2(1): 26–33.

Pathology

Riddhi Jaiswal, Priyanka Gogoi

INTRODUCTION

Obstructive lung disease is a heterogeneous group of diseases with clinical and histopathological overlap. Depending upon the anatomic location of disease and the extent of destruction it causes, obstructive lung diseases include distinct clinicopathological entities like emphysema, chronic bronchitis, asthma and bronchiectasis. Emphysema and chronic bronchitis are often clinically clubbed together as chronic obstructive pulmonary disease (COPD) under the umbrella definition of "decreased airflow that is not fully reversible". However, bronchial asthma and bronchiectasis are not included in COPD in view of the presence of bronchospasm which is reversible.

The underlying pathology of COPD is an exaggerated inflammatory response in the lungs incited by noxious particles or gases, particularly cigarette smoke that leads to irreversible and irreparable damage. Autoimmunity and ageing also play an important role in the genesis and progression of disease.

Besides lung cancer, COPD contributes substantially to the burden of morbidity and mortality. WHO predicts that it will become the third leading cause of death worldwide by 2030.

PATHOGENESIS OF COPD

The pathogenesis of COPD entails complex interactions among several factors (Fig. 3.1) including oxidative stress, inflammation, extracellular matrix destruction, alterations of cell growth and cell repair, and cellular apoptosis on exposure to air pollutants including cigarette smoke. Genetic factors, senescence, and infection further modify these interactions, contributing to the development and severity of the disease. An increasingly growing number of molecules are now being recognized as mediators of these pathogenetic processes (Fig. 3.2). The resultant pulmonary injury involves stages of initiation, progression and consolidation.

INITIATION

Role of Oxidative Stress and Inflammation

Bronchial inflammation on exposure to inhaled cigarette smoke and other noxious particles is the initiating event in the pathogenesis of COPD.

Irritative effects of noxious particulates deposited on the airway mucosa causes epithelial injury. This in turn leads to metaplasia of normal respiratory pseudostratified columnar epithelium to cuboidal or squamous and hyperplasia of bronchial mucous glands inducing wound-repair inflammatory responses. In addition to this breach in the airway barrier system, there is

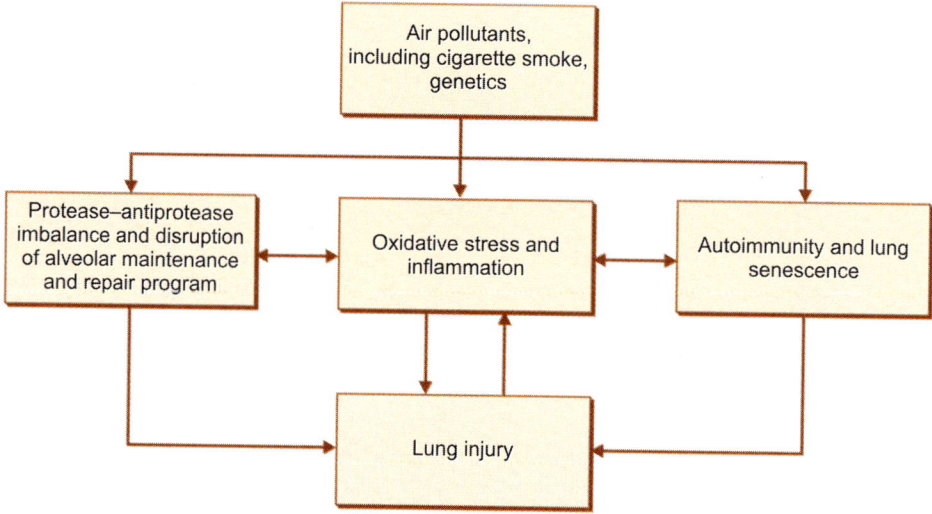

Fig 3.1: Pathogenesis of COPD

Components of cigarette smoke and potential mechanism of injury: *(Report of Surgeon General, 2010)*

a. Acrolein—cilia toxic

b. Formaldehyde—cilia toxic + irritant

c. Nitrogen oxides—oxidant activity

d. Cadmium—oxidative injury + emphysema

e. Hydrogen cyanide—affects oxidative metabolism of cells

The dose of inhaled toxic particles and gases received from each cigarette varies depending upon the nature of tobacco, volume and number of puffs of smoke, amount of air accompanying each puff, and local characteristic within the lung. Altogether they determine diffusion of toxic gases and deposition of particles.

Fig. 3.2: Molecules recognised as mediator of pathological process found in cigarette smoke

also disruption of the lung endothelial cell barrier function which increases the access of circulating proteins, plasma, and inflammatory cells to the interstitial and alveolar spaces. Together, these processes may synergize to promote inflammation in lung parenchyma.

Under physiological conditions, O_2 undergoes reduction by accepting four electrons, which result in the formation of water. During this process, reactive intermediates such as the superoxide (O_2^-) radical, the hydrogen peroxide (H_2O_2) radical and the hydroxyl (OH^-) radical reactive oxygen species (ROS) are formed. The reactive nitrogen species (RNS) are formed from the synthesis of nitric oxide (NO) through the conversion of L-arginine into L-citrulline by nitric oxide synthases.[16]

The production of reactive species is an integral part of metabolism. It is present under normal conditions, notably in the physiological processes involved in the production of energy, regulation of cell growth, phagocytosis, intra-cellular signaling and synthesis of important substances, such as hormones and enzymes. In order to offset this production and its potential negative effects, the body has an antioxidant system. In situations in which there is an imbalance between the pro-oxidant system and the antioxidant system, oxidative stress occurs. Oxidative stress plays an important role in the pathogenesis of COPD through direct injurious effects in lungs but also activates molecular mechanisms that initiate lung inflammation. Oxidative stress is the key mechanism involved in these pathogenetic processes.

Substances in tobacco smoke, in particular alkyl, alkoyl and peroxyl organic free radicals cause lipid peroxidation in plasma and organellar membranes leading to alterations in structure and membrane permeability and extensive membrane damage. In addition the lipid-free radical interactions yield peroxidases (including 4-hydroxynonenal, malonaldehyde and isoprostanes) which being unstable and reactive, set up an autocatalytic chain reaction and propagate it. The oxidant stress is also contributed by α, β-unsaturated aldehydes like acrolein and crotonaldehyde and superoxide, N_2O and nitric oxide present in tobacco smoke which causes oxidative modification of proteins with resultant damage to active sites of enzymes and disruption of conformation of structural proteins.

Oxidants in tobacco smoke and air pollutants also trigger NF-κB-dependant inflammatory responses (Fig. 3.3) which are acute and transient. This occurs via oxidant-induced inactivation of histone deacetylase-2 which increases acetylated or loose chromatin, thereby exposing NF-κB sites and its activation. NF-κB is a transcription factor which controls induction of inflammatory genes leading to the synthesis and secretion of mediators which are chemotactic (leukotriene B4, IL8), proinflammatory (TNF-α, IL-1β, IL6) and induce structural changes like fibrosis in small airways (growth factor TGF-β). There is also increased expression of adhesion molecules. This in turn leads to further recruitment and activation of leukocytes, including neutrophils, macrophages, and lymphocytes. The latter primarily include CD8-positive lymphocytes. NF-κB also enhances the activity of other cell-specific and signal-specific transcription factors.

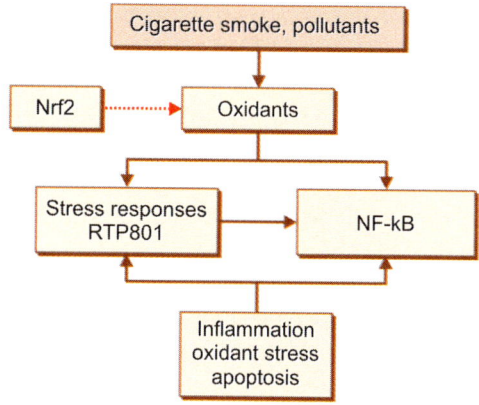

Fig. 3.3: Initiation: Air pollutants, including cigarette smoke trigger host cell responses, resulting in inflammation and oxidative stress largely via activation of the NF-κB pathway. RTP801 is activated by cigarette smoke, largely due to oxidants, mediating inflammatory responses, oxidative stress, and alveolar cell death. Nrf2, by activating a host of antioxidant mediators, protects the lung and may promote lung repair processes.

Several host responses have been implicated in sustaining and amplifying the initial inflammatory response induced by NF-κB. Activation of inducible nitric oxide synthase by cigarette smoke has been linked to alveolar damage by generation of oxidants like peroxynitrite. Engagement of the CXCR2 receptor of neutrophils by the collagen degradation product proline-glycine proline peptide amplifies the initial inflammation induced by cigarette smoke.

Recently, the role of stress response proteins in modifying the early response of the lungs to injury caused by cigarette smoke has been studied in experimental models in mice. Among these, the lung expression of RTP801, a stress-induced molecule which mediates apoptosis and increases oxidative stress by activating NF-κB was markedly increased on exposure to cigarette smoke. Further mice lacking RTP801 showed absence of acute inflammation, apoptosis and development of emphysema on exposure to cigarette smoke.

The role of oxidant stress in the initiation and progression of COPD is also supported by experimental studies on the Nrf2 gene. This gene encodes an antioxidant transcription factor Nrf2, which controls genes involved in antioxidant defenses, detoxification and cellular physiology. Mice lacking Nrf2 showed significant lung inflammation and upregulated RTP801 expression on exposure to tobacco smoke than normal mice. Further, genetic variants in *Nrf2*, *Nrf2* regulators, and *Nrf2* target genes are all associated with smoking-related lung disease in humans.

PROGRESSION

Role of Protease–Antiprotease Imbalance and Disruption of Alveolar Maintenance and Repair Program

Progression of alveolar injury in COPD has been linked to protease-induced extracellular matrix proteolysis for almost 30 years. The idea that proteases are important in the pathogenesis of COPD is based on two independent landmark observations.

The first is the markedly enhanced tendency of patients with a genetic deficiency of the antiprotease α_1-antitrypsin (A1AT) to develop pulmonary emphysema, which is compounded by smoking. A1AT is a glycoprotein molecule produced by hepatocytes and released into the blood and is the main protease (particularly neutrophil elastase) inhibitor in human serum. It is encoded by the proteinase inhibitor (*Pi/ SERPINA 1*) locus on the long arm of chromosome 14. The locus is polymorphic, and individuals homozygous for the Z allele or heterozygous for the Z and null allele (referred to as PiZ individuals) have severe A1AT deficiency. It has been observed that around 80% of PiZ individuals often develop early onset lower lobe dominant panacinar type of emphysema, which is greatly influenced by cigarette smoking.

The second was the induction of emphysema by intratracheal instillation of porcine pancreatic elastase in experimental animals coupled with the observation that neutrophil elastase null mice were significantly resistant to chronic cigarette smoke induced emphysema.

Based on these observations, it has been postulated that cigarette smoke upsets the normal protease–antiprotease balance by imposing an oxidant stress on the lungs resulting in an influx of and activation of inflammatory cells (Fig. 3.4). Both neutrophils and macrophages have been found to be increased in the lungs of cigarette smokers, persisting even after cessation of smoking. In the wake of this inflammatory onslaught, the body's antioxidants and antiproteases system remains largely inadequate resulting in degradation of the elastin framework of the lungs and subsequent alveolar destruction.

Neutrophil elastase and matrix metalloproteinases (MMP) play a significant role in the protease–antiprotease imbalance mechanism in the pathogenesis COPD. Elastin and other matrix components of the alveolar septum are degraded by these enzymes, resulting in destruction of alveolar tissue. Oxidants inactivate A1AT, the primary inhibitor of neutrophil elastase, thereby potentiating its effect. Treatment with a synthetic elastase inhibitor ZD0892 have been found to reduce neutrophils in bronchoalveolar lavage (BAL) fluid from smokers. Besides elastase, other neutrophil proteases including cathepsin G and MMP 9 are also implicated in the extracellular matrix proteolysis in COPD. Increased levels of several MMPs have been described in the emphysematous lungs. MMPs are a family of at least 20 proteolytic enzymes involved in tissue remodeling and repair by degradation of extracellular matrix components. *In vivo*, they are physiologically inhibited by α-2 macroglobulin and the tissue inhibitor of

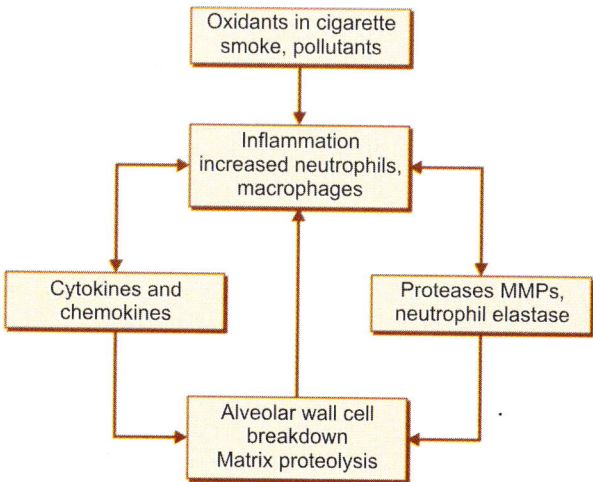

Fig. 3.4: Oxidative stress, Inflammation, and extracellular matrix proteolysis. Oxidants in air pollutants and cigarette smoke triggers inflammation, leading to the recruitment of macrophages and neutrophils. These inflammatory cells might be the source of cytokines (TNF-1α, IL-1β, IL8, MCP, MIP-1), chemokines (IFN-γ, IL-4, IL-13), perforins, oxidants and proteases. These stimuli result in alveolar wall cell breakdown and matrix proteolysis. Further inflammation might be triggered by elastin fragments. Cell injury decreases antioxidant and antiprotease defense so as to favour protease and oxidant-mediated alveolar wall destruction

metalloprotease (TIMP) family of proteins produced by several cell types. MMP-12, predominantly produced by alveolar macrophages, has been observed in the sputum, BAL, bronchial biopsies and peripheral lung tissues of patients with advanced emphysema. Also, higher expression levels of MMP-2, -9 and -12 transcripts in macrophages isolated from BAL of COPD patients were seen as compared to controls.

Polymorphisms of the TIMP-2 gene associated with downregulation of TIMP-2 activity identified in COPD patients support the role of MMP/TIMP imbalance in the MMP mediated destruction of lung extracellular matrix.

The remodeled extracellular matrix may modulate the alveolar inflammation. Proteolytic cleavage products of elastin serve as chemoattractant for monocytes. In addition, peptides derived from the breakdown of collagen results in neutrophils infiltration in lungs; both mechanisms acting in tandem to create a destructive positive feedback loop.

While extracellular matrix proteolysis remains a central mechanism in the pathogenesis of emphysema, it cannot wholly explain the complexity of alveolar destruction in COPD. The concept that alveolar maintenance is required for structural preservation of the lungs and that the disruption of this maintenance and repair program resulted in COPD led to the discovery of alternative molecular determinants and destructive processes in its pathogenesis. Central to this concept was the observation of decreased expression of vascular endothelial growth factor (VEGF) and VEGF receptor-2 (VEGFR-2) in COPD lungs as well as the finding that decreased VEGF or VEGF signaling caused experimental emphysema. Produced primarily by vascular endothelial cells and also by type II pneumocytes, VEGF maintains lung homeostasis. Phagocytosis of apoptosed endothelial cells by epithelial cells and migrated macrophages enhance production and release of VEGF that promote growth of adjacent cells and inhibit their apoptosis by upregulating expression of bcl-2. Besides VEGF, altered expression of other maintenance factors including Wnt signaling components and adiponectin have been found in lung samples from COPD patients.

Variability in the mechanisms involved in lung maintenance and repair could explain the diversity of clinical phenotypes and disease severity and progression seen in COPD as well as the 20–25% risk that smokers have of developing COPD.

Emphysema

In emphysema, disruption of the lung homeostasis program is associated with loss of alveolar cells by apoptosis. Lungs with advanced emphysema demonstrated increased apoptosis of septal endothelial and alveolar epithelial cells associated with a decrease in lung alveolar surface area.

Apoptosis of lung parenchymal cells on exposure to cigarette smoke have been variously attributed to oxidative stress injury, loss of growth factors or as an intracellular response to stress imposed by noxious stimuli present in the smoke. Moreover, cigarette smoke extract induces transient autophagy activation in lung epithelial cells, endothelial cells, fibroblasts and alveolar macrophages. Attenuation of this autophagy flux with insufficient autophagic clearance is postulated to increase cellular stress leading to caspase activation and apoptosis in COPD lungs.

Mediators and signaling pathways linking inflammation, oxidative stress, protease–antiprotease imbalance and apoptosis appears to intersect resulting in self-amplifying injury loops and alveolar destruction which is independent of ongoing tobacco exposure. Upregulation of pro-apoptotic membrane sphingolipids including ceramide directly by cigarette smoke or indirectly by VEGF deprivation or oxidative stress has been seen to amplify alveolar destruction by transducing stress related signals and mediating apoptotic cell death. In a feed forward mechanism, the accumulated ceramide caused further synthesis of ceramides, increased oxidative stress, induced inflammation with activation of extracellular matrix proteases and impaired alveolar macrophage clearance of apoptotic cells. Apoptotic cells express several caspases on their cell surface and release intracellular proteases which proteolytically activate endothelial monocyte activating protein II (EMAP II). EMAP II in turn causes caspase dependent apoptosis of endothelial cells as well as inflammation via monocyte chemoattraction and activation by engaging the CXCR3 chemokine receptor.

Emerging evidence suggests that the inflammatory cell activation and influx in the progressive phase is dependent on mechanisms which differ from that in the initial stage of the disease. As the disease progresses, the abnormal clearance of apoptotic cells, autoimmune processes and concurrent infections seems to drive the inflammatory response. Evolving phenotype of the inflammatory infiltrate is also seen in advanced emphysema. Macrophages show a switch from the proinflammatory M1 to the profibrotic M2 phenotype; thus enhancing fibrosis while limiting inflammation. Disease severity also correlates with presence of CD8+ T lymphocytes and oligoclonal CD4 cells detected in advanced disease suggest an autoimmune mechanism in alveolar destruction at this phase of the disease.

Although the association of respiratory infections with the initiation and progression of COPD remain to be proven, they are important causes of exacerbations and may affect the nature of the immune response in COPD patients.

Finally, the proteolytic cleavage products of elastin function as chemotactic peptides further augmenting the inflammatory response independent of the initiating noxious stimuli.

Inadequate lung repair mechanisms contribute to the progress of the disease (Fig. 3.5). In experimental models, cigarette smoke extract inhibits human airway epithelial cell chemotaxis, proliferation and contraction associated with inhibition of TGF-β and fibronectin synthesis. COPD patients also show significantly lower levels of TGF-β_1 and its receptor as compared to controls and reduced expression of decorin, a key TGF-β signaling target, suggesting the critical role of TGF-β signaling in repair mechanisms. Prolonged exposure to cigarette smoke has profound effects on bone marrow and circulating precursor cells. Cigarette smoke has an inhibitory effect on both the number as well as the function of these cells, thereby adversely affecting lung repair mechanisms.

Air pollutants inhibit production and release of growth and survival factors (most notably VEGF) from alveolar epithelial cells, endothelial cells, and interstitial cells. This, combined with oxidative stress and intracellular stress responses trigger apoptosis and autophagy. Impairment of efferocytosis causes decreases of growth factor release from cells involved in apoptotic cell clearance (macrophages as well as epithelial and endothelial cells), and thus might also contribute to persistent inflammation. Decreased circulating progenitor cells might delay replenishment of damaged lung epithelial and endothelial cells. Reduced production and function of TGF-β by cells involved in apoptotic cell clearance might delay repair processes and contribute to inflammatory cell activation. Apoptotic and inflammatory cells might be the sources of enzymes involved in extracellular matrix proteolysis.

Airway Disease

Excessive mucus production and chronic inflammation of the bronchial walls with chronic airflow obstruction are characteristically seen in airway disease. While the dominant site of chronic inflammation with

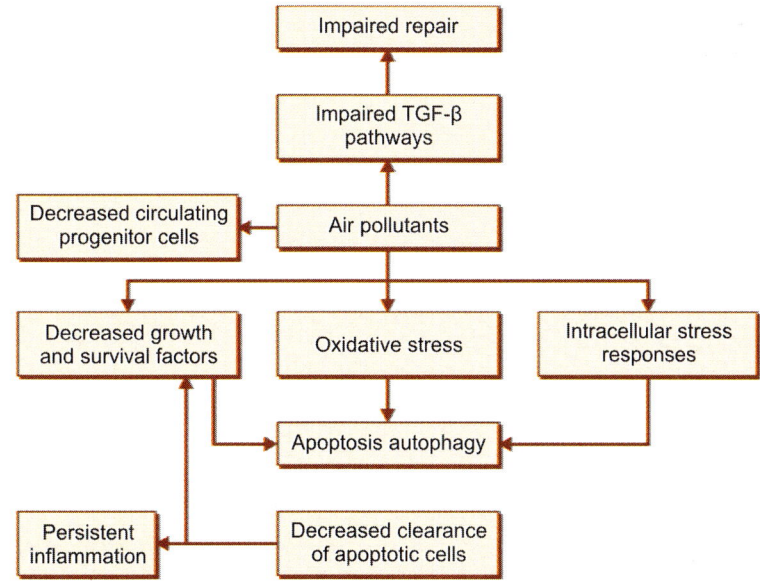

Fig. 3.5: Disruption of alveolar maintenance and repair program in emphysema

mucus secretion are the large airways, small airways (<2 mm) remain the major site of airflow resistance. Cigarette smoking induced inflammation is a critical factor affecting both the processes.

Airway inflammation: The principal inflammatory cell in chronic bronchitis is the CD8+ cytotoxic T lymphocyte, observed in the sputum. It diffusely infiltrates the bronchial tree. Actively involved in viral clearance, CD8 lymphocytes utilize contact-dependent effector mechanisms including release of perforin and FAS ligand to activate mediators of cell death. Interferon-γ (IFN-γ) and tumor necrosis factor-α (TNF-α), secreted by these cells in response to viral infection are the principal mediators of T cell induced lung injury. Disease progression and acute bacterial exacerbations in chronic bronchitis is also associated with neutrophils expressing high levels of myeloperoxidase (MPO) and leuketriene B_4 (LTB$_4$). Exacerbations in COPD were associated with an increased expression of cytokines and chemokines which functions to maintain the inflammatory response and activation of epithelial and endothelial cells. IL-6, IL-1β, TNF-α, growth related gene-α (Gro- α), monocyte chemoattractant protein-1 (MCP-1) and IL-8 were overexpressed in sputum, while bronchial epithelium over-expressed MCP-1 and its receptor CCR2, IL-8 and MIP-1α which correlated with airflow limitation.

Increased number of activated eosinophils in peripheral blood positive for IL-12 has also been linked to exacerbations in chronic bronchitis. It has been suggested that eosinophils might play a role in promoting Th-1 response (in contrast to the Th-2 response typically seen in asthma) by promoting the development of Th-1 cells, facilitating CD8+ T cell responses, enhancing the lytic activity of NK cells and inducing the secretion of IFN-γ from both T cells and NK cells.

Mucus: An increase in luminal mucus attributed to increased production of mucins, increased secretion from goblet cells, goblet cell hyperplasia and/or meta-plasia and accumulation of inflammatory cells and cell debris as described in chronic bronchitis. Intrathecal instillation of pancreatic elastase in mouse models have showed goblet cell hyperplasia and mucus hypersecretion suggesting a role of elastase proteolytic activity driven inflammatory process documented by an increase in IL-5 and Gro-α levels. Besides elastase, LPS, TNF-α, IL-1β also induces mucus hyper-secretion by activating various downstream signaling cascades. The role of various growth factors in goblet cell hyperplasia is well established. Signals induced by epi-dermal growth factor-α (EGF-α) and trans-forming growth factor-α (TGF-α) has been found to play important roles in mucin production in human airway epithelial cells.

Cigarette smoke or oxidative stress causes epidermal growth factor receptor activation (EGFR) via reactive oxygen species (ROS) and activation of the TNF-α converting enzyme (TACE) which releases TGF-α in epithelial cells leading to goblet cell hyper-plasia and increased mucus production. Increased levels of VEGF and IL-13 in COPD airways also contribute mucus gland hyperplasia and bronchial smooth muscle hypertrophy. Cigarette smoke has also been found to inhibit the expression of the cystic fibrosis transmembrane conductance regu-lator (CFTR), a cAMP regulated chloride channel leading to impaired anion transport, increased intracellular Ca^{2+} and activation of the NF-κB signaling. The net effect is abnormal mucus secretion which adheres to the cell surface, thereby reducing muco-ciliary clearance and enhancing retention of pollutant and pathogens.

Small airway remodeling: With disease progression, the small airways in COPD exhibit increased thickness, goblet cell metaplasia, and heightened inflammatory infiltrate, often with presence of lymphoid follicles within the walls of the affected bronchioles and obliteration of the lumen with mucus. All of this contributes towards airway obstruction. The mucus metaplasia is dependent on IL-13/IL-14 receptor signaling while inflammation and fibrosis is attributed to the overexpression of IL-1β and TGF-β. The role of TGF-β is supported by the beneficial effects of anti-TGF-β antibodies or its inhibition by the angiotensin receptor inhibitor Losartan on airway remodeling and airspace enlargement due to cigarette smoke (Fig. 3.6). Molecular and pharmaceutical inhibition of IL-1β also showed similar results. Signaling pathways involving fibroblast growth factor (FGF) and its receptor are also associated with airway and vascular modeling in chronic bronchitis. Smokers with airway limitation show increased expression of FGF in the bronchial glands suggesting that FGF may have a role in promoting mucus hypersecretion. Submucosal hypercellularity of endothelial cells in response to overexpressed VEGF is another mechanism causing small airway modeling and obstruction.

CONSOLIDATION (Fig. 3.7)

Role of Autoimmunity and Lung Senescence

It has been seen that end-stage lungs of COPD patients show exuberant and

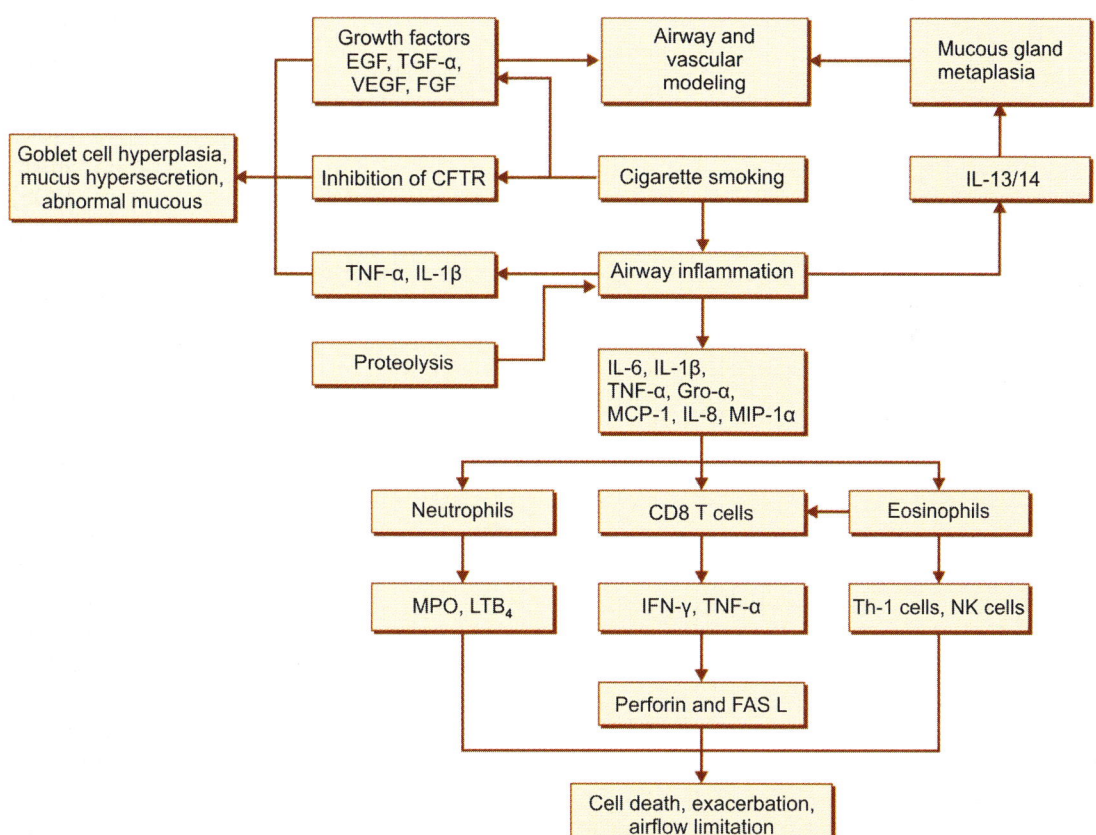

Fig. 3.6: Interplay of various cytokines, chemokines and growth factors in mucus hypersecretion and air remodeling (*see* text for details)

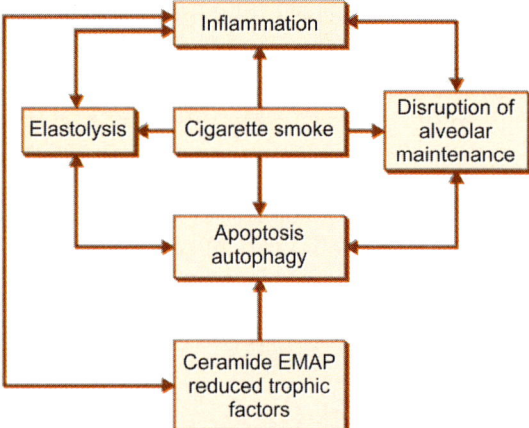

Fig. 3.7: Consolidation: Over decades of exposure to cigarette smoke and self-amplification of destructive processes, there is progressive lung aging, with telomere erosion leading to cell senescence. Autoinflammatory stimuli generated through self-antigens or microbial/viral agents mediate the autoimmunity process via autoreactive T cells together both the processes lead to a terminally injured lungs.

persistent inflammatory responses long after cessation of smoking. This suggests that mechanisms of cigarette smoke-induced inflammation that initiate the disease differ from mechanisms that sustain inflammation and perpetuate the disease. A growing body of evidence suggests the emerging role of autoimmunity and lung senescence in consolidating the disease in genetically susceptible individuals long after cessation of active smoking. Autoreactive T cells or auto-antibodies are thought to active an adaptive immune response. Studies in lungs of patient with COPD have demonstrated oligiclonal CD4 cells while mice exposed to cigarette smoke exhibit lung infiltration by CD8 T cell oligoclones. Autoantibodies have also been identified in the lungs of patients with advanced disease including autoantibodies directed against carbonylated proteins with avidity for pulmonary epithelium and the potential to mediate cytotoxicity. Also, elastin reactive T cells have been detected in the peripheral blood of patients

with established COPD. It has been postulated that the profound structural alteration occurring as a result of cigarette smoke expose or alter lung proteins which act as targets with resultant loss of tolerance to self epitopes. TH17 lymphocytes, often identified in other autoimmune processes, are found in increased numbers in COPD lungs and IL-17 RA knockout mouse showed protection against inflammation and emphysema, thereby suggesting the role of this subset of lymphocytes in alveolar destruction.

Several studies have demonstrated molecular signatures of aging in the lungs of patients with advanced emphysema. The telomerase enzyme, by preserving the shortening of ends of chromosomes during each cycle of mitosis controls the biological clock of cell turnover. Oxidative stress resulting from mitochondrial free radical generation along with potential exhaustion of lung protective mechanisms is the leading hypothesis in the pathogenesis of lung aging in COPD. Peripheral blood mononuclear cells of patients with advanced disease show decreased telomere lengths, a hallmark of senescing cells, as compared to healthy controls. Also, the alveolar epithelial and endothelial cells of emphysema patients exhibit increased expression of markers of cellular senescence. The significance of shortened telomeres was demonstrated by observations in telomerase reverse transcriptase knockout mice, which showed increased sensitivity to alveolar injury and airspace enlargement due to cigarette smoke.

PATHOGENESIS OF SYSTEMIC MANIFESTATIONS OF COPD

As the lung allows passage of oxidants into the blood stream, the pathogenetic processes involved in the systemic manifestations of COPD largely mirrors those in the lungs.

Right ventricular dysfunction in COPD patients is multifactorial, occurring due to pulmonary and systemic inflammation, chronic hypoxia by direct action on the myocardium and increased workload due to pulmonary arterial remodeling. The concomitant oxidative stress with reduced expression of vasodilators contributes to the ventricular dysfunction.

The effect of cigarette smoke on the **bone marrow hematopoietic progenitor cells** has already been referred earlier.

Increased apoptosis and decreased vascular regeneration has been linked to the **skeletal muscle wasting** and decreased physical activity typically described in COPD patients. The decreased mobility along with poor nutritional status and decreased levels of anabolic steroid contributes to the **osteoporosis** seen in these patients.

Panniculitis and **small vessel vasculitis** are both associated with A1AT deficiency. While unopposed elastolysis has been proposed as the mechanism for panniculitis, gene associated regulation of the inflammatory process may be involved in the pathogenesis of small vessel vasculitis.

Chronic Bronchitis

As the name suggests, obstruction is the cause and duration of obstruction is the key factor. It is a system complex, defined for the first time in 1950s by the British Medical Research Council, as the presence of chronic productive cough for most days of the month for at least three consecutive months in two consecutive years without any other explanation.

Anatomically, the larger airways are first involved while the smaller ones succumb later. Chronic inflammation, comprising of mucous gland enlargement and bronchial wall remodeling, reflects a deregulated healing processing tissue persistently damaged by the inhalation of tobacco smoke.

The dose of inhaled toxic particles and gases received from each cigarette varies depending upon the nature of tobacco, volume and number of puffs of smoke, amount of air accompanying each puff, and local characteristic within the lung. Altogether they determine diffusion of toxic gases and deposition of particles. In a person who starts smoking in young age and continues till old age in comparison to an elderly heavy smoker, the detrimental effect may be more pronounced because the number of pack-year of cigarettes is more.

As the smoke moves more deeply into the respiratory tract, more soluble gases are adsorbed and particles are deposited in airways and alveoli. High level exposures, when sustained, overwhelm lung defenses, thereby reducing their efficacy.

Studies indicate that the mass median aerodynamic diameter of particles sized 0.3 to 0.4 micrometers, penetrate to by sedimentation or diffusion and are deposited in the deep lung by impaction (*Martonen 1992; Bernstein 2004*).

The fluid lining the epithelium removes toxic gases by absorption, depending upon the gas solubility. Soluble gases are removed in the upper respiratory tract, while insoluble (e.g. carbon monoxide) may reach the alveoli and diffuse across the alveolar-capillary membrane. Such dosimetric considerations indicate a high potential for lung injury in active smokers.

Besides tobacco, industrial smoke, biomass fuels, and air pollutants containing various gases and dust also harm the lungs, although maximum numbers of COPD patients are found to be smokers.

Use of **electronic cigarettes** needs a mention here. They were earlier considered to be harmless, but are now shown to warrant development of COPD as well. Besides, there is no sufficient evidence to suggest that e-cigarettes help addicts quit smoking. Long-term harm is undocumented.

Pathology

Grossly the mucous membranes of the bronchi show hyperemia and oedema and are covered by mucinous or mucopurulent secretions. Occasionally, luminal obliteration by mucus plugging is noted.

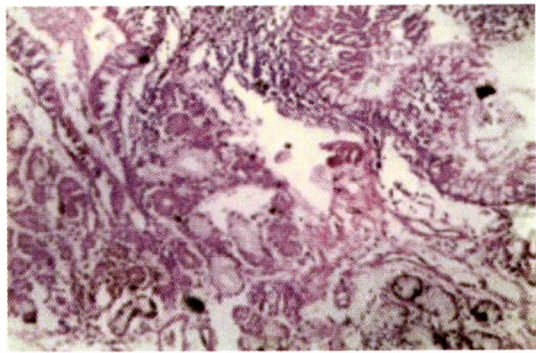

Fig. 3.8: Mucosal gland hyporplasia with chronic inflammatory cells surrounding hypertrophied respiratory epithelium

The bronchial mucosal pits are prominent representing dilated orifices of the bronchial mucous glands.

Cross sectional views of the bronchus shows thickening of bronchial wall with luminal narrowing.

Histologically, mucous gland hyperplasia (Fig. 3.8) is the most characteristic feature of chronic bronchitis characterized by marked increase in the size of the tracheal and bronchial submucosal mucus glands. This increase is commonly associated with disruption of bronchial lining (Fig. 3.9), broken pseudostratified columnar epithelium (Fig. 3.10) and assessed by the Reid index in which a section of a designated bronchus with a cartilaginous plate is selected and the ratio of maximum thickness of the bronchial gland to the thickness of the wall from the basement membrane to the perichondrium is calculated. The mean value of Reid index (normally 0.4) is increased in chronic bronchitis and correlates with the duration and severity of disease.

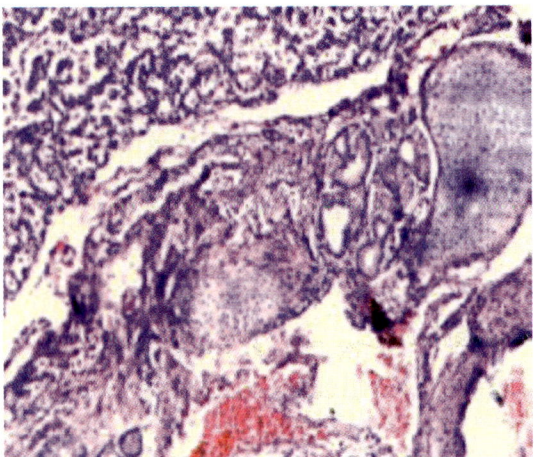

Fig. 3.9: Disrupted bronchial lining with surrounding mature cartilage with congested lumen along with part of uninvolved normal alveoli

Marked increase in the number of goblet cells in the surface mucosa with alteration of the goblet cell: Ciliated cell ratio is observed (normally one goblet cell to 20 cilated cells is seen in the trachea and the number of goblet cells progressively decreases in the lobar and segmental bronchi) leading to impaired

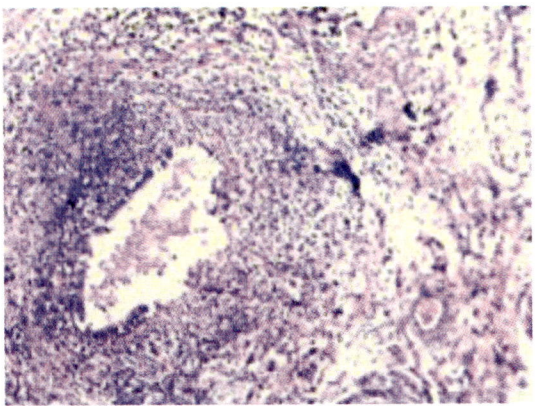

Fig. 3.10: Broken pseudostratified columnar epithelium infiltrated by dense chronic inflammatory cells

mucociliary clearance. Occasionally the surface epithelium exhibits squamous metaplasia and dysplasia.

The submucosa shows infiltration by a mixed inflammatory infiltrate (Fig. 3.11) composed of lymphocytes, plasma cells and macrophages along with oedema and fibrosis.

Smooth muscle hypertrophy (Fig. 3.12) may be variably present.

Clinical Features

Patients cough a lot with increased production of thick sputum, succumb to

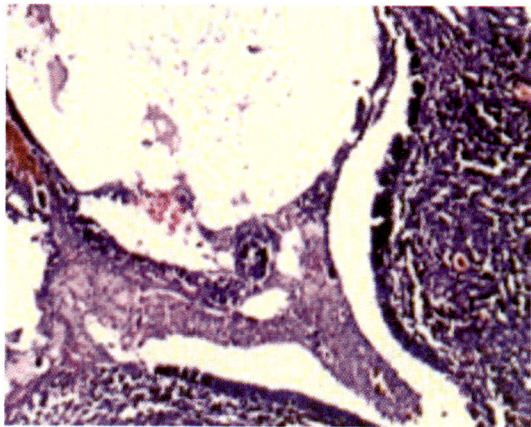

Fig. 3.11: Chronic inflammatory cells aggregated into lymphoid follicles

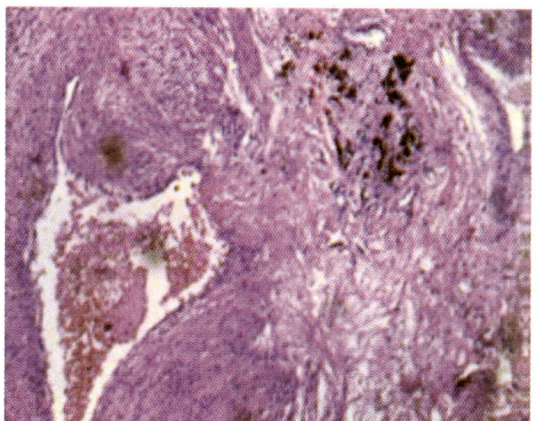

Fig. 3.12: Smooth muscle hypertrophy and intimal fibrosis with carbon deposits and inflammatory infiltrate

respiratory tract infections and allergies frequently and get breathless even on minimal physical activity. Respiratory drive is reduced causing hypercapnia (increased carbon dioxide retention) and hypoxemia along with cyanosis in severe cases. In obese patients, these symptoms earn them the name 'blue bloaters'.

Emphysema

Irreparable damage to the alveolar walls, with superadded inflammation, in the region distal to terminal bronchioles, i.e. involving acini and lobules, characterise emphysema. Fibrosis is not usually seen in the affected parenchyma, as the supporting connective tissue is lost. Bronchoconstriction initially is reversible but worsens with time thus limiting airflow. Based on the segment of small airway involved, the various morphological types of emphysema are:

a. **Centriacinar/centrilobular:** Focal distribution limited to central portions of acini in the proximal alveoli. Distal alveoli are spared. Apical segments of upper lobe of lung are seen to be commonly affected. This distribution is commonly seen in heavy smokers and is often associated with chronic bronchitis.

b. **Panacinar/panlobular:** Uniform enlargement of acini occurs from respiratory bronchiole to the terminal alveoli. Lower zones of lungs are commonly affected. This distribution is seen in association with genetic deficiency of α_1 anti-trypsin deficiency. More than 80% patients with congenital α_1 anti-trypsin deficiency develop symptomatic panacinar emphysema, smoking typically exaggerating the symptoms.

c. **Distal acinar/ paraseptal:** Frequently seen in young adults. Opposite to the centriacinar type, distal airway, sacs, ducts and alveoli are affected sparing the proximal portions. It is the least commonly encountered entity. When the disease is localised to fibrous septae or pleura, multiple contiguous, enlarged air spaces (ranging from 0.5 to 2.0 cm) known as 'bullae' may erupt resulting in 'bullous emphysema' or sometimes even ending into pneumothorax.

d. **Irregular/paracicatricial:** Emphymetous destruction occurs adjacent to pulmonary scars and is associated with prior pulmonary inflammation. Any part of lobule may be disproportionately involved.

e. **Compensatory:** Some patients show dilation of unaffected alveoli in compensation to lost parenchyma elsewhere either due to disease or surgical removal of diseased lung.

f. **Obstructive overinflation:** Occurs as a life-threatening condition in response to blockade by a foreign body or tumour, expanding the air within it; as an improportionate area of uninvolved parenchyma may be compressed.

g. **Interstitial:** When air leaks from the destroyed lung parenchyma and enters mediastinum, connective or subcutaneous tissue. Usually results from a rib fracture or whooping cough, and normalises once the site of air entry is sealed.

Pathology

Gross morphological features of emphysematous lungs are best demonstrated on lungs fixed in an expanded position. Early in the disease, fenestrations are discernible in the alveolar septa which are distinguished from the normal pores of Kohn by their larger and variable sizes. As the disease progresses, the fenestrations enlarge, becomes numerous with destruction of the alveolar septum and formation of bullae by coalescence of multiple emphysematous spaces resulting in voluminous lungs. Emphysematous area also shows pigment deposition and is

traversed by fine strands representing the original vasculature which had supplied the area of destruction.

Histologically, airspace dilatation and destruction characterizes emphysema (Fig. 3.13). There is collection of cells of inflammation like lymphocytes and macrophages as around congested blood vessels and broken alveolar septa (Fig. 3.14) and swollen up epithelial cells with edemal fluid in interstitial space (Fig. 3.15). Alveolar destruction manifests as loss of its attachment of the alveolar septa to outer wall of small airways. Frequently, pigmented alveolar macrophages are seen. Changes of pulmonary arterial hypertension with thickening of the media of small muscular pulmonary arteries with or without intimal thickening are observed.

Subsequently failed attempt at regeneration and repair leading to permanent loss of lung parenchyma (Fig. 3.16).

Clinical Features

Breathlessness or dyspnoea accompanied by cough and wheezing are early symptoms, worsening over time in unattended patients. Associated loss in weight may prompt the treating doctor to investigate for a malignant pathology. Reduced FEV_1 (due to lost elastic

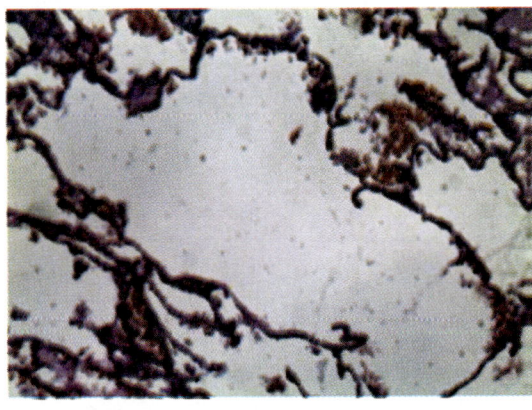

Fig. 3.13: Dilated alveoli with damaged walls without much fibrosis

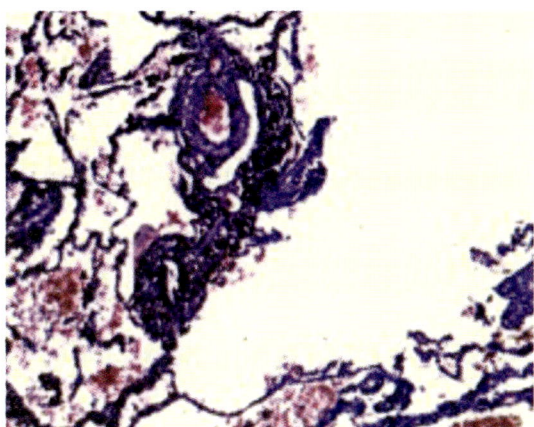

Fig. 3.14: Collections of lymphocytes and macrophages around congested blood vessels and broken alveolar septa

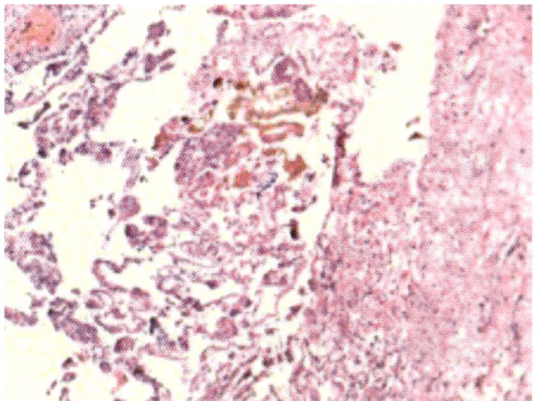

Fig. 3.15: Swollen up epithelial cells with oedema fluid in the interstitial spaces

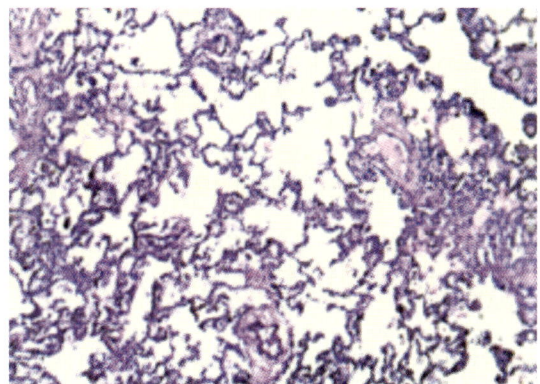

Fig. 3.16: Failed attempt at regeneration and repair leading to permanent loss of lung parenchyma

recoil) prolongs expiration while near normal FVC, decreases the FEV_1/FVC ratio (to below 0.7 on spirometry). Due to hyperventilation in compensation and prominent dyspnoea, blood gas analysis and haemoglobin oxygenation are reasonably normal until late in disease; giving a pinkish appearance to patients earning them the name 'pink puffers'.

Alveolar destruction reducing the capillary perfusion bed area with spasm of pulmonary vessels may cause secondary pulmonary hypertension leading to respiratory acidosis and culminating into cor pulmonale.

SUMMARY

The lungs have myriad protective mechanisms against chemical and biological injuries. However, persistent exposure to smoke and other pollutants cause debilitating alterations in the anatomy and physiology of respiratory tract leading to permanent damage of the gas exchange surface in the functional units of respiration.

Depending upon the anatomic location of disease and the extent of destruction it causes, obstructive lung diseases include distinct clinicopathological entities like emphysema, chronic bronchitis, asthma and bronchiectasis. Emphysema and chronic bronchitis are often clinically clubbed together as chronic obstructive pulmonary disease (COPD) under the umbrella definition of "decreased airflow that is not fully reversible".

The pathogenesis of COPD entails complex interactions among several factors including oxidative stress, inflammation, and extracellular matrix destruction, alterations of cell growth and cell repair, and cellular apoptosis, on exposure to air pollutants, including cigarette smoke. Genetic factors, senescence, and infection further modify these interactions contributing to the development and severity of the disease.

Oxidative stress not only produces direct injurious effects in lungs, but also activates molecular mechanisms that initiate lung inflammation. The underlying interactions of various mediators of chronic inflammation, production of chemicals in response to offence faced, disturbance of the normal tissue repair and remodelling are multistep processes that clinically manifest as COPD.

Smoking cessation remains the only proven strategy for reducing the pathogenetic processes leading to chronic obstructive pulmonary disease. In unattended patients, with no modification in lifestyle, pulmonary hypertension and right-sided heart failure may result in death.

BIBLIOGRAPHY

1. Agusti A, Vestbo J: Controversies and future perspectives in COPD. Am J Respire Crit Care Med 184: 507, 2011.

2. Beasley MB: Smoking related small airway disease—a review and update. Adv Anat Pathol 17: 270, 2010.

3. Charo IF, Ransohoff RM: The many roles of chemokine and chemokine receptors in inflammation. N Engl J Med 354: 610, 2006.

4. Cosio MG, Saetta M, Agusti A: Immunologic aspects of COPD. N Engl J Med 360: 2445, 2009.

5. Galli SJ: The development of allergic inflammation. Nature 454: 445, 2008.

6. Gartner GC, Werner S, Barrandon Y, et al: Wound repair and regeneration. Nature 453: 314–21, 2008.

7. Hogg JC: A pathologist's view of airway obstruction in COPD. Am J Respire Crit Care Med 186: 2012.

8. Hogg JC, Timens W: The pathology of COPD. Annu Rev Pathol 4: 435, 2009.

9. Holt PG, Sly PD: Viral infections and atopy in asthma pathogenesis: New rationales for asthma prevention and treatment. Nat Med 18: 726, 2012.

10. Husain AN: Obstructive Lung diseases, E, Thoracic pathology, Philadelphia, Elsevier Saunders, 2012, 46–61.

11. Husain AN: Lung, Chapter 12, Robbins Basic Pathology, 9th edition, New Delhi, Reed Elsevier India Private Limited, 2014, 462–72.

12. King PT: Pathogenesis of bronchiectasis. Paediatric Respir Rev, 12: 104, 2011.

13. King PT: The pathophysiology of bronchiectasis. Int J Chron Obstruct Pulmon Dis 4: 411, 2009.

14. Martonen TB: Deposition patterns of cigarette smoke in human airways. Am Ind Hyg Assoc J 53: 6–18.

15. Meyers DA: Genetics of asthma and allergy: what have we learned? J Allergy Clin Immunol 126: 439, 2010.

16. Mitzner W: Emphysema—a disease of small airways or lung parenchyma? N Engl J Med 365: 1637, 2011.

17. Nathan C, Ding A: Non-resolving inflammation. Cell 140: 871, 2010.

18. Novak ML, Koh TJ: Macrophage phenotypes during tissue repair. J Leukoc Biol 93: 875–81, 2013.

19. Pag-McCaw A, Ewald AJ, Werb Z: Matrix metalloproteinases and the regulation of tissue remodelling. Nat Rev Mol Cell Biol 8: 221, 2007.

20. Papayannapoulos V, Zychlinsky A: NETs a new strategy for using old weapons. Trends Immune 30: 513, 2009.

21. Ricklin D, Lambris JD: Complement in immune and inflammatory disorders. J Immune 190: 3831–8, 3839–47, 2013.

22. Robinson RJ, Yu CP: Deposition of cigarette smoke particles in the human respiratory tract. Aerosol Science and Technology 34: 202–215, 2001.

23. Rock KL, Kano H: The inflammatory response to cell death. Annu Rev Pathol 3: 99, 2008.

24. Schultz GS, Wysocki A: Interactions between extracellular matrix and growth factors in wound healing. Wound Repair Region 17: 153, 2009.

25. Tuder RM, Petrache I: Pathogenesis of COPD. J Clin Invest 122: 2749, 2012.

26. US Department of Health and Human services. How Tobacco Smoke Causes Disease: The Biology and Behavioral Basis for Smoking Attributable Disease: A Report of the Surgeon General, Atlanta (GA): Centres for Disease Control and Prevention. National Centre for

Chronic Disease Prevention and Health Promotion. Office on Smoking and Health, 2010.

27. Van Dypen SJ, Locksley RM: Interleukin 4 and 13 mediated alternatively activated macrophages: roles in homeostasis and disease. Annu Rev Immunol 31: 317–43, 2013.

28. Vercelli D: Discovering susceptibility genes for asthma and allergy. Nat Rev Immunol 8: 169, 2008.

29. Wynn TA: Cellular and molecular mechanisms of fibrosis. J Pathol 214: 199, 2008.

30. Zlotnik A, Yoshi O: The chemokine superfamily revisited. Immunity 36: 705–16, 2012.

Diagnosis

Anand Kumar, Shraddha Singh, Amit Kumar Verma

INTRODUCTION

Chronic obstructive pulmonary diseases (COPD) is a chronic respiratory condition affecting a large population all over the world. Its incidence and prevalence is progressively increasing and it is supposed to be 3rd common cause of mortality globally.[1] Although incidence and prevalence vary widely in different countries and even in different regions and population of the same country. It is also well-understood that it is under-reported all over the world because less than 6% of the patients are labelled with the diagnosis of COPD.[2] Various methods are being used for the collection of data regarding incidence and prevalence of COPD in previous years because of non-uniformity of the diagnostic criteria. After the formation of Global initiative for chronic obstructive lung diseases (GOLD) program in 1998 and its first report "global strategy for diagnosis management and prevention of COPD" in 2001 there has been tremendous progress in understanding the diseases burden, pathophysiology, precipitating factor and validation and standardization of diagnostic tool for COPD. Today spirometry is considered essential for the diagnosis and prognosis of COPD. Radiological specially CT thorax has also increased the awareness and diagnostic accuracy of the diseases.

DEFINITION

According to GOLD 2016 criteria:

Chronic obstructive pulmonary disease (COPD) is a common, preventable and treatable disease that is characterized by persistent respiratory symptoms and airflow limitation that is due to airway and/or alveolar abnormalities usually caused by significant exposure to noxious particles or gases.[3]

According to ATS 2015 criteria:

The ATS and ERS define COPD as a preventable and treatable disease state characterized by airflow limitation that is not fully reversible. The airflow limitation is usually progressive and associated with a chronic inflammatory response of the lungs to noxious particles or gases. Cigarette smoking is the most common risk factor for COPD, but others are increasingly being recognized (e.g. biomass fuels, α_1 antitrypsin deficiency). Dyspnoea and exacerbations represent the most prominent respiratory manifestations of COPD. In most patients, COPD represents the pulmonary component of a chronic systemic multimorbidity. It is particularly common among the elderly and associated with many common risk factors, such as smoking, pollution, aging, inactivity, and diet.[4]

Diagnosis of COPD is easy to suspect but difficult to establish. Easy to suspect because of non-availability of any etiological factor but presence of multiple risk factors that can lead to development of this chronic respiratory disorder.

COPD can be suspected by a physician when the patient presents with:

- Complaint of dyspnoea which is progressively increasing and/or which worsen on exertion
- Chronic cough with expectoration, or
- History of exposure to risk factor, or
- Had family history of COPD

But difficult to confirm because of non-availability of gold standard confirmatory test and there are multiple comorbidities and associated complications. Establishing a diagnosis further become difficult when a patient comes to the hospital for the first time in acute exacerbation and with associated comorbidities.

Hence a systemic approach may be helpful in reaching the diagnosis of COPD.

HISTORY

Common symptoms of patient of COPD are:

- Cough with expectoration
- Breathlessness on exertion
- History of smoking
- History of exposure to biomass fuel or working in environment of heavy smoke.

History of exposure to heavy vehicle traffic either due to long duration of travels or having residence/workplace on busy road.

COPD patients are usually diagnosed late as it is slow progressive disease and presentation are subtle in the initial years. No etiological agent is known and precipitating factors are many so exact duration of illness cannot be timed. Among the precipitating factors smoking is most consistent and environmental pollution, particularly exposure to biomass fuel exposure, is well established.[5] People who are working in heavily polluted environment like factories or area of heavy vehicular traffic were also found to be more prone to develop COPD.[6]

Usual presentation is after the age of 40 years and most common presentation is chronic cough with expectoration which they co-relate with their smoking habit called 'smokers cough' or to exposure of biomass fuel exposure. The sputum is usually mucoid but may turn into purulent or mucopurulent in between. These symptoms are more common during winter season or change of seasons. The intensity and duration of cough keeps on increasing over time and ultimately patient starts feeling breathless in any of such episode, mostly this is the time when he consults his physician. These patients are often diagnosed as patients of chronic bronchitis by the physician.

Second most common symptoms in patients of COPD or rather first symptom in predominantly emphysematous patients is gradual onset dyspnoea which keeps on increasing in severity over the time in spite of treatment. These patients are smokers but more having exposure to environmental smoke. These symptoms exacerbate in between and resolve with treatment but never return to normal level or to the level before exacerbation. The severity of dyspnoea as defined by mMRC (modified Medical Reserch Council) is grading of dyspnoea as given in Table 4.1.

While asking history one should ask in details about duration of smoking, type of smoking and amount of smoking. One should also ask about other inhalation addictions present in our society as these can also lead to COPD. Severity of smoking can be calculated in smoking index which is

Table 4.1: Grades of dyspnoea

Grade	Description

0. Not troubled with breathlessness except with strenuous exercise

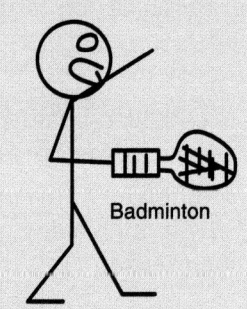

Badminton

1. Troubled by shortness of breath when hurrying on the level or walking up in a slight hill

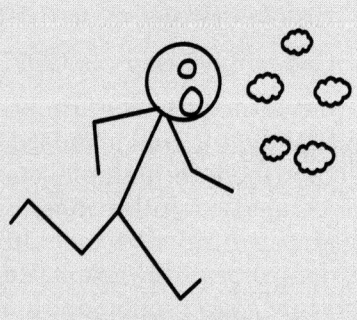

2. Walks slower than people of the same age on the level because of the breathlessness or has to stop for breath when walking at own pace on the level

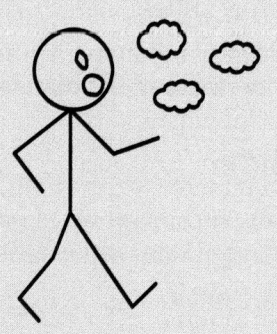

3. Stops for breath after walking about 100 yards or after a few minutes on the level

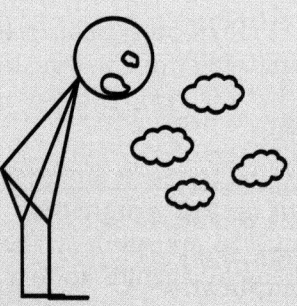

Table 4.1: Grades of dyspnoea *(Contd.)*

Grade	Description
4.	To breathless to leave the house or breathless when dressing or undressing.

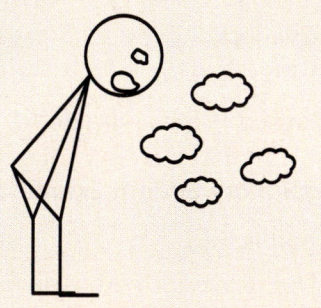

calculated by multiplying the number of packs of cigarettes smoked per day for the numbers of years the person has smoked. There might be patients who have left smoking, in these patients also details of smoking habit should be noted and also the time of quitting. Similarly specially in family history of biomass fuel exposure be explored in the form of type of kitchen in the home, type of fuel used for cooking and duration of exposure to biomasss fuel in days and years and if there were symptoms of cough during such exposure in detail. Every patient should also be asked for the nature of his job which might give an idea about the possibility of environmental smoke at his workplace or occupational lung diseases. He should also be asked about the association of cough at his workplace.

Although chronic bronchitis and emphysema invariably coexist unless it is caused by any congenital anomaly, it is the predominant symptoms search which might give an idea of the phenotypic variants. They have been classified as blue bloaters and pink puffers in earlier literature depending upon the presentation and the possible complication that might occur or pre-dominate.

Along with cardinal symptoms patients might present with associated symptoms like generelized fatigue, vague chest pain or feeling of weakness. Weight loss and exercise limitation are important symptoms in these subjects, this is because of dyspnoea on exertion or leg fatigue or combination of the two. One should also look for presence of pedal oedema or facial puffiness suggestive of corpulmonale or chonic use of oral steroid which is common in our country. In advance stage of the diseases chronic hypoxia is responsible for the peripheral muscle atrophy, highly related to deconditioning and poor nutrition of the patients. High wasted ventilation and oxygen cost of the ventilation may further be responsible for the weight loss. Sometimes patients might present with altered sensorium because of hypercarbia. Patients also present with complaint of swelling of feet and palpitation suggestive of feature of corpulmonale.

EXAMINATION

Examination findings are also vary from minimal finding to the feature of emphysema. Common examination findings are:

General Examination

Tachycardia

Tachypnea with pursed lip breathing

Cyanosis

Pedal oedema

Raised JVP if associated with CHF.

Respiratory System Examination

a. Inspection

Use of accessory muscle of respiration

Tracheal tug

Barrel-shaped chest

In drawing of supraclavicular fossa and subcostal

Intercostal recession.

b. Palpation

Normal situated trachea with tracheal tug present with deep inspiration

Decreased chest expansion (normal values—for Indian male: 84 cm and +5 cm on expansion, for Indian female: 79 cm and +5 cm on expansion)

Ratio of anteroposterior to lateral diameter of chest is altered.

Masked apex impulse or a parasternal heave.

c. Percussion

Overall hyper-resonant note

Level of diaphragm and tidal percussion is low.

Masking of cardiac dullness and liver dullness.

d. Auscultation

Presence of rhonchi all over the chest.

Overall decreased breath sound or sometimes silent chest

Presence of crepts in a few cases

Cardiac auscultation may reveal loud P2 and murmur at pulmonic area.

Physical findings depend on the stage of the diseases and predominant variant of phenotype. A patient of chronic bronchitis may present with tachypnea tachycardia and no other abnormality except for basal crepts on auscultation. Patients of emphysema may have barrel-shaped chest with kyphosis and increased anterior posterior diameter, ribs are placed more horizontally, prominent sternal angle and wide subcostal angle. These changes are permanent. There will be decreased movement of chest wall and patient might be using accessory muscle of respiration. There will be in drawing of the suprasternal and supraclavicular fossae and of intercostals muscle, predominantly in the axillary area. Percussion will low level of diaphragm and tidal percussion will also be low. Auscultation finding will reveal rhonchi as well as crepts. There might be universally decreased breath sound or silent chest in advance stage of the diseases.

Apart from finding of respiratory system patients might present with other sequelae or complications of the diseases or might presents with features of comorbid conditions, for example, right parasternal heave, presence of loud P2 on cardiac auscultation, presence of systolic murmur at pulmonic or tricuspid area pedal.

Oedema, hepatomegaly and hepato-jugular reflex as sign of corpulmonale. Patients might also present with feature of irritability, anxiety tremors, hypersolmence, or altered sensorium because of chronic hypoxia or hypercarbia. During examination one should also keep in mind the possibility of other diagnosis, for example, a patient of diabetes mellitus or hypertension with chronic CHF may also have signs and symptoms of COPD but can be differentiated by presence of bilateral basal crepitations. Tuberculosis is a major health problem in our country.

Tuberculosis and post-tuberculosis fibrosis and fibrocavitatory lesion obstructive airways symptoms may be a diagnostic challenge and can be differentiated by presence of harsh vesicular breath sound or fine crepts or decreased breath sound over the area.

Patients of occupational lung diseases may present with marked symptoms and radiological feature with minimal examination findings.

DIFFERENTIAL DIAGNOSIS

Common differential diagnosis of COPD is chronic persistent asthma, bronchiectasis, ACOS, congestive heart failure, tuberculosis and associated complications, obliterative bronchiolitis and diffuse panbronchilitis (Fig. 4.1).

Among these asthma and ACOS are most difficult to differentiate at times. GOLD 2015 and GINA 2015 has jointly published document and have following differentiating features that can be helpful. These differentiating features have been given in Table 4.2.

INVESTIGATION

Diagnosis is confirmed with the relevant investigations. Investigations are also required to rule out other possible causes of dyspnoea and to assess the severity of these diseases. Important investigations for the diagnosis of COPD are:

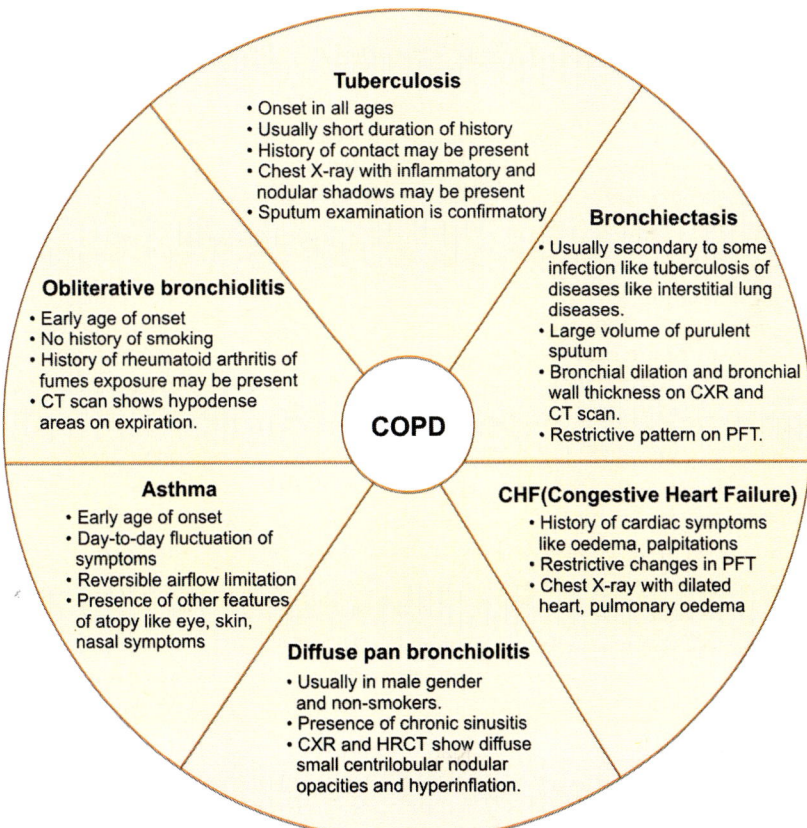

Fig. 4.1: Differential diagnosis of COPD

Table 4.2: Differentiating features of COPD, asthma and ACOS

Feature	Asthma	COPD	ACOS
Age of onset	Usual childhood onset but can commence at any time	Usually after the age of 40 years	Usually age>40 years but may have had symptoms in childhood or early adulthood.
Pattern of respiration	Symptoms may vary over time (day-to-day or over longer period) often limiting activity, and triggered by exercise, emotions including laughter, dust of exposure to allergen.	Chronic usually continuous symptoms particularly with exercise with better and worse days.	Respiratory symptoms include exertional dyspnoea are persistent but variability is prominent.
Lung function	Current of historical variable airflow limitation, e.g. bronchodilator reversibility	FEV_1 may improve with therapy but post bronchodilator FEV_1/FVC <70% persist	Airflow limitation not fully reversible but often with current of historical variability
Lung function between symptoms	May be normal between the symptoms	Persistent airflow limitation	Persistent airflow limitation
Past history or family history	Many patients have allergies and a personal history of asthma in childhood and/or family history of asthma	History of exposure to noxious particle and gases (mainly tobacco smoke and biomass fuel)	Frequently a history of doctor diagnosed asthma, current or previous allergies and family history of asthma and/or history of exposure of noxious exposure.
Time onset	Often improves spontaneously or with treatment but may result in fixed airflow limitation	Generally slowly progressive over the years despite treatment	Symptoms are partly but significantly reduced by treatment, progression is usual and treatment needs are high.
X-ray chest	Usually normal	Severe hyperinflation and other changes of COPD	Similar to COPD
Exacerbation	Exacerbation occurs but the risk of exacerbation can be considerably reduced by treatment	Exacerbation can be reduced by treatment. If present comorbidities contribute to the impairment.	Exacerbation are more common than in COPD but are reduced by treatment, comorbidities may contribute to the impairment.
Airway inflammation	Eosinophilic and/or neutrophilic	Neutrophilic ± eosinophilic in sputum, lymphocyte in airways may be systemic inflammation.	Eosinophilic and/or neutrophilic in sputum.

Pulmonary function test.

Radiological investigation.

Arterial blood gas analysis.

ECG and ECHO.

Pulmonary Function Test

Pulmonary function test had several components like forced expiratory volumes, gas diffusion studies, respiratory muscle functions and cardiopulmonary exercises. Most important component is forced expiratory manoeuvre which is used to confirm the diagnosis of COPD. Spirometry is not only essential for the diagnosis of COPD but also helps in differentiating COPD from bronchial asthma, interstitial lung diseases and other possible causes of dyspnoea.

It is desirable to perform spirometry in all individuals with unexplained dyspnoea, or patients with risk of developing COPD or working in the environment that can lead to abnormal lung function.

Spirometry

Common measurements which are done with the spirometers and their description are given in Table 4.3.

Procedure: Patients are asked to take maximum inhalation followed by forceful and complete exhalation till he can exhale and again inahale to the maximum capacity (Fig. 4.2). This act is repeated to achieve at least three comparable volume and flow results fulfilling the repeatability and acceptable criteria. Reversibility test is done by giving patient 200 to 400 microgram of salbutamol inhaler and same forced expiratory procedure is repeated to look for the change of the FVC and FEV_1. Reversibility is done at least 30 minutes after the bronchodilators therapy. Reversibility is calculated as:

Table 4.3: Common measurements of PFT	
Measurement variable	*Description*
VC	Vital capacity is the volume that can be expired after full inspiration of the patients
FVC	Forced vital capacity is the volume that can be expired with maximum effort by the patients after full inspiration. (May be equal or less than VC)
FEV_1	Forced expiratory volume in one second that is volume of air exhaled in the first second of FVC manoeuvre.
FEF_{25-75}	Forced expiratory flow between 25% to 75% is the average flow during the middle half of the FVC manoeuvre.
PEFR	Peak expiratory flow rate is the maximum flow attained during the FVC manoeuvre.
MVV	Maximum ventilatory ventilation is the volume of air a patient can breath rapidly and forcefully over a specified period of time.

%Change = {(post-bronchodilator volume – prebronchodilator volume) ÷ (prebronchodilator volume)} × 100

Spirometer display: There are two ways to display the spirogram:

A. Volume time curve

B. Flow time display

The volume time curve puts volume in litres on the vertical axis and time in seconds on the horizontal axis. Display is useful in assessing the duration of expiration viewing the terminal portion of the spirometry to assess whether a plateau was achieved and patients exhale fully (Fig. 4.3).

The flow volume display puts flow in litre/sec on the vertical axis and volume in

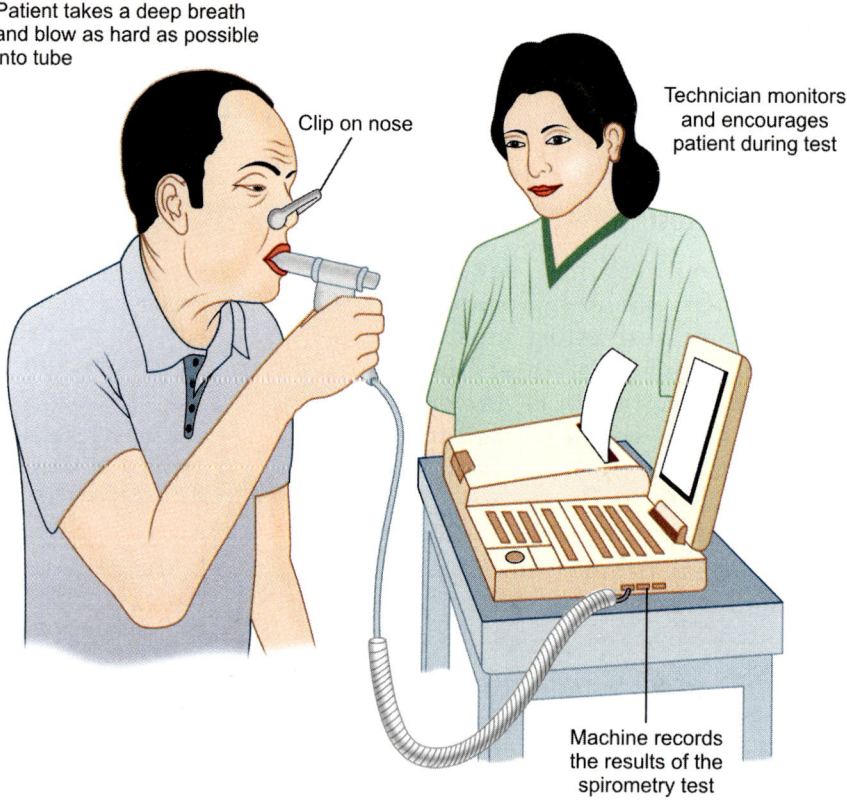

Patient takes a deep breath and blow as hard as possible into tube

Clip on nose

Technician monitors and encourages patient during test

Machine records the results of the spirometry test

Fig. 4.2: Procedure of performing PFT

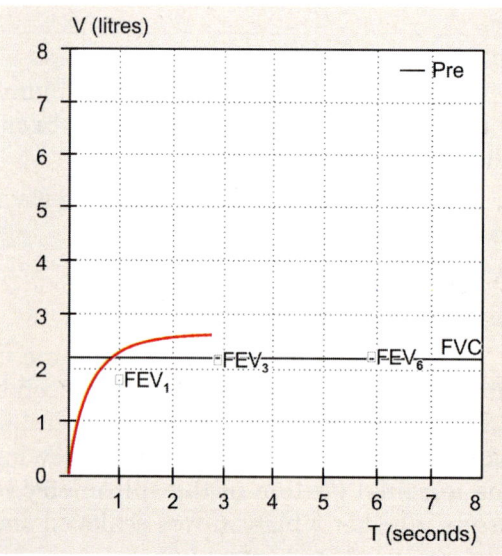

Fig. 4.3: Normal volume time graph. Time is on X axis and volume on Y axis. Graph represents achievement of FVC at 5 sec and plateau level

litre on horizontal axis. This display is most useful in assessing the initial portion of spirometry and peak expiratory flow. Scaling are done in such a manner that scale for flow is double to the scale of volume (Fig. 4.4).

Interpretation: Interpretation of the spirometry results should be started with looking at the flow and loop. These flow should be smooth and expiratory time should be of 6 sec. However, a minimum of 3 seconds manoeuvre is accepted but less than that is rejected for interpretation. First one should look for FEV_1/FVC followed by FVC followed by FEV_1. A post-bronchodilator FEV_1/FVC of less than 70% and FEV_1 of less than 80% is considered to be the diagnostic feature of obstructive airway diseases (Figs 4.5 and 4.6).

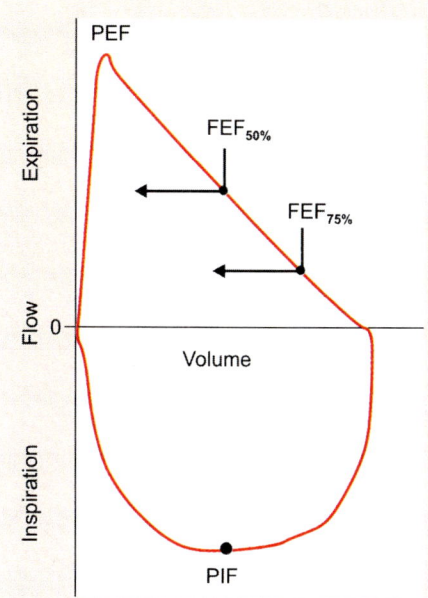

Fig. 4.4: Normal flow volume loop showing volume at X axis and flow at Y axis. Above 0 line is expiration while loop below 0 line shows inspiratory effort. Highest point in expiratory phase should be peaked and depicts peak expiratory flow rate, while lowest point in inspiratory phase is indicative of peak inspiratory flow rate

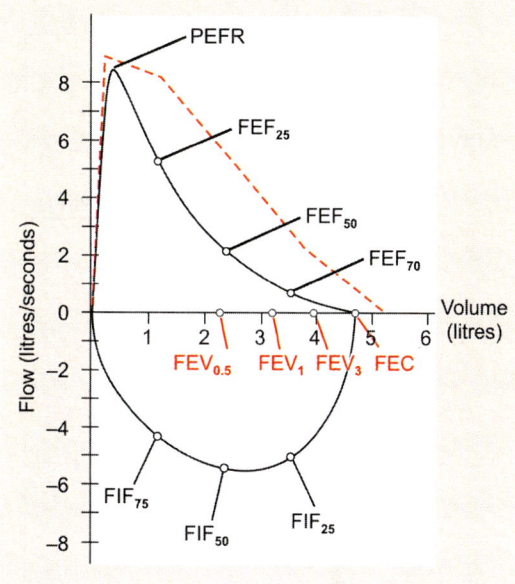

Fig. 4.6: Flow volume loop of a patient of obstructive airway diseases

To differentiate asthma from COPD, reversibility test is helpful. A patient of bronchial asthma shows good reversibility in FEV_1 (Figs 4.7 and 4.8) which is defined as

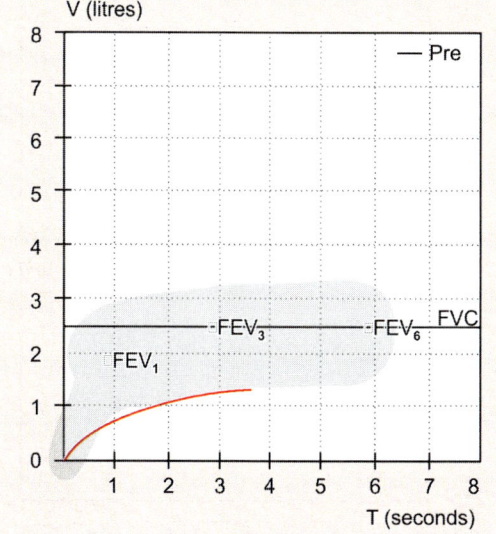

Fig. 4.5: Volume time graph of patients with obstructive airway diseases. Graph shows a steep pattern and non-achievement of plateau

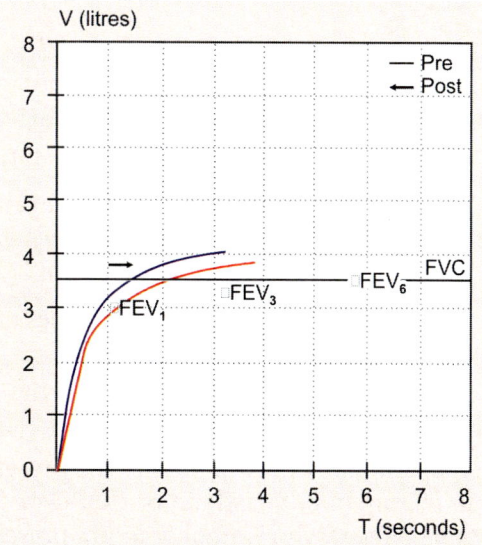

Fig. 4.7: Volume time graph of patient of obstructive airway diseases with good reversibility. Change in volume at 1 sec (FEV_1) is significant

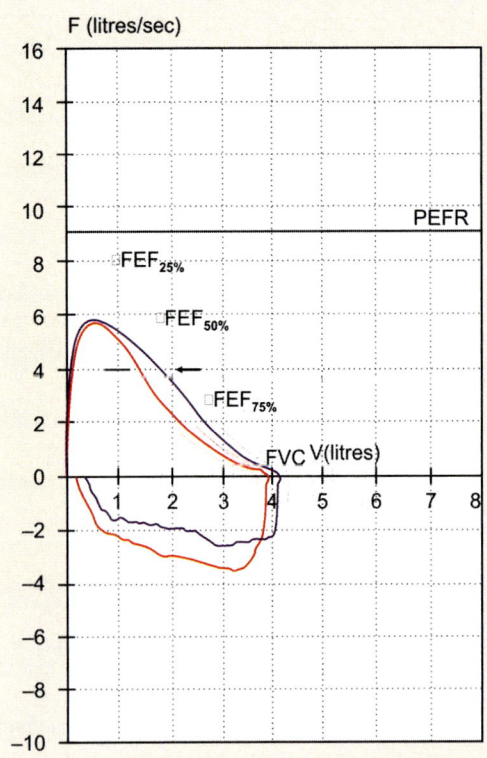

Fig. 4.8: Flow volume loop of patient with obstructive airway diseases with good reversibility

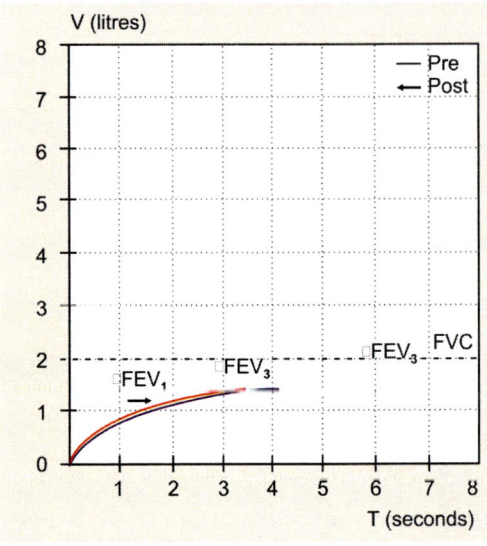

Fig. 4.9: Volume–time graph of patient of obstructive airway diseases with poor reversibility. Change in volume at 1 sec (FEV$_1$) is minimal

change in FEV$_1$ of 200 ml and 12% of the pre-bronchodilator value. While a patient of COPD will have poor reversibility (Fig. 4.9).

When FVC and FEV$_1$ both are reduced and FEV$_1$/FVC is more than 80%, it is suggestive of restrictive lung pathology (Fig. 4.10).

And a restrictive lung pathology does not show reversibility in any of the value.

Summary of PFT interpretation is given in Figs 4.11 and 4.12, Table 4.4.

There might be a few patients who present with feature of both asthma or COPD or an asthma patient who is smoker might present with clinical features of COPD and his spirometric parameters are also does not fit into asthma or COPD pattern. These patients

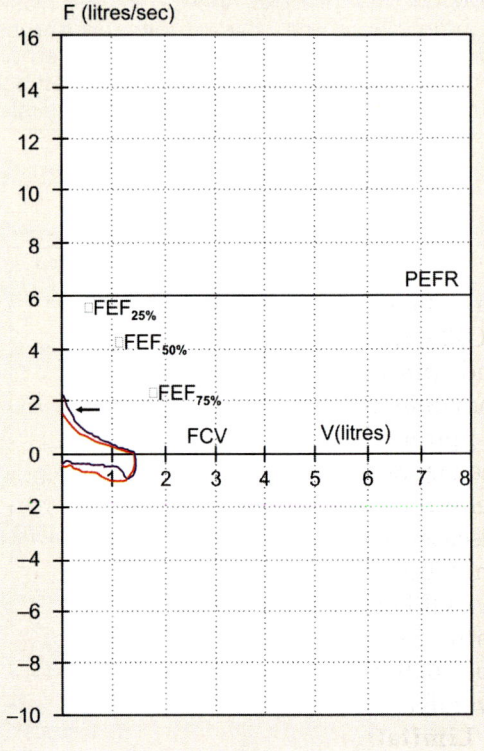

Fig. 4.10: Flow volume loop of patients with restrictive lung diseases showing both FVC and FEV$_1$ are markedly reduced and almost no reversibility

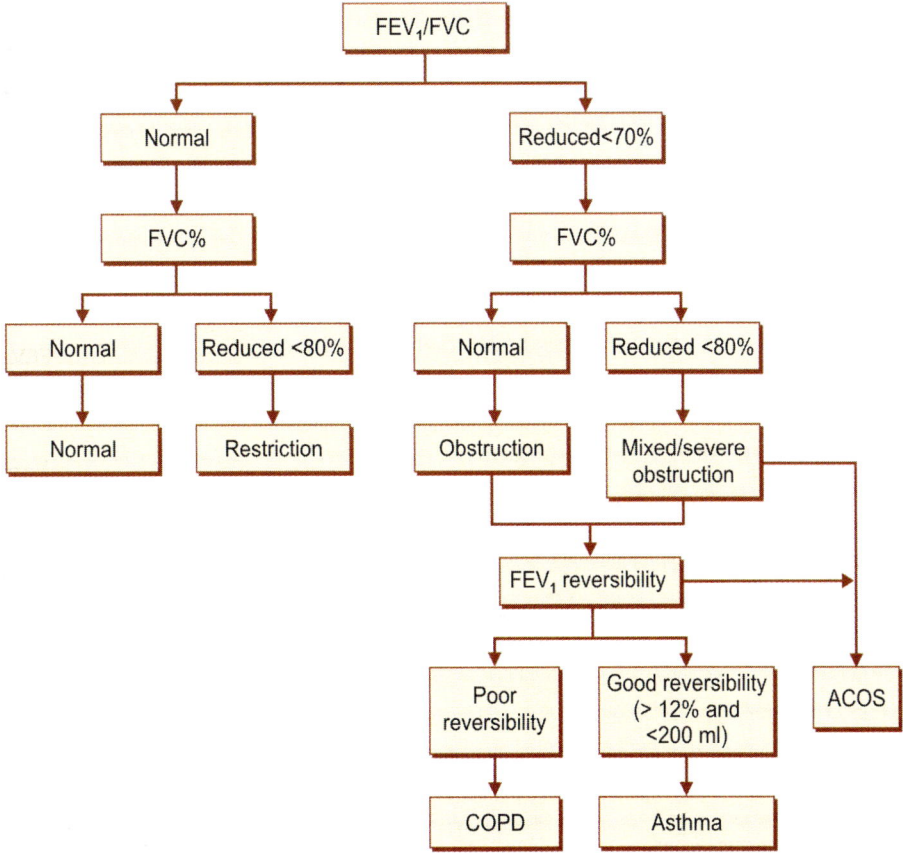

Fig. 4.11: PFT interpretation summary

have been categorize as ACOS (asthma, COPD overlap syndrome). Clinical features and spirometric differentiation features are shown in Tables 4.2 and 4.5 respectively.

Spirometry not only help to differentiate the diagnosis of COPD from asthma but also helpful in assessment of the severity of the diseases by assessing the severity of airflow limitation. The severity of airflow limitation in COPD is based on FEV_1/FVC and FEV_1 value. Assessment of severity of airflow obstruction is an important component of overall assessment of the diseases severity.

Limitations of spirometry: Though spirometry is essential step for the diagnosis and severity assessment of COPD, spirometry is exhaustive investigation to perform.

It needs a lot of effort from the instructor as well as patients. Instructor should be versed with the local language and must have good communication skill. Moreover, it is a diagnostic tool which needs a lot of co-operation from the patients. It is not like ECG, EEG where patient has to lie straight on bed and to do nothing, there are prerequisite before performance of spirometry and relative contraindication like recent MI, CVA, surgery, pregnancy aneurysm, recent pneumothorax. Spirometry cannot be performed in acute exacerbation as patient might not be able to perform and even if he can, the result will not be accurate and true reflective of his stable lung status. This limitation of spirometry has lead to search of

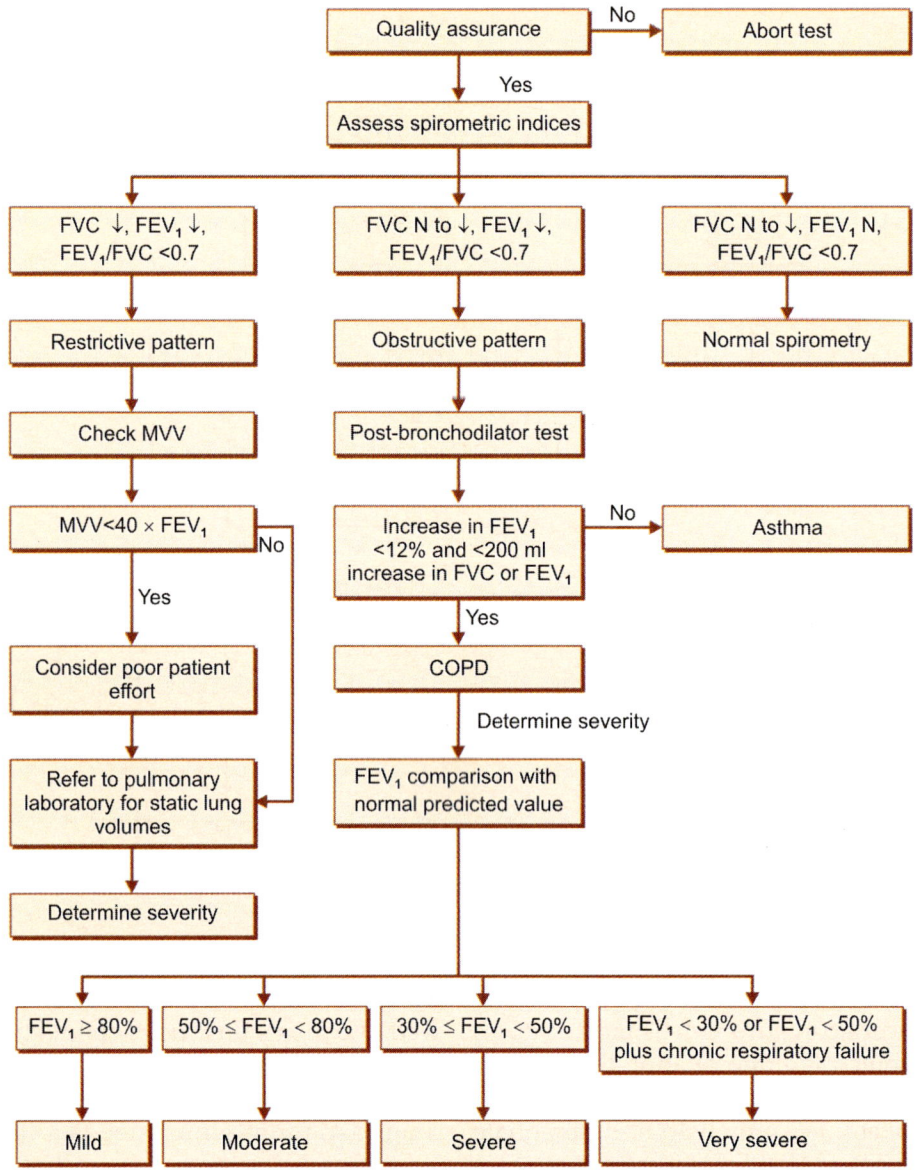

Fig. 4.12: Algorithm of interpretation of PFT

questionnaire-based diagnostic tool for COPD. Various questionnaires have been developed and validated for the diagnosis of COPD. Among all these CAT score and COPD diagnostic questionnaire have been accepted to have good accuracy and sensitivity and specificity.

Radiography

A plane X-ray chest PA view is necessary for the evaluation of the patients of COPD. The lateral view is also helpful some times. A plane X-ray chest may be within normal limit in patients or sometimes may present only

Table 4.4: FEF_{25-75}, forced expiratory flow rate over the middle 50% of the FVC; FEV_1, forced expiratory volume in 1 second; FVC, forced expiratory vital capacity; MVV, maximal voluntary ventilation; N, normal; PEF, peak expiratory flow; ↓, decreased; ↑, increased.

Typical patterns of impairment		
Measurement	*Obstructive*	*Restrictive*
FVC (L)	N to ↓ than 80% of predicted value	↓ than 80% of predicted value
FEV_1 (L)	↓ than 80% of predicted value	↓ than 80% of predicted value to N
FEV_1/FVC	<.7	>.7
FEF_{25-75} (L/s)	↓	N to ↓
PEF (L/s)	↓	N to ↓
MVV (L/min)	↓	N to ↓

with hilar prominence or with increased bronchovascular marking especially if the patient is having chronic bronchitis type of phenotype.

However, in emphysematous phenotype the classical sign of increased lucency of the lung field, tubular heart shadow and low and flat diaphragm may be seen in isolation or in combination with each other. Increased lucency can be detected by decreased bronchovascular marking in the periphery. The maximum curvature of the right dome of diaphragm is less than 1.5 cm and is placed of the extent that 7½ of the anterior part of the rib and 11th rib at the vertebral level can be seen. This is defined as low and flat diaphragm. Presence of regional hyperlucency (bulla) or vascular attenuation are the confirmatory sign of emphysema. A bulla is defined as small (less than 1 cm) hyperlucent space with hairline margins. The bulla may remain of the same size or occasionally it progresses in size and

gradually compress most part of the lung so that most part of the hemi thorax is seen as hyperlucent without any recognizable normal lung parenchyma. This is known as "vanishing lung syndrome".

On a lateral film there may be increased retrosternal space below the manubrium. A retrosternal space of greatest diameter from the sternum to the anterior heart is more than 2.5 cm. Fluoroscopic examination of the diaphragm may reveal decreased or paradoxical movement.

CT Thorax: CT thorax is nowadays important diagnostic tool for the diagnosis of COPD in early stage and it has shown a good correlation with morphological difference among the patients with airway obstruction. It also reflects important differences in the underlying pathophysiology and genomic profile of the patients diagnosed with COPD. Presently two dominant CT phenotypes have been proposed.

a Emphysema predominant diseases

b Airway predominant diseases, resulting from chronic airway inflammation and resulting airway remodeling and narrowing.

Emphysema predominant disease is usually defined by presence of bulla and hyperlucent area and can be divided according to the type of emphysema present into centrilobular, pan lobular and paraseptal and bullous emphysema. In contrast to emphysema predominant COPD, airway predominant COPD is defined by relatively minor degree of emphysema associated with marked degree of airways wall abnormalities and in particular airway wall thickening. Nakano et al have shown that CT measurement of airway wall area coupled with measurement of luminal dimension can be used to differentiate patients with asthma (increased airway wall area but normal luminal dimension) to patients of COPD (increased airway wall area and decreased

Table 4.5: Comparison of various spirometric indices in asthma, COPD and ACOS

Spirometric	Asthma	COPD	ACOS
Normal FEV_1/ Variable FVC pre- or Post BD	Compatible with the diagnosis	Not compatible with diagnosis	Not compatible unless other evidence of chronic airflow obstruction present
Post-BD FEV_1/ FVC <70%	Indicate airflow limitation but may improve spontaneously or on treatment	Required for the diagnosis (GOLD)	Usually present
$FEV_1 \geq 80\%$ predicted	Compatible with diagnosis (good asthma control or interval between the symptoms)	Compatible with GOLD classification of mild airflow obstruction	Compatible with diagnosis of mild ACOS
$FEV_1 < 80\%$ predicted	Compatible with diagnosis, risk factor for asthma exacerbation	An indicator of severity of airflow limitation (mortality and COPD exacerbation)	An indicator of severity of airflow limitation and risk of future events (mortality and exacerbation)
Post-BD increase in FEV_1 >12% and 200 ml from base line	Usual at sometimes in the course of asthma but may not be present when well controlled or on controllers.	Common and more likely when FEV_1 is low	Common and more likely when FEV_1 is low
Post-BD increase in FEV_1 ≥12% and 400 ml from base line (marked reversibility)	High probability of asthma	Unusual in COPD Consider ACOS	Compatible with diagnosis of ACOS

luminal dimension). Inflammatory small airways diseases can be directly identified on CT scan by presence of peripheral micronodular opacities, obstructive airways disease is identified by gas trapping on expiratory CT. In the absence of emphysema, other supportive features which can be seen on CT are presence of tracheobroncho-malacia, saber sheath trachea, tracheobronchial out pouching, patchy ground glass opacities, enlargement of pulmonary artery suggestive of pulmonary hypertension and bronchiectasis.

CT clearly demonstrates that the degree of airways obstruction co-relate poorly with the anatomical extent of emphysema specially if it is predominantly in upper lobe and is centrilobular. CT evidence of emphysema is frequently found in the patients who even do not meet the spirometric criteria of COPD. CT can serve to complement clinical and physiological phenotype and may potentially provide in site in underlying genetic pattern of the diseases.

Other Investigations

The detection of secondary polycythemia suggests chronic hypoxia and indicates to assess the need of oxygen therapy. The degree of polycythemia may be related to the level of carboxyhaemoglobin due to smoking and the value lessen after stopping smoking. However, in Indian subcontinent polycythemia may not be present because of poor nutritional status of the patients. On cardiological evaluation electrography may show right axis deviation and presence of P pulmonale (Fig. 4.13).

The ECG below is from a 58-year-old man with a recent diagnosis of COPD. Echocardiogram showed neither right atrial nor right ventricular dilatation. P wave axis is +80 degrees (P wave verticalization). The P wave is negative in lead aVL. Low voltage and incomplete right bundle branch block are also seen.

On echocardiography there may be dilated RA and RV and there might be presence of mild tricuspid regurgitation and increased contractility of the right heart. However, these findings may be seen late in the disease.

Patients should be screened for presence of alpha 1 antitrypsin deficiency as alpha 1 antitrypsin deficiency is an important cause of emphysema. Persons who have following features should be screened for alpha1 antitrypsin deficiency.

a. Early onset emphysema

b. Emphysema in nonsmokers

c. Emphysema predominance at lung bases

d. Necrotizing panniculitis

e. C-ANCA positive vasculitis

f. Family history of early onset emphysema

g. Bronchiectasis without any etiology.

Recurrent chest infection is also common in COPD patients although nonspecific to COPD it has significance in the treatment as it may progress to pneumonia and that may further worsen the lung function.

An arterial blood gas analysis should be done in patients of COPD specially when

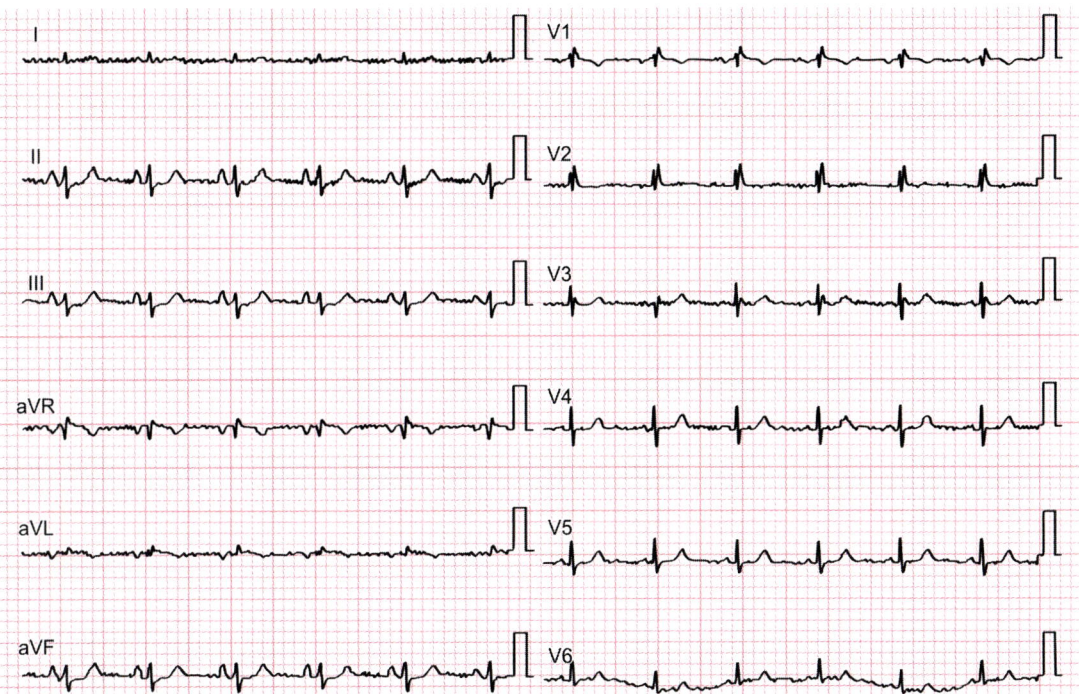

Fig. 4.13: ECG changes in COPD

they come in acute condition. Arterial blood gas analysis may show respiratory acidosis because of hypercarbia suggesting type II respiratory failure. There may be presence of hypoxia associated with hypercarbia.

ASSESSMENT OF SEVERITY OF COPD

Over the years severity of COPD was classified only on the basis of severity of airflow obstruction but with recent literature and evidence it was found that severity of airflow obstruction has poor co-relation with overall prognosis of the patients. In GOLD 2015 severity of the diseases is been changed to a combined assessment including level of dyspnoea, degree of airflow obstruction, and number of exacerbation over last one year.

Severity of airflow obstruction as per GOLD criteria:

Presence of obstruction—FEV_1/FVC ≤70% (diagnostic criteria of COPD)

Severity of Obstruction

GOLD 1	Mild	FEV_1 <80% of the predicted
GOLD 2	Moderate	FEV_1 50–80% of predicted
GOLD 3	Severe	FEV_1 30–50% of predicted
GOLD 4	Very severe	FEV_1 <30% of predicted of <50% with feature of cor pulmonale

Overall severity assessment of the COPD patient and his categorization in stage ABCD has three steps.

Step 1   Find level of dyspnoea as per mMRC of CAT score

Step 2   Find level of airflow obstruction as GOLD 1, 2, 3, 4

Step 3   Find number of exacerbations over last one year

Step 4   Categorize as Table 4.6

Assessment of Severity (Table 4.7)

GOLD established criteria assess the COPD severity based on a physiological variable, post-bronchodilator FEV_1% predicted as mild>80, moderate 50–80, severe 30–50 and very severe <30, "rule of 30–50–80".

Table 4.7: Assessment of severity

GOLD spirometric criteria for COPD severity. FEV_1/FVC <0.7 after bronchodilator test is required for the diagnosis of COPD.

Mild COPD	FEV_1 ≥80% predicted
Moderate COPD	50% ≤FEV_1 < 80% predicted
Severe COPD	30% ≤FEV_1 < 50% predicted
Very severe COPD	FEV_1 < 30% predicted or FEV_1 < 50% predicted with chronic respiratory failure

Table 4.6: Categorization of COPD patients

Group	Characteristic	Spirometric grade	No. of exacerbation	CAT Score	mMRC
A	Low risk low symptoms	1	<1	Less than 10	0–1
B	Low risk high symptoms	2	<1	10 or more	2 or more
C	High risk low symptoms	3	2 or more	Less than 10	0–1
D	High risk more symptoms	4	2 or more	10 or more	2 or more

The systemic manifestations of COPD are not reflected by the FEV_1. Hence, the BODE (body mass index, obstruction, dyspnoea, and exercise tolerance) index has been used to assess the respiratory and systemic manifestations of COPD. The BODE index score (Table 4.8) helps in predicting hospitalisation for COPD. A BODE index of 0–2, 3–4, 5–6 and 7–10 is thought to be associated with a 52 months mortality rate of approximately 10, 30, 50 and 80% respectively.

SUMMARY

Any patient presenting with complaints of chronic cough with expectoration, breathlessness on exertion and having history of smoking or exposure to environmental smoke should be suspected for the possibility of COPD. It becomes difficult sometimes to establish a diagnosis of COPD and to differentiate it from other respiratory conditions. Careful history and detailed examination is essential before going for the investigation. Spirometry and radiology is necessary for the diagnosis of COPD. Flow sensor spirometer are portable and are commonly used. FEV_1/FVC <70% is indicative of obstructive airway diseases and reversibility of FEV_1 helps in differentiating COPD from asthma and ACOS. Radiological findings are helpful to differentiate different phenotypic presentation and to look for complication and CT thorax is far more sensitive than simple X-ray chest. Spirometry is essential for confirmation of the diagnosis and for assessment of severity and prognosis of the diseases. Though spirometry has some limitation and it cannot be performed in every patient, such patients should be screened through COPD diagnostic questionnaire. Arterial blood gas analysis and echocardiography should be done in selected patients. Patients should also be screened for alpha-1 antitrypsin deficiency if patients young or had family history of COPD.

Table 4.8: BODE index

Variables	Points			
	0	1	2	3
FEV_1 (% Predicted)	>65	50–64	36–49	<35
Walk distance in 6 min (m)	>350	250–349	150–249	<149
Modified Medical Research Council (mMRC) Dyspnoea Scale	0–1	2	3	4
Body mass index (BMI= weight in kg/height in m^2)	>21	<21	-	-

mMRC scale uses the same clinical descriptors as the original MRC scale (1–5), although values are denoted as 0–4 in the calculation of the BODE index

BIBLIOGRAPHY

1. An Official American Thoracic Society/ European Respiratory Society Statement: Research Questions in Chronic Obstructive Pulmonary Disease American Journal of Respiratory and Critical Care Medicine Volume 191 Number 7 | April 1 2015.
2. GOLD REPORT 2015.
3. Halbert RJ, Natoli JL, Gano A, Badamgarav E, Buist AS, Mannino DM. Global burden of COPD: systematic review and meta-analysis. Eur Respir J 2006; 28: 523–32
4. Hnizdo E, Sullivan Pm, Bang KM, Wagner G. Airflow obstruction attributable to work in industry and occupation among US Race/ Ethanic group: A study of NHANES III data AM J Ind Med 2004; 46: 126–35.
5. Lozano R, Naghavi M, Foreman K, Lim S, Shibuya K, Aboyans V, Abraham J, Adair T, Aggarwal R, Ahn SY, et al. Global and regional mortality from 235 causes of death for 20 age groups in 1990 and 2010: a systematic analysis for the Global Burden of Disease Study 2010. Lancet 2012; 380: 2095–2128.
6. Oroczo-Levi M, Gracia Aymerich J, Villarj, Ramirez, Sermiento A, Anto JM, Gea J. Wood smoke exposure and risk of chronic obstructive pulmonary diseases. Eur Respir J; 2006; 27: 542–6.

Comorbidities

Chapter

5

Ashok Kumar Singh, Amit Kumar Verma

INTRODUCTION

In a ECLIPSE (2008) study including a cohort of 911 COPD patients, it has been found that COPD patients dies due to its comorbidities more than COPD itself.

Table 5.1 shows that only 35% of these patients died because of respiratory causes, among them 8–9% are non-COPD causes. Hence it can be concluded from this study, that in 60–70% instances cause of death in COPD patients is its comorbidities. A good knowledge, understanding and management of these comorbidities will definitely improve prognosis in COPD.

Table 5.1: Classification of cause of death in 911 COPD patients on salmetrol/fluticasone therapy in a randomized controlled trial over 3 years

System	Proportion of death (%)
Cardiovascular (ischemic heart disease, CHF, hypertension, stroke, etc).	26
Respiratory	35
COPD	27
Pneumonias	8
Others	<1
Cancers	21
Lung	14
Other	7
Other causes	10
Unknown	8

Out of the top 5 causes of death in India reported by WHO, COPD is one of that. From ECLIPSE study we found that the cause of death in COPD patients has been largely because of co-morbidities associated with it.

All the above reasons signify the importance of chapter, **comorbidities in COPD.**

Hence a good knowledge of co-morbidities to all practicing physicians, will definitely improve outcome in the disease.

Conventionally comorbidity is defined as "a disease co-existing with primary disease of interest".

In COPD, however, it is little different in a way that certain co-existing illness may be consequences of chronic systemic inflammation in pathogenesis of COPD itself or may be consequences of prolong treatment with oral or inhaled corticosteroids or certain diseases may be due to shared common risk factors, e.g. age, smoking, poor physical activity (sedentary life).

COMORBIDITIES

Cardiovascular diseases are the most common comorbidities in COPD. It includes hypertension, ischemic heart diseases and congestive heart failure. After CVD, osteoporosis has been found 2nd most common coexisting condition in COPD.

Other major comorbidities are gastro-esophageal-reflux diseases (GERD), skeletal muscle dysfunction, depression, anaemias, and diabetes mellitus in decreasing order of prevalence.

List of major co-morbid diseases in COPD with prevalence (%) found in different studies (Table 5.2).

Table 5.2: Major comorbidities in COPD	
Name of disease	*Prevalence in COPD (%)*
Cardiovascular	55–90
Hypertension	40–60
Ischaemic heart disease	10–23
Congestive heart failure	5–7
Osteoporosis	50–70
GERD	30–60
Skeletal muscle dysfunction	25–32
Depression	20–25
Anaemia	10–17
Diabetes mellitus	12–14

Minor comorbidities (Table 5.3) are those diseases which are less prevalent in COPD or they do not significantly affect the mortality in COPD. These include arrhythmias, chronic renal failure, stroke, obstructive sleep apnoea, pneumonia, tuberculosis, pneumothorax, oral candidiasis or cushingoid disease.

Major Comorbidities

Hypertension

Hypertension is the most common co-morbid condition in COPD. Indeed COPD and hypertension share the two most prevalent conditions in middle age and later part of life. Since age is significant common

Table 5.3: Minor comorbidities in COPD
Pneumothorax
Obstructive sleep apnoea
Stroke
Tuberculosis
pneumonia
Oral candidiasis
Cushingoid disease
Chroinc renal failure

risk factor in these two conditions, they are often co-morbid to each other. Prevalence of hypertension in India in normal subjects is reported raised to 25–35% but in COPD patients it is 40–60%. This shows that hypertension has somewhat more strong relation with COPD than normal population.

Definite pathological mechanism of link between these two conditions is not described clearly in literatures but accelerated ageing, loss of connective tissues and increased arterial stiffness may have a role, suggested in many literatures.

How to suspect hypertension in COPD: Hypertension should be screened out in all patients of COPD. Mostly early stages of hypertension is always asymptomatic, hence, best way to screen out hypertension in COPD is to check blood pressure all the time patient visits to you.

The blood pressure of more than 140 mmHg systolic and 90 mmHg diastolic, on regular/daily basis or on most of the days of a week is considered hypertension in COPD. It should be managed to maintain at less than 120 mmHg systolic and 80 mmHg diastolic.

Before starting treatment for hypertension we must rule out causes of secondary hypertension that found in this age group.

Insomnia, headache, tingling sensations in limbs, dizziness are some of the common symptoms of hypertension for which a practitioner should be careful and vigilant.

Ischaemic Heart Disease

It is clearly revealed in various studies that ischaemic heart disease (MI and angina) are more common in COPD patients than normal population.

Link between ischaemic heart diseases with COPD can be explained with common risk factors like age and smoking. Chronic persistent systemic inflammatory process in COPD may also be the cause of ischaemic heart disease.

It has been shown that patients with COPD and heart disease have worse health status and have the highest hospital visits. So, presence of ischaemic heart disease should be detected at the earliest.

How to Suspect IHD

1. Obese COPD patients (chronic bronchitis phenotype)

2. Regular symptom of chest pain or locations like shoulder/jaw/arm/back. It may start anywhere on the chest and radiates to these locations. It may feel like pressure over chest or squeezing on chest. Pain tends to worse with activity and go away with rest.

3. Any previous history of severe chest pain associated with nausea, vomiting and/or perspiration.

4. Regular complaint of no relief in dyspnoea even after full bronchodilation and proper management of COPD.

Patients presenting with above mentioned symptoms should be investigated thoroughly and if diagnoses of having IHD, should be managed with the help of a cardiologist or general medicine doctors.

Congestive Heart Failure

It can be either right side or left side heart failure or both together. COPD is more commonly associated with right-sided heart failure. Right side heart failure in COPD is mediated by raised pulmonary artery pressure which often happens in advance stage COPD.

Isolated right side heart failure in COPD is called cor pulmonale. Elevated pulmonary artery pressure, in COPD, is generally driven by persistence of hypoxia, vascular remodelling and epithelial dysfunction.

Cause of left-sided heart failure is maximally due to presence of hypertension since long duration and recent onset IHD or due to the presence of chronic anaemia. Chronic hypertension and anaemia increase the work load of the heart, whereas IHD cause contractility dysfunction. Increase work load over the heart and contractility dysfunction both lead to pooling of blood in the left ventricle and increased back pressure to pulmonary veins and cause lung congestion and hence increase the proportion of dyspnoea to the COPD patients.

Suspecting RHF in COPD

1. COPD patients complaining of on and off pedal oedema. Pedal oedema specially in the evening, gradually progressing in nature. On examination, JVP found raised.

2. Chronic bronchitis phenotype of COPD patients more prone to have RHF

Suspecting LHF

1. No relief in dyspnoea even after full COPD therapy with which the patient had history of getting complete relief previously.

2. History of orthopnea: Dyspnoea increase on lying down.

3. History of recent paroxysmal nocturnal dyspnoea: Patient has history of awak-

ening in the night due to breathlessness, which was earlier not noticed by the patient, but now this has developed repeatedly to patient.

4. History of early morning: Dyspnoea more than the other hours of the day.

5. On examination—basal crepts are heard on auscultation.

Osteoporosis

Osteoporosis should be suspected in all COPD patients, with long history of diagnosed COPD, that is more than 5 years, especially in those COPD patients who have long history of treatment with oral corticosteroids.

Link between these two conditions can be explained with:

a. Excessive proteolytic activity in emphysematous phenotype of COPD

b. Persistent systemic chronic inflammatory process in COPD patients

c. Smoking history of COPD patients

d. Low sex hormone at COPD age

e. Systemic steroid treatment given to COPD patients by multiple practitioners

CT-bone densitometry is best investigation for early diagnosis.

Gastroesophageal Reflux Diseases (GERD)

It should be suspected with COPD patient having frequent history of exacerbations.

Studies show that GERD is associated more with COPD patients than normal population.

Link Between the GERD and COPD can be explained with:

1. Hyperinflated COPD leads to low lying diaphragm, which increases the intra-abdominal pressure and

Pressure on the stomach, which increases reflux of liquid and food material in the oesophagus.

2. Persistent regular coughing exerts pressure over stomach.

3. Increase work of abdominal muscle in COPD patients for ventilation.

4. Transient relaxation of lower oesophageal sphincter, allows stomach content to spill in oesophagus. This spilled stomach content may rise as high as larynx because of presence of increased intra-abdominal pressure in COPD patients.

Link between GERD and COPD exacerbation has arouses curiosity into the medical professionals and require further research on this.

Skeletal Muscle Dysfunction

Skeletal muscle dysfunction is prominent in emphysematous phenotype of COPD.

Pathophysiology of skeletal muscle weakness is multifactorial. A few of the likely factors are listed below, but exact cause is still not definitely understood.

1. Reduce activity in COPD (because of exertional dyspnoea) causes disuse atrophy.

2. Protein catabolism, more than the anabolism in COPD patients because of chronic persistent hypoxia and oxidative stress and hence, lead to muscle wasting.

3. Poor nutritional intake and unmatched calorie expenditure (more calorie expenditure against airway resistances contributes to muscle wasting).

4. Systemic chronic inflammatory process may cause cachexia itself.

Low BMI (<18.5) with quadriceps wasting obvious in these patients and hence, diagnosis is not difficult. This is quite common in emphysematous and hyperinflation phenotype of COPD.

Depression

Depression is a common co-morbid condition in most symptomatic chronic diseases. It has been suggested in many of the studies that COPD patients are particularly more susceptible to depression.Up to quarter of the COPD patients has depression. Hence it is important to screen out.

Depression can by screened out with PHQ-2 (patients health questionnaire-2), whereas severity of a depression should be assessed by PHQ-9 (patient health questionnaire-9) (Table 5.4).

First two questions of PHQ-9 can be used for screening of depression and called PHQ-2, to screen out depression.

Interpretation of PHQ-2 (screening): First two questions can be used for screening depression in COPD patients. Total score range from 0 to 6. Score 3 or more than 3 is considered as depressive symptoms and hence particular attention required.

Interpretation of PHQ-9

1–4: Minimal depression

5–9: Mild depression

10–14: Moderate depression

15–19: Moderate severe depression

20–24: Severe depression

Depression is an under recognized condition in COPD patients and screening (PHQ-2) may be useful tool to clinical diagnosis, upon which management should be based.

Pathophysiology of depression in COPD is not very clear, but systemic inflammation, perhaps via TNF-α and oxidative stress have been implicated by K. AI-shair, Morris JD Singhetal in their study in 2011.

Table 5.4: Patient health questionnaire -9				
Over the last 2 weeks, how often have you been bothered by any of the following problems?	Not at all	Several days	More than half the days	Nearly every day
1. Little interest or pleasure in doing things	0	1	2	3
2. Feeling down, depressed, or hopeless	0	1	2	3
3. Trouble falling or staying asleep, or sleeping too much	0	1	2	3
4. Feeling tired or having little energy	0	1	2	3
5. Poor appetite or overeating	0	1	2	3
6. Feeling bad about yourself—or that you are a failure or have let yourself or your family down	0	1	2	3
7. Trouble concentrating on things, such as reading the newspaper or watching television	0	1	2	3
8. Moving or speaking so slowly that other people could have noticed. Or the opposite—being so fidgety or restless that you have been moving around a lot more than usual	0	1	2	3
9. Thoughts that you would be better off dead, or of hurting yourself in some way	0	1	2	3

Total score: 1–4 minimal depression; 5–9 mild depression; 10–14 moderate depression; 15–19 moderately severe depression; 20–27 severe depression

Anaemia

Anaemia prevalence has been described variably in COPD outdoor patients and indoor patients.

Its prevalence has been found 10% in outdoor COPD patients and 17% in indoor COPD patients. This shows that prevalence of anaemia increases as the COPD severity progresses.

Anaemia in COPD has a special characteristic that is decreased haemoglobin with increased RBC count (anaemia with polycythemia).

Hb<13 gm/d/in male is considered anemia and

Hb<11 gm/d/in female is considered anaemia.

Link between COPD and anaemia can be explained as:

i. Chronic nutritional deprivation because of chronic inflammatory disease condition.

ii. One more hypothesis of development of anaemia in COPD patients: A persistent chronic inflammation causes elevation of interleukin which interferes the response of erythropoietin.

Suspecting Anaemia in COPD

1. Persistence of dyspnoea even after best of COPD control effort
2. Fatigue, lethargy more than proportion to COPD stage
3. Abnormal heart rhythm with *ghabrahat*
4. Pulse rate more than the usual

We should always keep in mind, whenever there is anaemia to a COPD patients associated with restlessness, nausea and vomiting, we must investigate for chronic renal failure.

Diabetes Mellitus

Prevalence of diabetes in COPD has been found 10–14% as seen in ECLIPSE study and many other studies. Whereas it is <6% in normal population. This shows that diabetes mellitus is more associated with COPD than normal population.

However, long-term systemic corticosteroid therapy by many practitioners in COPD patients may cause hyperglycemia, hence association of incident diabetes with COPD is still a matter of debate.

The association of multiple risk factors like hypertension, hyperglycemia, hyperinsulinemia, abdominal obesity, atherogenic dyslipidemia, prothrombotic and proinflammatory state known as metabolic syndrome is an early step in the development of diabetes and vascular disease, with low level of lung function has been well-established entity now.

Common mediator for this association of metabolic syndrome with COPD is IL-6, TNF and adipokins as recent research indicates.

Suspecting Diabetes Mellitus

- More common in chronic bronchitis phenotype
- Recurrent complaints of dryness of mouth and tongue
- Frequent urination
- Increased appetite
- Non-healing of any ulcer or injury on the body

Steroid should be withhold one week to 10 days before final blood sugar-fasting/post-prandial conclusive report to level the patient as diabetic.

Minor Co-morbidities

Three minor co-morbidities that worth description in brief here are commonly encountered in day-to-day practice of COPD management. These three are described here.

Table 5.5: Summary of prevalence, impact, phenotypic association and areas of uncertainty among reviewed COPD comorbidities

Comorbidity	Preva-lence	Impact on COPD outcome	Mechanistic pathway	Associated phenotype	Area of uncertainty
1. Cardiovascular	55–90%	• Mortality • Quality of life • Frequency and • Duration of exacerbation	CRP, TNF	• Airway predominance • Chronic bronchitis	• Effect of cardiovascular medications on COPD control. • Risk of COPD medication on cardiac disease
2. Osteoporosis	55–70%	Quality of life	Metallo-proteinase proteolytic activity	Emphyse-matous	Mechanism
3. GERD	30–60%	• Quality of life • Exacerbations	• Weak oesophageal sphincters • Increased intra-abdominal pressure • Aspirin	Frequent exacerbations	Mechanism
4. Skeletal muscle dysfunction	25–35%	Quality of life	• Catabolic state • Energy expenditure • Disuse atrophy	Emphyse-matous	Therapy
5. Depression	20–25%	Quality of life	Unclear	—	Mechanism
6. Anaemia	10–17%	• Quality of life • Mortality	IL-1, poor response to erythropoietin	—	Mechanism
7. Diabetes	12–14%	• Mortality • Quality of life	IL-6, TNF, adipokine	Airway predominance (chronic bronchitis)	Role of adipokine

Obstructive Sleep Apnoea Syndrome

More common in chronic bronchitis phenotype with obesity and metabolic syndrome. Should be suspected when there is history of snoring with daytime sleepiness, and inability to concentrate. These symptoms in a patient of chronic bronchitis, obesity, metabolic syndrome and sometime diabetes strongly suggests OSAS.

Pneumothorax

Quite common in COPD with emphysematous phenotype.

Suspected when there is typical history of sudden bouts of cough followed by chest pain and rapidly progressing dyspnoea. On examination, you may find:

1. Markedly diminished or absent breath sound to one side of chest
2. Hyper-resonant note on percussion
3. Decrease *vocal fremitus* to the affected side

Oral Candidiasis

White coating over the tongue and oral ulceration in COPD patients due to prolong inhaled corticosteroid therapy or systemic corticosteroid therapy.

SUMMARY

With the current socio-economical environment in India incidence and prevalence of COPD is expected to be on rise. Most of the time in COPD patients have other diseases, which are due to common inflammatory mechanism exacerbated in this disease due to its effect. To name a few are cardiovascular diseases, GERD, diabetes mellitus, osteoporosis, depression, anaemia, skeletal muscle dysfunction, etc. In the view of authors due to this reason COPD should be termed chronic obstructive respiratory syndrome, to highlight the importance of management of these co-morbidities along with that of respiratory part.

BIBLIOGRAPHY

1. Antonelli Incalzi R, Fuso L, De Rosa M et al. Co-morbidity contributes to predict mortality of patients with chronic obstructive pulmonary disease. Eur. Respire. J. 10(12), 2794–2800 (1997).
2. Barr RG, Celli BR, Mannino DM, et al. Comorbidities, patient knowledge, and disease management in national sample of patients with COPD. Am. J. Med. 122 (4), 348–55 (2009).
3. BTS Guidelines 2003 for management of Primary spontaneous pneumothorax.
4. Calverley PM, Anderson JA, Celli B, et al. Salmeterol and fluticasone proportionate and survival in chronic obstructive pulmonary disease. New Engl. J. Med. 2007; 365(8): 775–89.
5. Curkendall SM, DeLuise C, Jones JK et al. Cardiovascular disease in patients with chronic obstructive pulmonary disease, Saskatchewan Canada cardiovascular disease in COPD patients. Ann. Epidemiol. 16(1), 63–70 (2006).
6. Feary JR, Rodrigues LC, Smith CJ, Hubbard RB, Gibson JE. Prevalence of major comorbidities in subjects with COPD and incidence of myo-cardial infarction and stroke, a comprehensive analysis using data from primary care. Thorax 65(11), 956–62 (2010).
7. Feldman G, Siler T, Prasad N, et al. Efficacy and safety of indacaterol 150 microg once-daily in COPD: a double-blind, randomized, 12-week study. BMC Pulm. Med. 2010; 10: 11. Doi: 10.1186/1471-2466-10-11
8. Gershon A, Croxford R, Calzavara A, et al. Cardiovascular safety of inhaled long-acting bronchodilators in individuals with chronic obstructive pulmonary disease. JAMA Intern Med. 2013; 173(13): 1175–85.
9. Gottlieb SS, McCarter RJ, Vogel RA, Effect of beta-blocker on mortality among high-risk and low-risk patients after myocardial infarc-tion. New. Engl. J. Med. 339(8), 489–97 (1998).
10. Joint National Committee report 2007 for management of hypertension.
11. Kessler R, Faller M, Weitzenblum E, et al. Resp. crit. care. Med. 164(2), 219–224 (2001)." Natural

history " ofpulm. Hypertension 131 patients with COPD.

12. Mannino DM, Thorn D, Swensen A, Holguin F. Prevalence and outcomes of diabetes, hypertension and cardiovascular disease in COPD. Eur. Respir. J. 32(4), 962–9 (2008).

13. McGarvey LP, John M, Anderson JA, Zvarich M, Wise RA. Ascertainment of cause specific mortality in COPD, operations of the TORCH Clinical Endopoint Committee. Thorax 62(5), 411–5 (2007).

14. Mills NL, Miller JJ, Anand et al , Thorax 63(4) 306–11 (2008). Increased arterial stiffness in COPD for increased cardiovascular risk.

15. RSSDI Guidelines for diagnosis and management of diabetes mellitus 2.

16. Rutten FH, B-Blocker and their mortality benefit, underprescribed in heart failure and COPD. Future cardiol. 7(1), 43–53 (2011).

17. Rutten FH, Zuithoff NPA, Hake E, Hoes AW. Beta-blocker may reduce mortality and risk of exacerbation in patients with COPD. Arch. Intern. Med.

18. Salpeter S& E, Ormiston T, Cardiovascular beta-blockers for chronic obstructive pulmonary disease. Cochrane Database Syst Rev. 2005; (4): CD003566.

19. Salpeter S, Ormiston T, Salpeter E, Cardio-selective Beta-blockers for chronic obstructive pulmonary disease. Cochrane Database Syst. Rev. (4), CD003566 (2005).

20. Sin DD, Man SFP. Why are patients with chronic obstructive pulmonary disease at increased risk of cardiovascular diseases?The potential role of systemic inflammation in chronic obstructive pulmonary disease. Circulation 107(11), 1514–19 (2003).

21. Soriano JB, Visick GT, Mulellerova H, Payvandi N, Hansell AL. Patterns of comorbidities in newly diagnosed COPD and asthma in primary care. Chest 128 (4), 2099–2107 (2005).

Section II
Management of COPD

Stable COPD

Arun Sampath, Amit Kumar Verma

COPD is characterized by persistent respiratory symptoms and chronic airflow limitation, which is caused by combination of medium-sized airways disease (chronic bronchitis), small airways disease (obstructive bronchiolitis) and parenchymal destruction (emphysema). Hence the intensity of symptoms (such as breathlessness, cough and/or sputum production) varies with individual COPD patient depending upon the predominance of each factor. Though smoking is the most important risk factor for development of COPD, indoor or outdoor air pollution also contributes to COPD. Various studies have found direct relation of biomass cooking (burning wood/cow dung/crop residues/coal in open fires or poorly functioning stoves) to development of COPD.[1,2] About 70–80% of population in India belong to rural or semi-urban regions, where use of biomass fuel for cooking is still prevalent and hence the prevalence of COPD in non-smokers may be high. However, data is still insufficient regarding the natural course of COPD in non-smokers. COPD is still largely underdiagnosed in India, and patients may under-report their symptoms. Patients may perceive breathlessness as normal for their age or may limit indirectly their activities and hence do not feel breathless. Airflow limitation is usually measured by spirometry as this is the most widely available and reproducible lung function test. However, chronic respiratory symptoms may precede the development of airflow limitation[3] and hence COPD could be underdiagnosed if spirometry test alone is taken into consideration. Recent GOLD guidelines thus focus more on the symptoms based assessment approach, rather than only on spirometry based diagnosis and classification.

STABLE COPD

The term 'stable' should be a misnomer as it does not equate to 'no symptoms'. There is no particular definition for stable COPD, however, any COPD patient who has no exacerbation of symptoms in the preceding 5–6 weeks can be considered as stable.

In order to guide proper therapy, COPD patients have to be assessed in terms of:

i. *Level of airflow limitation* (spirometric assessment).

ii. *Impact of disease on patient's health status* by

  a. Modified Medical Research Council (mMRC) Questionnaire for breathlessness assessment

  b. COPD Assessment Test (CAT)[4]—an 8-item unidimensional measure of health status impairment in COPD—which includes self-reported grading scale of severity of cough, sputum production, chest tightness, breathlessness, limitation of activities, sleep quality and perception of energy level. Each parameter has scores from 0 to 5 and the total score can be anywhere between 0 and 40. Larger the score, worse the symptoms.

c. Other comprehensive questionnaires such as SGRQ (St. George's Respiratory Questionnaire), CRQ (Chronic Respiratory Questionnaire) are too complex to use in primary level/ routine practice.

d. Assessment of presence of co-morbidities such as cardiovascular disease, skeletal muscle dysfunction, malnutrition, osteoporosis, depression, anxiety and lung cancer.

iii. *Risk of future events* (such as exacerbations/hospital admissions/death) depends on:

a. History of previous exacerbations

b. Severity of airflow limitation (more severe the COPD, more risks for future exacerbations)

c. Deteriorating airflow limitation

d. Higher blood eosinophil count (especially in patients not on ICS)—scientific data is controversial at present time

However, none of the above assessment tools are perfect. There is only a week correlation between FEV_1, symptoms and impairment of a patient's health status.[5] The more comprehensive SGRQ is well validated and scores <25 are uncommon in diagnosed COPD patients and scores ≥25 are very uncommon in healthy persons. The equivalent cut-point for the CAT is 10 and score < 10 or ≥10 can be used to classify as less or more symptoms to guide therapy.[6] On the other hand, mMRC scores do not exactly correlate with overall COPD symptoms. Though more symptomatic patients (SGRQ ≥25) will usually have an mMRC of ≥1, patients with mMRC<1 may also have other symptom and hence a comprehensive assessment tool is recommended over mMRC. Since the use of mMRC is universal, a mMRC score ≥2 can be taken as threshold for separating 'less breathlessness' from 'more breathlessness'. Recent GOLD 2017 guidelines recommend using revised combined COPD assessment (Fig. 6.1), wherein the COPD treatment groups are

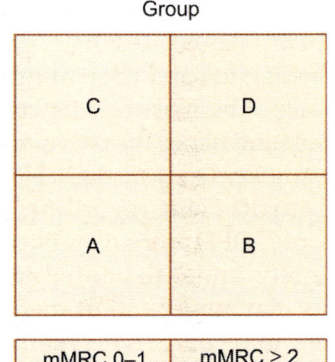

Spirometry classification		Exacerbation history	Group	
FEV₁% Predicted		≥ 2 Exacerbation/year or ≥ 1 exacerbation leading to hospital admission	C	D
GOLD 1	≥80%			
GOLD 2	50–76%			
GOLD 3	30–49%	0 to 1 exacerbation/year Not leading to hospital admission	A	B
GOLD 4	<30%			
			mMRC 0–1 CAT < 10	mMRC ≥ 2 CAT ≥ 10
			Symptoms	

Fig. 6.1: Revised combined COPD assessment*

* Global Initiative for chronic obstructive lung disease (GOLD)—2017 Report

classified based on symptoms (mMRC or CAT scores) and history of exacerbation. The spirometric classification (based on FEV_1) of COPD (GOLD stages) has been separated from the combined assessment as it leads to confusion in exactly defining the COPD groups.

ABCD groups (which guide therapeutic recommendations) will be derived exclusively from patient symptoms and exacerbation history.

Spirometry-based severity classification (**GOLD 1–4 stages**) is used to prognostication and consideration for other therapeutic approaches, e.g lung volume reduction or lung transplantation as shown in Table 6.1.

Table 6.1: Prognostication of COPD patients based on GOLD classification

Group A	Low risk[#]	Less symptoms
Group B	Low risk[#]	More symptoms
Group C	High risk[#]	Less symptoms
Group D	High risk[#]	More symptoms

[#] Risk for future exacerbation

MANAGEMENT GOALS

Important goals of management of stable COPD include: a. to reduce risk factors (e.g. smoking/environmental tobacco smoke); b. to achieve symptomatic control and hence improve exercise tolerance and quality of life; c. to reduce future risk (by preventing and treating exacerbations); d. to manage co-morbidities simultaneously and e. to minimize the adverse effects of medications. This could be done by appropriate pharmacotherapy according to disease severity, supportive non-pharmacological measures and health education. Until now, the only interventions that can change the natural course of COPD are smoking cessation, and oxygen supplementation in COPD patients with chronic resting hypoxemia.[7–9] Therefore, pharmacotherapy is used to decrease symptoms and complications. Recent clinical trials have demonstrated that certain pharmacological treatments can prevent acute COPD exacerbations and can slow decline in lung function over time.[10,11] Hence, identifying and treating patients at early COPD stage can lead to better control of disease and improve patients' quality of life. Recent standard guidelines (GOLD 2015-16) emphasise the change in treatment approach from 'disease severity basis' to 'symptoms basis treatment'. Various available options for COPD are detailed in Table 6.2.

Bronchodilators

The term 'bronchodilator' denotes any medicine that can alter airway smooth muscle tone and thus increase expiratory flow and volumes (FEV_1) and other spirometric variables. Since lung elastic recoil is permanently affected in COPD, any improvement in expiratory flow by bronchodilator is due to widening of airways. In severe to very severe COPD patients, though they may have subjective benefit from bronchodilators, the improvement in FEV_1 is minimal. Dose-response relationship between FEV_1 and any class of bronchodilators is relatively flat and hence increasing the dose is not helpful in stable disease. Toxicity is also dose related. Bronchodilators are given either as needed basis or a regular basis to reduce symptoms. The effectiveness of bronchodilator therapy should not be assessed by lung function alone but should include a variety of other measures such as improvement in symptoms, activities of daily living, exercise capacity and rapidity of symptom relief. Inhaled bronchodilators are considered as central to the symptomatic management of all stages of COPD, even when symptoms are intermittent or minimal. Patients who remain symptomatic should have their

Table 6.2: Therapeutic options for stable COPD

I. Pharmacologic therapy
  A. Bronchodilators
    i. β₂-agonists: Short acting (SABA), long acting (LABA)
    ii. Anti-muscarinics: Short acting (SAMA)/long acting (LAMA)
    iii. Methylxanthines
  B. Anti-inflammatory agents
    i. Corticosteroids: Inhaled (ICS)/ parenteral
    ii. Phosphodiesterase-4 (PDE4) inhibitors (Roflumilast)
    iii. Macrolide antibiotics
  C. Mucolytic/Mucokinetics: N-acetylcysteine/erdocysteine/ carbocysteine
  D. Alpha-1 antitrypsin augmentation therapy
  E. Vaccinations
II. Non-pharmacologic therapy
  A. Reduction of risk factors: Smoking cessation/measures to reduce exposure to indoor/outdoor pollution
  B. Pulmonary rehabilitation
  C. Patient's education and self care
  D. Nutrition
III. Other treatment
  A. Oxygen therapy
  B. Non-invasive ventilator support
IV. Surgery
  A. Lung volume reduction surgery (LVRS)
  B. Bullectomy
  C. Lung transplantation
V. Endobronchial interventions (endoscopic LVRS)
  A. Endoscopic unidirectional valves
  B. Thermal vapour ablation
  C. Nitinol coil placement
VI. Palliative care/therapies
VII. End of life care

inhaled treatment intensified to include combination of two classes of short acting bronchodilators or long acting bronchodilators.

β₂ AGONISTS (Fig. 6.2)

Stimulate β₂ adrenergic receptors (β₂AR) and increase cyclic AMP and which finally reduce myosin light chain kinase activity, which precludes its interaction with contractile protein myosin and promotes relaxation of airway smooth muscle. Also, β₂ agonists can interact with plasma membrane potassium channels, which result in hyperpolarisation of the cell membrane and inhibition of calcium influx and decrease airway smooth muscle tone. Short acting β₂ agonists (e.g. salbutamol, terbutaline, fenoterol) have a rapid onset of action within 5–10 minutes and extend up to 4–6 hours. Albuterol is a racemic mixture containing equal parts of R and S salbutamol. The S isomer binds to β₂AR weakly and may have pro-inflammatory effects, whereas R isomer (levalbuterol) is more active and produces greater bronchodilation over a longer period.

Unlike salbutamol, which is hydrophilic, both long acting β₂ agonists (LABA: Salmeterol, Formoterol) possess liphophilic properties which allow them to remain in airway tissues in close proximity to β₂AR and hence duration of action lasting more than 12 hours. In addition to being liphophilic, formoterol is also water soluble, ensuring rapid access to β₂AR and thus have rapid onset of action. It has been demonstrated that inhaled formoterol 12 and 24 µg and inhaled salbutamol 400 and 800 µg are equi-effective doses in inducing a rapid onset of action in stable COPD patients.[12] Evidences show that LABA significantly improve FEV₁, lung volumes, dyspnoea, health related quality of life and reduce exacerbation rate and the need for hospitalization, but have no effect on decline in lung function and mortality.[13] Ultra long acting β₂ agonists (Ultra LABA: Indacaterol, vilanterol) have bronchodilator effect for 24 hours and has significant effects greater than LABAs on dyspnoea, health

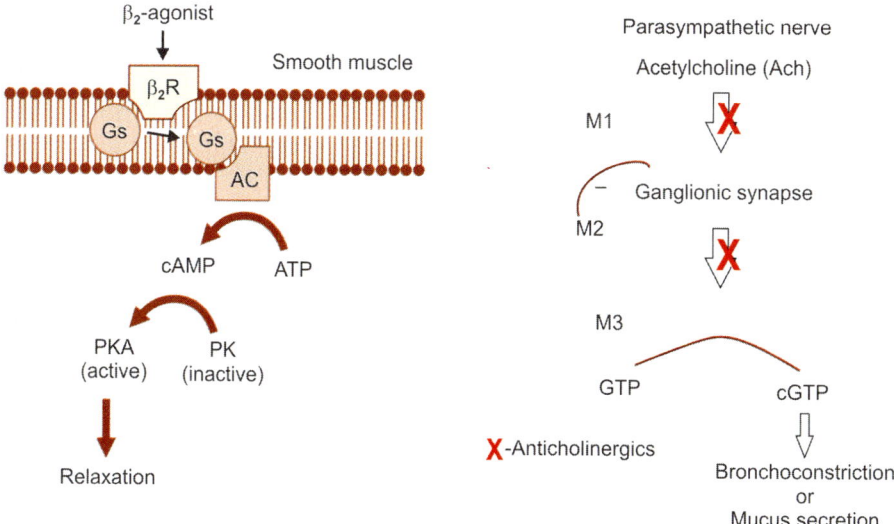

β₂-agonists interact with β₂-receptors in bronchial smooth muscles to activate coupling of stimulatory G protein (Gs) with adenylcyclase (AC). This in turn leads to increased production of cAMP which activates protein kinase A (PKA) and finally results in smooth muscle relaxation

Anti-cholinergics inhibit muscarinic receptors (M1 or M2) and inhibit production of cGMP and hence inhibit bronchoconstriction. M2 receptor autoregulates at anticholinergics (e.g. ipratropium) which also inhibit M2 may limit their activity.

Fig. 6.2: Mechanism of action at cellular level of different class of bronchodilators

status and exacerbation rates.[14] Generally, the maximum bronchodilator response to inhaled β₂ agonists in COPD occurs significantly later to that observed in asthmatics and the magnitude of response is also less in COPD. The increase in vital capacity is higher than that of change in FEV_1 and often it is associated with a symptomatic improvement. Formoterol elicited a greater acute increase in inspiratory capacity (IC) and this is closely correlated with the improvement of dyspnoea sensation. Part of the symptomatic benefit of these agents might be mediated through the reduction of dynamic hyperinflation, as this makes breathing more comfortable. LABAs can increase the level of cAMP in neutrophils, thereby inhibiting neutrophil adhesion, accumulation and activation and inducing apoptosis and can exert anti-inflammatory effects[15] which may be termed non-broncholytic effects of LABAs (Table 6.3).

Table 6.3: Non-broncholytic effects of LABAs
Reduced lung hyperinflation
Increased diaphragm and intercostals muscle function
Increased mucociliary transport
Anti-neutrophil activity
Mucosa cytoprotection
Inhibition of inflammatory mediator release

Since β₂ agonists also have mild pulmonary vasodilator effects and theoretically can cause ventilation–perfusion imbalance (shunt like effect) and hence mild fall in PaO_2 can occur with any class of SABA or LABAs. Despite the concerns raised some years ago related to hypoxemia caused by β₂ agonists in asthma, further detailed studies have found no such association between β₂ agonists and increased mortality in asthma or in COPD patients. Some important adverse effects of β_2 agonists include sinus tachycardia, precipitation of arrhythmia, exaggerated somatic tremor, hypokalemia and muscle weakness. Cardiac arrhythmias are common in COPD patients with respiratory failure, since factors such as hypoxemia, hypercarbia and acidosis are arrhythmogenic. In particular, hypoxemic COPD patients have autonomic neuropathy that has been associated with a prolongd QTc and risk of ventricular arrhythmia. Though some of these adverse effects could be troublesome and can be a limiting factor to use β_2 agonists, these effects usually occur with high doses and usually show tachyphylaxis.

Anticholinergic Agents

Normally in humans, parasympathetic system provides the predominant basal bronchoconstrictor tone. In fact, anticholinergics are the bronchodilator of choice in treatment of COPD as cholinergic vagal tone appears to be the only reversible element of airway narrowing.[16] Anticholinergics are also effective in reducing neurogenic control of mucus hypersecretion in chronic bronchitis. Anticholinergics block acetylcholine's effects on muscarinic (M1, 2, 3) receptors and hence bronchomotor tone. M2 pre-ganglionic receptor autoregulate other post-ganglionic receptors and hence short acting (SAMA) drugs (ipratropium, oxitropium) which block non-selectively all muscarinic receptors have short duration of action which lasts up to 8 hours. On the other hand, long acting (LAMA) drugs (tiotropium, glycopyrronium) selectively block M1 and M3 receptors and have bronchodilator effects more than 24 hours. Tiotropium (LAMA) improves FEV_1, symptoms, health status, reduces exacerbations and related hospitalizations and improves effectiveness of pulmonary rehabilitation.[17,18] Tiotropium is more effective when given once daily than

ipratropium given four times daily[19] and also tiotropium is more effective than LABA in preventing exacerbation.[20] However, there is no effect of anti-cholinergics on reducing the rate of lung function decline. In general, the inhaled anticholinergic drugs, which are positively charged quarternary ammonium compounds are poorly absorbed, which limits the troublesome systemic effects. The common side effects are dry mouth and metallic taste. Reports of paradoxical bronchoconstriction with ipratropium bromide, especially when given by nebulizer, were largely explained by the hypotonicity of the solution. However, inhlaed ipratropium can cause occasional bronchoconstriction due to the fact that it also suppresses M2 receptors. Anticholinergics can precipitate arrhythmias very occasionally. Nebulised anticholinergics can induce acute angle closure glaucoma in susceptible individuals due to direct topical effect by nebulising vapours. This is not a possibility with inhaled formulations. Although occasional urinary obstruction symptoms can occur in patients with prostatic hypertrophy, there are no exact data to prove the true causal relationship.

Methylxanthines

They are non-selective phosphodiesterase inhibitors which prevent degradation of cAMP and hence increase their levels and cause bronchodilation. However, compared to other bronchodilator drugs, methylxanthines have weak bronchodilatory effect. They have a lot of non-bronchodilator effects such as enhancement of diaphragmatic contractility, respiratory centre stimulant, mucociliary sweep, anti-inflammatory properties, inotropic and chronotropic cardiac effects. The clinical significance of such actions is still controversial. Also, they increase the histone deacetylase activity (HDAC) and hence enhance the effects of inhaled corticosteroids in COPD patients, especially those who continue to smoke cigarettes. The toxicity is dose-related and the fact that serum toxicity levels overlap therapeutic levels explains the high incidence of toxic side effects. Hence recommended dose schedule (Table 6.4) should be properly followed. Common side effects include nausea, gastritis, headache, tremors and insomnia. Less frequent but sometimes fatal adverse effects include arrhythmias (atrial/ventricular) and grand mal seizures and can happen within therapeutic range of serum levels. Though the risk of such serious adverse effects can be reduced by monitoring of drug's serum levels, such tests are not widely available and expensive. Theophylline, the most common methyxanthine is metabolized by cytochrome P_{450} oxidase and hence can have a lot of interactions with many drugs which can either increase or decrease its drug levels. Compared to all other bronchodilator drugs, theophylline is widely used in Indian set up as it is much cheaper. Various studies have proven the beneficial effect of theophylline (sustained release pre-parations), when combined with other class of bronchodilators in improving FEV_1, symptoms score compared to individual drugs alone. A new methylxanthine (doxofylline) may have less affinity for α_1 and α_2 receptors and does not antagonize calcium channels and have less effect on heart rate/rhythm, gastric secretions and

Table 6.4: Dose recommendations of various xanthines			
Xanthine	*Dose*	*Therapeutic dose range*	*Available dose formulations*
Theophylline Deriphylline (theophylline + etophylline)	**Non-smokers:** 10 mg/kg/day, maximum 900 mg/day **Smokers:** 16 mg/kg/day, max 900 mg/day **Congestive cardiac failure/cor-pulmonale/liver dysfunction:** 5 mg/kg/day, max 400 m/day **Intravenous:** 10 mg/kg loading dose or 5 mg/kg loading dose (if already on theophylline)	10–20 µg/ml	100, 150, 200, 300, 400, 600, 800 mg oral tablets/capsules 46.5 mg theophylline + 14 mg Etophylline/5 ml syrup
Aminophylline (theophylline + ethylenediamine)	**Loading dose** (patient not already receiving theophylline): 6 mg/kg in 100–200 ml of IV fluid over 20–30 minutes **Maintenance dose:** 0.7 to 0.9 mg/kg/hr continuous infusion *CCF/cor pulmonale/liver disease:* 0.25 mg/kg/hr		25 mg/ml in 10 ml or 20 ml ampoule
Acebrophylline (theophylline-7-acetic acid with ambroxol)	100 mg bid, 200 mg SR OD		100 mg, 200 mg SR capsules, 10 mg/ml syrup
Doxophylline (doxofylline)	200 to 400 mg bid to t.i.d		200, 400 mg tablet, 100 mg/ml syrup

CNS stimulation. Another methylxanthine (acebrophylline), which contains ambroxol and theophylline-7 acetic acid, has been claimed to improve ciliary clearance in addition to bronchodilation. In some very severe COPD patients with significant hyperinflation and thus very low inspiratory efforts, the inhaled bronchodilators could not achieve adequate effect as they may not inhale efficiently. In such patients, theophyllines can be used as it is given parenterally, and can reach lung tissues through plasma distribution. However, in view of low therapeutic window and potential fatal side effects, methylxanthines should be carefully used in selected patients, where other bronchodilator drugs are not affordable or not available.

Combination Therapy with Bronchodilators

COPD is not homogeneous anatomically. This may create a particularly important advantage for combination bronchodilator therapy.

Rationales for combination therapy include:

- Airflow limitation in COPD results from several distinct histophysiologic processes that are present in varying degrees of severity.

- All airways have some degree of resting smooth muscle tone that slightly narrow airways. Bronchodilators, therefore, improve modestly about 3–5% of airway muscle tone even in normal individuals and different class of bronchodilators have different degree of improvement.

- Studies have shown that proximal airways are relatively endowed with cholinergic receptors, while the distal airways with β_2-receptors and hence β_2-agonists and anticholinergics can produce different bronchodilation effect. Thus greater bronchodilator effect is possible with the combination of both drugs.

- The three classes of bronchodilators cause smooth muscle relaxation by different mechanisms and hence can have synergistic action when used as combination therapy.

- Inhaled bronchodilators may not effectively reach areas within the lung that are severely airflow limited. Theophylline, because it reaches the lung through circulation could bronchodilate such regions and also by improving airflow, it could improve the distribution of inhaled bronchodilators into such airways.

The long acting bronchodilators (LABA or LAMA) achieve their long duration of action by interacting with the cell surface and/or receptors differently than do the short acting bronchodilators (SABA or SAMA). Hence any β_2-agonists (SABA or LABA) can be combined with any anticholinergics (SAMA or LAMA). Combining different bronchodilators may increase the degree of maximal bronchodilation with a lower risk of side effects compared to increasing dose of a single bronchodilator.[21-23] Given the much higher benefits of both long acting agents (LABA and LAMA) as compared to their short acting counterparts (discussed above), it is rationale to combine LABA and LAMA for achieving maximal bronchodilation. Combination treatment with a LABA and LAMA increases FEV_1, reduces symptoms and improve health status in COPD.[24] Combination of LABA/LAMA reduces exacerbations to a greater extent compared to monotherapy[25] or to ICS/LABA combination[26].

Anti-inflammatory Drugs

Inhaled Corticosteroids

Since the inflammation in COPD is predominantly due to neutrophilic pathway, corticosteroids usually have less effect in COPD. Although it is well known that corticosteroids are effective at suppressing airway inflammation in asthma, their effects on lower airways inflammation in COPD is still controversial. Some studies suggest that inhaled corticosteroids (ICS) attenuate neutrophilic recruitment, activation and chemotactic activity and reduces neutrophil elastase activity, myeloperoxidase levels, but other studies have found ICS actually increase sputum neutrophils levels and have no effects on inflammatory mediators (TNFα, IL-8, MMP9) and alveolar macrophages activities. The relative lack of ICS response could be linked to oxidative stress induced by smoking, which influence glucocorticoid receptors translocation, suppression of histone deacetylase (HDAC) expression (HDAC is important for ICS mediated nuclear events in inflammatory cells). Hence ICS alone have no beneficial effect in COPD and neither modify the long-term decline in FEV_1 nor reduce mortality. Studies show controversial evidences regarding the outcomes of ICS in COPD and their role in the management of stable COPD is limited to specific indications. Responsiveness to ICS may be severity-dependent.[27] Thus, treatment of severe COPD patients with ICS results in improved exacerbation rates and quality-adjusted life expectancy without substantial additional cost compared to other therapies.[28] ISOLDE study reported that regular treatment of high dose inhaled fluticasone for 3 years resulted in fewer exacerbations, higher FEV_1 and improved health status in moderate-severe COPD.[29] On contrary, in TORCH trial, ICS alone had been shown to be associated with more mortality compared to ICS+LABA combination or placebo.[30] Cochrane systematic reviews[31] have shown that ICS combined with LABA compared with either component alone, is more effective in improving lung function, health status and reducing exacerbation rates. However, present guidelines recommend to use ICS in combination with other bronchodilators in severe COPD ($FEV_1<50\%$) and in patients with frequent exacerbations. ICS use is associated with side effects such as hoarseness of voice, oropharyngeal candidiasis, skin bruising and increased prevalence of pneumonia. The incidence of pneumonia is more with ICS-fluticasone furoate even in lower doses. The risk of developing pneumonia is higher in COPD patients aged ≥55 years, current smokers, low BMI <25, severe airflow limitation and those who have history of previous exacerbations or pneumonia.[32] As with any steroids, ICS has been observed with increased risk of cataract, diabetes, mycobacterial infections and osteoporosis but the data is not strong. While long term treatment with triamcinolone acetonide is associated with risk of reduced bone mineral density, the evidence with other ICS is controversial. Increase in symptoms and/or exacerbation rate had been observed upon withdrawal of ICS, but some studies did not find such correlation. However, withdrawal of ICS should be attempted only in stable COPD with adequate control of symptoms and regular use of long acting bronchodilators should be continued even after ICS withdrawal.

In view of well-known side effects of long-term use of oral corticosteroids, their use in stable COPD is not recommended. Steroid-induced myopathy and related muscle weakness, an important side effect of steroids, can actually worsen dyspnoea, effort tolerance and affect quality of life significantly.

Phosphodiesterase-4 Inhibitors

PDE-4 is abundant in inflammatory cells and selective PDE-4 inhibitors (cilomilast, roflumilast) can reduce inflammation by inhibiting breakdown of intracellular c-AMP. They have no practical bronchodilator effects. Both the drugs share similar pharmacokinetic characteristics, but clinical evidences show that Roflumilast has better tolerance and therapeutic index as compared to cilomilast and hence the former drug is preferred in COPD patients. Studies have shown that roflumilast reduce moderate and severe exacerbations in patients with chronic bronchitis, severe and very severe COPD and those with previous history of exacerbations.[33] Roflumilast (500 µg) is given once daily orally and has to be prescribed along with other bronchodilator drugs. Since roflumilast itself a PDE inhibitor, there is no rationale to use in combination with theophylline. The most frequent side effects include gastrointestinal issues (such as nausea, diarrhoea, abdominal pain, reduced appetite and weight loss), headache and sleep disturbances. Adverse effects happen more frequently with PDE4 inhibitors and lead to poor drug compliance. Roflumilast should be used with caution in low BMI, depression and gastritis.

Antibiotic as Anti-inflammatory Agent

The macrolide antibiotic group has been demonstrated to have good anti-inflammatory effects, which have been proven to be effective in certain bronchiolitis, ILD and bronchiectasis. Older studies did not show any benefit in giving prophylactic continuous antibiotic on frequency of exacerbation[34] and previous guidelines did not recommend it. However, more recent studies have shown that regular use of macrolide antibiotics (erythromycin 500 mg twice daily or azithromycin 250 mg/day or 500 mg three times/week) for one year may reduce exacerbation rate.[35, 36] However, such long-term antibiotic use lead to increased bacterial resistance and azithromycin particularly lead to impaired hearing. Hence the safety of such chronic antibiotic therapy is still under debate. Such practice especially in Indian setup is not possible due to financial implications and high frequency of community infections.

Treatment Algorithms

The recent GOLD guidelines recommend the preferred treatment strategies according to the group of COPD patients (group A to D) (Table 6.5). However, the patients have to be regularly re-assessed (by using 'revised combined assessment tool') whether the patient has improvement or worsening of symptoms and/or further exacerbations with present treatment strategy and hence the treatment has to be modified. Though patient may be stable as per symptoms/exacerbations, the disease severity (based on FEV_1 criteria) should also be kept in mind before advising any change in treatment strategies.

- For patients with severe breathlessness, initial therapy with LAMA+LABA may be considered.

- Associated co-morbidities could contribute to the symptoms and impact their prognosis and they should be carefully assessed during each visit and managed appropriately.

- In some group D patients with findings suggestive of ACOS or with high blood eosinophil count (still controversial), initial therapy with ICS+LABA may be preferred.

- ICS use is associated with higher risk of developing pneumonia (especially in group D patients).

- In very advanced COPD with significant hyperinflation lungs, domiciliary nebulized therapy can be considered to inhalers, as patient cannot generate adequate inspiratory airflow. All about nebulization therapy can be seen in Table 6.6.

- Theophyllines can be considered if the preferred inhaled therapy is not available, not affordable or patients with poor inspiratory capacity (severe airflow

Table 6.5: Treatment algorithms according to COPD groups

COPD patient group	Preferred treatment	Simplified version	Escalation therapy (if persistent symptoms/further exacerbations)	Simplified version
Group A	A single inhaled bronchodilator (either a short acting or long acting drug)	MDI or rota cap salbutamol/ levosalbutamol Or MDI or rota cap salmeterol/ formoterol alone	—	—
Group B	A long acting bronchodilator (LABA or LAMA). LAMA is preferred to LABA	MDI or rota cap tiotropium or salmeterol/ formoterol	LABA+ LAMA combination	Tiotropium + formoterol combinations
Group C	A long acting bronchodilator **LAMA** is preferred to LABA	MDI or rota cap tiotropium or salmeterol/ formoterol	LAMA + LABA or LABA + ICS	Tiotropium + formoterol combinations Or Salmeterol + fluticasone/ formoterol + fluticasone/ salmeterol + budesonide
Group D	LAMA+ LABA	MDI or rota cap tiotropium or salmeterol/ formoterol	**LAMA + LABA + ICS** If patient on triple therapy still have exacerbations, then 1. Consider macrolide in former smokers 2. Consider roflumilast if $FEV_1 < 50\%$ predicted and patient has chronic bronchitis	MDI or rota cap tiotropium + MDI or rota cap Salmeterol + fluticasone/ formoterol + fluticasone/ Salmeterol + budesonide Add 1. Tablet azithromycin/ clarithromycin if in former smokers 2. Tablet rofumilast 500 μg OD if $FEV_1 < 50\%$ predicted and patient has chronic bronchitis

limitation with significant dynamic hyperinflation).

- To add on various preparations for management of COPD available in India are detailed in Table 6.7.

Adjunctive Therapy

Mucolytic agents reduce sputum viscosity and improve secretion clearance. Viscous lung secretions in patients with COPD consist of mucus-derived glycoproteins and

Table 6.6: Nebulizer therapy for stable COPD patients

I. Pre-requisites for ideal nebulizer

- Alleviating hand-breath co-ordination
- Lack of dependence on high inspiratory flow rates
- Use of mechanical energy for actuation
- Generation of fine particle aerosol
- Stable liquid formulation
- Propellant free function

II. Whom to prescribe nebulizer therapy in stable COPD?

- Moderate to severe COPD patients with very low PIFR (unable to generate inspiratory flow to use DPIs/high-resistance breath actuated devices)
- Elderly patients
- Cognitive or visual impairment
- Diminished manual dexterity
- Chronic muscle weakness
- Patients discharged from hospital after an acute exacerbation

III. Types of nebulizers

- **Conventional Jet nebulizer:** Uses compressed air to generate a fine mist of drug. Easy to use, no co-ordination required. But it has drawbacks such as: Cumbersome, longer administration time (>10 minutes), device preparation, daily cleaning requirement and may not readily aerosolize drug. Newer portable jet nebulizer **(Trek® S, PARI, USA)** has been developed.

- **Ultrasonic nebulizer (Aeroneb GO®-Philips Healthcare, USA):** Uses ultrasonic vibrations passed through the drug to generate a fine mist. Offers a very consistent particle size and virtually silent. Drawbacks: Medication restrictions because heat is transferred to medication; high cost; device preparation; daily cleaning requirement.

- **High efficiency vibrating mesh nebulizer (MicroAir® NE-U22 Omron, USA; eFlow® PARI, USA):** Portable (battery operated), quiet, ultrafast treatment. Drawbacks: High cost; requires disassembly and cleaning after each use to prevent clogging of the mesh apertures; not all medications are available in this format; optimal doses need to be defined by additional studies to avoid overdosing.

- **Automatic aerosol delivery (AAD) nebulizer (Akita Jet®Vectura, UK; I-neb® Philips Healthcare, USA):** AAD monitors duration and peak inspiratory flow of the first three breaths and then AAD pulses aerosol during the first 50–80% of inspiration in subsequent breaths. This automated timing of aerosol delivery, based on the patient's breathing pattern improves the precision and reproducibility of dosing. It is light weight, silent and ultra fast. Drawback: Expensive, ideal dosing not yet determined.

- **Soft Mist Inhaler (Respimat® SMI, Boehringer Ingelheim, Germany):** Delivers a slow moving mist via the release of stored energy from a tensed spring when the tension is released by pushing a button. It is a compact, hand held, slow velocity aerosol generated, multiple-dosing (~1 month) device. It is not actually a nebulizer, but meets some of the requirements of nebulizer. Aerosol persists for 1.5 seconds, increasing ease of synchronizing inhalation with actuation.

(Contd.)

Table 6.6: Nebulizer therapy for stable COPD patients *(Contd.)*

IV. Drugs available for Nebulizer therapy:

- **Short acting:**
  - o SABA (albuterol sulfate, levalbuterol hydrochloride)
  - o SAMA (ipratropium bromide)
  - o SABA-SAMA

- **Long acting:**
  - o LABA (Formoterol fumarate, arfomoterol tartrate, olodaterol hydrochloride)
  - o LAMA (Tiotropium bromide)
  - o LABA-LAMA (Tiotropium bromide—olodaterol hydrochloride)
  - o Newer LAMA [SUN-101 (soluble glycopyrrolate bromide); TD-4208 (Revefenacin) in Phase II-III trials]

- **Inhaled corticosteroids:**
  - o Budesonide, fluticasone propionate
  - o ICS-LABA (Formoterol fumarate-budesonide)

leukocyte derived DNA. Regular treatment with mucolytics, such as carbocysteine, erdosteine, N-acetylcysteine (NAC), ambroxol, iodinated glycerol have been shown to decrease cough and chest discomfort and may reduce exacerbations.[37,38] However, the efficacy of mucolytic agents in the treatment of COPD remains controversial. Mucolytics can be considered for use through the winter months at least, in patients with moderate to severe COPD (especially chronic bronchitis) in whom ICS is not prescribed. When used as an inhalational therapy, N-acetylcysteine should be administered along with a bronchodilator such as albuterol in order to counteract potential induction of bronchospasm.

High flow humidified air delivered via nasal canulae for up to 2 hours daily reduced annual exacerbation days and day to first exacerbation but not exacerbation frequency and has no impact on lung function and quality of life.[39] Such humdification therapy is not recommended.

Statins (HMG-CoA reductase inhibitors), apart from its lipid lowering action, have also shown to have pleiotropic and anti-inflammatory properties. Though some studies have shown that statin reduce exacerbation frequency in COPD, such effects are noted only in patients with cardiovascular comorbidities. Recently, large prospective clinical trials (STATCOPE)[40] concluded statins are not beneficial in COPD and current guidelines are against using statins in COPD as adjuvant therapy. However, in patients with multiple exacerbations despite optimal medical management, especially those with cardiovascular comorbidities, statins can be prescribed. But to get anti-inflammatory effects, statins should be given in relatively higher dose (atorvastatin 80 mg or rosuvastin 40 mg). Caution is warranted when using high dose statins due to the potential risk for statin related myopathies which can affect exercise tolerance.

Data is insufficient regarding chronic use of montelukast in COPD. However, it may be beneficial if associated with allergic symptoms and in asthma-COPD overlap syndrome (ACOS). Present guidelines do not recommend their regular use in COPD.

Table 6.7: Commonly available pharmacological drugs for COPD in India

Drug	Dose/formulations	Duration of action
Short acting β₂-agonists (SABA)		
1. Salbutamol (albuterol)	MDI: 100 µg DPI: 200 µg Tablet: 2, 4 mg, 8 mg SR Syrup: 2 mg/5 ml Nebulizer solution: 5 mg/ml Nebules: 5 mg/2.5 ml Injection: 50 µg/ml	4–6 hours
2. Levalbuterol	MDI: 50 µg DPI: 100 µg Tablet: 1, 2 mg Syrup: 1 mg/5 ml Nebulizer respules: 0.31 mg or 0.63 mg/2.5 ml (pediatric dose) or 1.25 mg/2.5 ml (adults)	4–6 hours
3. Terbutaline	MDI: 250 µg DPI: 500 µg Tablet: 2.5, 5 mg Syrup: 2.5 mg/5 ml Injection: 0.5 mg/ml	4–6 hours
Long acting β₂-agonists (LABA)		
1. Salmeterol	MDI: 25 µg DPI: 50 µg	12 hours
2. Formoterol fumarate	MDI: 4.5/6 µg DPI: 6 µg Respules: 20 µg	12 hours
3. Arfomoterol tartarate	Respules: 15 µg/2 ml	12 hours
4. Indacaterol	DPI: 75, 150, 300 µg	12 hours
Anti-muscarinics: **Short acting (SAMA)**		
1. Ipratropium bromide	MDI: 20 µg DPI: 40 µg	6–8 hours
Long acting (LAMA)	Respule: 500 µg/2 ml	
1. Tiotropium bromide	MDI: 9 µg DPI: 18 µg	24 hours
2. Glycopyrronium bromide	DPI: 50 µg	12–24 hours
SABA/SAMA combination	Salbutamol/ipratropium (DPI/MDI/respules) Levalbuterol/ipratropium (DPI/MDI/respules) Formoterol/tiotropium (MDI/DPI) Indacaterol/glycopyrronium (DPI)	6–8 hours
LABA/LAMA combination	Formoterol/glycopyrronium (DPI)	12–24 hours 12–24 hours 12 hours

(Contd.)

Table 6.7: Commonly available pharmacological drugs for COPD in India *(Contd.)*

Drug	Dose/formulations	Duration of action
Inhaled Corticosteroids		
1. Beclomethasone	MDI: 50/100/200 µg DPI: 100/200/400 µg	12 hours
2. Budesonide	MDI: 50/100/200 µg DPI: 100/200/400 µg	
3. Fluticasone	MDI: 50/125/250 µg DPI: 100/250/500 µg Respules: 0.5 mg or 2 mg/2 ml	
LABA/ICS combination	Salmeterol/fluticasone Formoterol/fluticasone Formoterol/budesonide Formoterol/mometasone Formoterol/beclamethasone Vilanterol/fluticasone furoate	12 hours
Methylxanthines		
1. Theophylline	Tablet: 150 mg, 300 mg, 400 mg, 600 mg Inj: Etophylline 84.7 mg + theophylline 25.3 mg/1 ml Syrup: Theophylline 14 mg+ Etophylline 46.5 mg per 5 ml	12–24 hours
2. Acebrophylline	Tablet: 100 mg, 200 mg (SR) Syrup: 50 mg/5 ml	
3. Doxophylline	Tablet: 400 mg	
4. Aminophylline (theophylline + ethylenediamine)	Injection: 250 mg/10 ml	12–24 hours
Phosphodiesterase-4 inhibitors Roflumilast	Oral: 500 µg	
Antioxidant: N-acetylcysteine	Tablet: 600 mg	

DPI: Dry powder inhaler; MDI: Meter dose inhaler

α_1-Antitrypsin Augmentation Therapy (α_1-AAT)

α_1-antitrypsin deficiency should be suspected in young COPD (<45 years age) and especially with pan acinar emphysema. Treatment of such AATD patients includes the standard treatment as in any COPD. α_1-AAT has been proved to be beneficial in reducing the disease progression and preserve lung tissue. Current guidelines recommend using intravenous α_1-AAT for AATD patients with FEV_1 ≤65% and those with disease progression. However, α_1-AAT is not possible in India due to its high cost and lack of availability. Also, AATD is not screened in India widely due to non-availability of such genetic tests.

Vaccinations

Influenza is associated with significant adverse health effects in elderly COPD and about 27% of AECOPD were associated with respiratory viruses. Influenza vaccination has been found to reduce serious lower respiratory infections, frequent exacerbations and hospitalization. Influenza vaccines containing either killed or live attenuated viruses are recommended for elderly patients with COPD.[41] Influenza vaccine could be either trivalent or quadrivalent (not available in India). Trivalent vaccines could be either split virion or subunit vaccine types, the former is more immunogenic. Influenza vaccination should be given during September-October in north Indian regions (peak season in winter) and during pre-monsoon April-May in rest of India.

Pneumococcal vaccination has been shown to prevent vaccine-type community acquired pneumonia (45%) and serious pneumococcal pneumonia (75%) among elderly COPD patients age ≤65 years and the efficacy persist for 4–5 years.[42] There are two types of pneumococcal vaccines available: 23-valent pneumococcal polysachharide vaccine (PPSV23) for young COPD (<65 years age) with an FEV_1 <40% and 13-valent conjugated pneumococcal vaccine (PCV13) for elderly individuals (≥65 years age). Pneumococcal vaccine has to be given once in 5 years.

Reduction of Risk Factors

Smoking cessation is the only intervention which has been proved to alter the natural course of COPD. Though more benefit from smoking cessation occur in patients with early stages of COPD, this intervention still can improve symptoms such as cough in severe patients. Patients who smoke should be counselled and encouraged to quit the habit permanently. The reported success rates vary between 10 and 30%.[43] Even brief counselling (~3 minutes) by treating physician could lead to successful smoking cessation in about 5–10% patients. Studies have shown that abrupt quitting lead to more success than gradual reduction of smoking. Patient's motivation influences smoking cessation, as long-term cessation can be achieved only in such motivated patients. More intense the cessation program, higher the quit rates. If possible, group therapy, cognitive behavioural sessions could be offered to influence the long-term cessation. However, relapse is common and reflects the chronic nature of tobacco dependence and addiction. A standard five-step program can be followed: **ASK** every patient during every visit about various tobacco product use; **ADVICE** all tobacco users to quit; **ASSESS** the willingness to make a quit attempt; **ASSIST** the willing patient with a quit plan, provide counselling, social support, recommend pharmacotherapies except in those with contraindications and **ARRANGE** subsequent follow-up visits for monitoring and aiding long-term cessation. Nicotine replacement therapies (nicotine chewing gum, transdermal patch, sublingual tablet, lozenge, nasal spray or inhaler) can be used to increase long-term cessation.[44] The other second line drugs include varenicline, bupropion and nortriptyline have also been shown to improve long-term abstinence rates[44, 45] (Table 6.8).

Reduction of exposure to smoke from biomass fuel is important and can be minimised by the use of smokeless chullahs, efficient ventilation, use of non-polluting cooking stoves, use of LPG, reducing the duration of stay in kitchen cooking. Exposure to environmental tobacco smoke

Table 6.8:	Pharmacologic agents for aiding smoking cessation			
NRT	Available dose formulations	Peak plasma level	Dose regime	How to use
Nicotine chewing gum	2 mg/4 mg	20 to 30 minutes	Chew one piece every 1 to 2 hours For heavy smokers: 4 mg strength should be used Therapy duration: 12 weeks or more Maximum dose: 24 nicotine gums/day	1. Chew nicotine gum slowly until you can taste the nicotine or feel a tingling sensation in your mouth. Stop chewing and park the piece between your cheek and gums. After about a minute, when the tingling is almost gone, start chewing again. Repeat this process until the tingle is gone (about 30 minutes). 2. Make sure to avoid eating or drinking anything for 15 minutes before using nicotine gum, and while you are using it. Even mildly acidic food and beverages can inhibit nicotine absorption into your bloodstream.
Nicotine transdermal patch	21/14/7 mg patches 15/10/5 mg patches	5 – 10 hours	**> 10 cigarettes/day:** 21 mg patch OD for 6 weeks, then 14 mg patch OD for 2 weeks, then 7 mg patch OD for 2 weeks (OR) 15 mg patch OD for 6 weeks, then 10 mg patch OD for 2 weeks, then 5 mg patch OD for 2 weeks **≤ 10 cigarettes/day:** 14 mg patch OD for 6 weeks, then 7 mg patch OD for 2 weeks (OR) 10 mg patch OD for 6 weeks, then 5 mg patch OD for 2 weeks	1. Apply to clean, dry, non-hairy area of skin (upper arm/shoulder) 2. Do not cut patch 3. Apply new patch daily 4. If vivid dreams/sleep disturbances, remove patch before night sleep and apply new in next morning
Nicotine nasal spray	10 mg/ml	5–7 minutes	1–2 doses/hour for 3 months **Max dose:** 5 doses/hour or 40 doses/day	* One dose: One spray in each nostril * By applying the spray directly into the nostril, nicotine is rapidly absorbed providing

(Contd.)

Table 6.8: Pharmacologic agents for aiding smoking cessation (*Contd.*)

NRT	Available dose formulations	Peak plasma level	Dose regime	How to use
				quick relief from cravings * Fast, powerful relief for heavy smokers * High nicotine dependence can occur
Nicotine lozenges	2 mg/4 mg	20–30 minutes	Use at least 9 lozenges/day **Duration:** 12 weeks **Max dose:** Not more than 5 lozenges in 6 hours or more than 20 lozenges/day	1. Place the lozenge in the mouth, occasionally moving side to side 2. Do not chew or swallow the lozenge 3. The medicine continues to work even after the lozenge is gone
Nicotine inhaler	10 mg/cartridge (4 mg delivered)	15 minutes	Regime: 6–16 cartridges/day for 12 weeks More than 12 weeks: Gradually reduce number of cartridges use per day Max: 16 cartridges/day	1. Line up the markers and pull each end in the opposite direction. 2. Insert the cartridge into the mouthpiece and twist to close securely. 3. Bring the mouthpiece to your mouth and inhale deeply into the back of your throat. Or puff in short breaths. Each cartridge lasts for approximately 20 minutes of frequent puffing.
Bupropion hydrochloride	150 mg SR tablet	NA	150 mg OD for 3 days then 150 mg bid for 6–12 weeks	Oral
Varenicline	0.5 mg/1 mg tablet	NA	Days 1 to 3: 0.5 mg OD Days 4 to 7: 0.5 mg BD Day 8 onwards: 1 mg BD (total duration: 12–24 weeks)	Oral
Nortryptiline			Days 1 to 3: 25 mg OD Days 4 to 7: 50 mg OD Day 8 onwards: 75 mg OD (total duration: 12–24 weeks)	Oral
Other pharmaco-therapies	Smoking aversive: Silver acetate Other agents: Clonidine, naltrexone, mecamyline Medicine to reduce withdrawal symptoms/replace positive effects of nicotine: Fluoxetine (SSRI), anxiolytics, stimulants, anorectics			

(ETS) can be reduced by stopping indoor smoking, especially in front of children and stopping smoking in public places. The other general measures include: Avoiding burning of crop residue, use of respirators at dusty workplace, avoiding constant exposure to potential irritants, if possible.

Oxygen Therapy

Chronic hypoxemia in COPD patients lead to pulmonary arterial hypertension and thus reduce their survival rate. The long-term administration of oxygen (LTOT) for at least > 15 hrs/day have been shown to improve survival in COPD patients with chronic resting hypoxemia.[46, 47] LTOT definitely improves exercise endurance, improvement in walking distance and ability to perform daily activities. The survival benefits have been seen only after 500 days of regular use of LTOT. Scientific data have shown that nocturnal dip in SPO_2 is deep with increasing severity of COPD, and hence the LTOT hours should cover the nocturnal sleep time. Protocol for oxygen therapy can be seen in Table 6.9.

Nutrition Assessment and Therapy
(Table 6.10)

COPD is a systemic inflammatory disorder which is often characterized by a progressive deterioration in nutritional status caused by protein calorie malnutrition with loss of muscle mass. Factors involved in lean body mass depletion in COPD are: 1. Inadequate energy intake (limited diaphragm movements cause increase in dyspnoea while eating, anorexia due to inflammatory mediators like TNF-α, depression); 2. Increased energy expenditure (due to increased RR, oxidative stress) and 3. Alteration of protein synthesis and turnover. About 25% of clinically stable COPD patients demonstrate a marked loss of muscle mass.[48] This lean body mass deterioration can happen without decrease in overall body weight (BMI) and hence it is possible that a normal or increased body weight could mask changes in lean body mass. Though various studies have reported poor outcome in COPD patients with low BMI, it would be better to evaluate various body composition by more reliable methods. One such method is bioelectrical impedance analysis (BIA), which is a reliable, less expensive and easy-to-use method to accurately detect Fat mass (normal value: 22–31%), fat free mass (Normal value: 69–78%), body cellular mass (normal value: 40–49%) and phase angle (normal value: 6–8°). Fat free mass index (FFM/height squared) <16 kg/meter squared in males and <15 kg/meter squared is considered FFM depletion. The consequences of body weight loss and muscle wasting are: Increased dyspnoea, reduced exercise capacity, worsening quality of life and susceptibility to infections. All about nutrition in COPD can be seen in Chapter 11 of this book.

Pulmonary Rehabilitation

COPD patients usually have chronic disabilities with limitation of activities and social interactions and have poor quality of life. Pulmonary rehabilitation improves exercise capacity; perception of breathlessness; overall health related quality of life; relieves anxiety, depression associated with COPD and reduces the number of hospitalisations among patients who have had a recent exacerbation. Pulmonary rehabilitation programs usually include exercise training, smoking cessation, education, nutritional advices, social and psychological support. Though pulmonary rehabilitation has been demonstrated to improve functional exercise capacity and

Table 6.9: Oxygen therapy for COPD patients

I. Whom to prescribe oxygen therapy*?
- COPD patients with resting PaO_2<55 mmHg or SPO_2<88%, with or without hypercapnia
- Resting PaO_2: 55 to 60 mmHg or SpO_2 88–92%, provided it is associated with either pulmonary arterial hypertension, cor pulmonale or polycythemia (hematocrit >55%)

II. How to prescribe oxygen therapy?
- **Long term (LTOT):** Oxygen therapy for at least 15–18 hours/day. Oxygen flow (litres/minute) should be titrated to achieve resting SpO_2>90–92%
- **Nocturnal:** All patients receiving LTOT should include nocturnal use of oxygen (especially if nocturnal SpO_2<88% in repeated occasions) and for selective patients [e.g. overlap syndrome (COPD with OSA) with significant nocturnal fall in SpO_2 in spite of using CPAP]
- **Short burst/ambulatory oxygen therapy**: For palliative care in very advanced COPD patients having severe exertional breathlessness with O_2 desaturation dip >4–6%. [This is still under debate]
- Prescription should clearly give instructions about flow of oxygen/minute; duration; O_2 device
- Oxygen is usually given by nasal prongs or by face mask/venturi mask (if high flow required)
- Humidification is not required when low flow oxygen is required
- Reassess the patient after 2–3 months, whether oxygen supplementation is effective and to assess whether oxygen is still indicated

III. Which type of oxygen delivery device?
- **Oxygen cylinders** (pressurized liquid O_2/cryo-oxygen) are cumbersome, more expensive (on long term use) and have to be refilled frequently. Also, safety is a concern to keep O_2 cylinders at home. But they deliver 100% FiO_2 and can be relied to the most and do not depend on electricity.
- **Oxygen concentrators** work on the principle of "Rapid pressure swing adsorption" of atmospheric nitrogen on to a molecular sieve incorporating zeolite (synthetic aluminium silicate) and is capable of concentrating >90% oxygen from air. They can supply oxygen from 5 to 10 litres O_2/minute. They can give 'pulsed flow or demand flow—only during inhalation' or 'continuous flow' oxygen. Pulsed flow saves oxygen and can be less irritating to the patient but continuous flow is preferred during sleep hours or in breathless patient. Oxygen concentrator is safe, relatively less expensive (over long period), can work in either AC or DC electrical output and can be carried even in commercial airlines.
- **Trans-fill unit:** Gaseous oxygen can be produced in the home by a concentrator and stored in a refillable, small and light weight 'M' tanks. The length of time these small portable tanks last varies on the O_2 litre flow/minute used and depends on the pressure (psi) with which these tanks are filled from O_2 concentrator.

IV. Oxygen therapy for air travel
- The cabin pressure of commercial aircraft usually equals to the altitude of 2100–2400 m sea level. At this pressure, alveolar PO_2 for healthy individual can decrease up to 64 mmHg and SaO_2 can decrease up to 93%. Hence, for COPD patients even with marginal SpO_2 drop at sea level can de-saturate much higher.

* Assessment for oxygen therapy (ABG or pulse oximetry) should be taken in stable phase COPD (no exacerbation in last 4 weeks), all potentially reversible factors have been treated and the patient must have stopped smoking at least for one month previously. It would be better if ABG/SpO_2 parameters are confirmed twice over a three-week period.

(Contd.)

Table 6.9: Oxygen therapy for COPD patients *(Contd.)*
• If sea level PaO$_2$ is < 70 mmHg, then the PaO$_2$ at 2300 meters will be less than 50 mmHg. The ATS currently recommends oxygen supplementation during flight, if sea level PaO$_2$ is < 70 mmHg
• Those COPD patients already on LTOT, an increase in flow rate of 1–2 litre/min during flight is needed
• Patients who recently had exacerbation or increase in symptoms should delay their air travel
• COPD patients who have co-morbidities (e.g. cardiac impairment, anemia) that can impair tissue oxygen delivery, may develop further worsening of hypoxemia during flight and hence they must be carefully assessed
• Patients must be warned about possible aggravation of hypoxemia if they walk along the aisle in flight

health related quality of life in all severity of COPD, more benefits tend to occur in moderate to severe cases and those who are self motivated. However, patients who are wheel chair bound or with mMRC-4 do not have much benefit from pulmonary rehabilitation. Patients must be assessed about their goals, specific health needs, exercise capabilities and limitations due to associated comorbidities (e.g. arthritis, impaired vision), nutritional status, psychological status and feasibility to attend such programs. Exercise training could include endurance training, walking/aerobic exercises, upper and lower limbs strength training, inspiratory muscle training. Training programs could be daily to weekly, with gradual increment in duration from 10 minutes to 30–45 minutes per session, based on the patient's tolerance or up to 60–80% of the symptom limited maximum is achieved. The rehabilitation programs should be at least for 6 to 8 weeks to get optimum benefit. Such rehabilitation programs require dedicated place and trained person to monitor/training, which could not be possible in primary level health care. In Indian setup, where most of COPD patients still seek primary health care, simple corridor exercise training (incremental walking alternating with rest for at least 20 minutes) can be advised. Breathing training such as pursed-lips breathing, diaphragmatic breathing, forward bending posture can also be done during rehabilitation. A few studies have found that certain yoga techniques could be beneficial in COPD patients (discussed in other Chapter 12). Relaxation techniques (deep breathing, meditation), psychological counselling and group counselling (behavioural therapies) can also be included in pulmonary rehabilitation programs.

Education and Self Management

COPD patients must be educated about basic information of the disease; importance of avoidance of risk factors (such as smoking, biomass fuel exposure, indoor pollution); specific aspects of medical treatment; adherence to therapy; proper inhaler techniques; self-management skills and advice about when to seek help and discussion about end of life issues. Patients should be preferably educated during each visit (if possible) or at least combined with rehabilitation programs. It would be better to discuss and educate each aspect in their own vernacular language and audio-visual mediated teaching could be helpful. Patient

Table 6.10: Nutritional management for COPD patients
1. Take energy dense supplements well divided in smaller portions spread over the day (5–6 small meals/day) to avoid adverse metabolic and ventilator effort from a high caloric load.
2. Concerns about adverse effects of carbohydrate supplementation in COPD due to increased carbon dioxide production have not been substantiated in recent studies.
3. High fat diet can actually produce increase in dyspnoea due to significant delay in gastric emptying time.
4. Ideal diet: ~30 calories/kg, carbohydrates: 50–55%; protein: 20%; fat: 25–30%. However, ideal daily calorie requirement should be calculated based on REE (resting energy expenditure) and TDEE (total daily energy expenditure).
5. Eat calcium and Vitamin D rich foods, high fibre foods (~20–35 gm fibre/day).
6. Diet rich with polyunsaturated fatty acids (PUFA) such as fish oils have been proven to reduce inflammatory mediators in lungs (e.g. leukotrienes).
7. Avoid gas producing foods, caffeine, junk foods and limit salt intake.
8. Drink adequate fluids (2–3 L/day) unless fluid restriction has been advised due to co-morbidities (e.g. cardiac failure).
9. Eat slowly and chew foods thoroughly to avoid swallowing air while eating.
10. Always eat in sitting upright posture to avoid pressure on lungs. Rest before and after meals.
11. Pulmonary rehabilitation/endurance training coupled with nutritional supplementation yield better results
12. Role of anabolic steroids (e.g. oral stanazolol, intramuscular nandrolonedecanoate) is still controversial. They can be used in selected COPD patients along with nutritional therapy and rehabilitation program.

education can improve their ability to cope with illness and health status but have no impact on lung function or exercise performance. Educating patients about "self-management skills" is still in nascent stage in India, as it depends upon patient's understanding capabilities. Also, certain applications (apps) have been recently developed for 'smart phones', which can be used by COPD patients for self-assessment of their disease status, warning signs and to take decision when to report to health care provider. With the utility of such tools, the treating physician can even assess the patient's report remotely and give appropriate advices. 'End of life' care directives is still not legally approved in India, however, patients and their families can be allowed to make informed decisions about the kind of care they want at the terminally advanced stage of the disease.

Interventional Therapy

COPD patients with severe emphysema and not adequately stabilizing with medical management can be considered for interventional therapy.

Lung volume reduction surgery (LVRS): The basic concept of LVRS is to resect areas of non-functioning lung to reduce hyperinflation and hence allow other areas to function more effectively. Best candidates for LVRS are those with bilateral upper lobe pattern of emphysema with poor exercise tolerance and LVRS has been demonstrated to improve survival in such patients.[49] Older patients (>70 years age), patients with FEV_1 ≤20%, DLCO ≤20% predicted or with homogeneous emphysema have increased risk of mortality with a little chance of benefit.[50] Hence, only fewer percent of severe COPD cases would actually be indicated for LVRS. It is usually done as a bilateral staple procedure through either a median sternotomy or VATS. However, unilateral LVRS can still be done in exceptional case with unilateral hetero-geneous emphysema or in patients with pleural adhesions on one side (due to previous interventions/disease). Patients can develop post-operative complications like air leak, pneumonia, progressive respiratory failure and carries about 5% mortality risk.

Bullectomy is a surgical procedure involving removal of either a large non-functioning bulla or bulla with frequent complications (e.g. pneumothorax). The pre-requisite for bullectomy is that the surrounding lung parenchyma should be relatively preserved (with perfusion but no ventilation). In carefully selected patient, bullectomy has been found to improve lung function and exercise tolerance.[51]

Lung transplantation: Criteria for listing for lung transplantation include BODE index > 7 and at least one of the following: FEV_1 <15–20% predicted with DLCO <20% predicted; ≥3 severe exacerbations during the previous year; one severe exacerbation with acute hypercapnic failure; significant pulmonary hypertension/corpulmonale not improving despite oxygen therapy; not candidate for LVRS. In appropriately selected severe COPD patients, lung transplantation improve functional capacity and quality of life, but not prolong survival.[51, 52] Bilateral lung transplantation is associated with increased median survival time as compared to single lung trans-plantation (7 years vs 5 years). Compli-cations of lung transplantation include acute rejection, bronchial dehiscence, bronchiolitis obliterans, opportunistic infections, lym-phoproliferative disorders and mortality. Major limiting factors for transplantation include non-availability of matched donor organs, financial restraints and only very few centres are doing lung transplantation in India.

Bronchoscopic LVR

The objectives of various bronchoscopic LVR methods are to decrease lung volume so as to improve dynamic hyperinflation. The choice between various procedures depends upon the presence of collateral ventilation (either thorough interlobular septa or fissures), which is evaluated by fissure integrity on HRCT or by endoscopic balloon occlusion and flow assessment.

1. Endobronchial unidirectional valve (allows expiration alone) placement for those with the absence of collateral ventilation. Though EB valves have been demonstrated to show improvement in FEV_1 and exercise capacity in some studies, the results are not uniform in various studies.[53,54] Also, such pro-cedure can complicate with pneumo-thorax, pneumonia, valve displacement, spontaneous expulsion on coughing and requirement of replacement.

2. Lung volume reduction coil (nitinol coils–self-retractable coils which tend to collapse and reduce the volume of that particular lung region where it has been placed) for those with the presence of collateral ventilation. Studies have shown improvement in exercise performance, quality of life with slight increase in FEV_1 with nitinol coil placement.[55,56] But more frequent exacerbations occurred in coil therapy and may develop complications such as pneumothorax, pneumonia and hemoptysis.

3. Targeted thermal vapour ablation to induce fibrosis and reduction of lung volume in more diseased segments have been shown to improve lung function and health status.

4. Previous techniques such as bronchial stents (creating additional pathway through bronchus to reduce air-trapping) and endobronchial sealants were dis-continued from clinical trials due to high morbidity and mortality

Though these bronchoscopic procedures seem to be promising semi-invasive lung volume reduction (LVR) techniques as compared to surgical LVRS, present data regarding their exact benefit is insufficient.

Palliative care in COPD: Although with all available modalities of management COPD patients responds well, but in some cases particularly when they are with end stage disese, need of something extra is felt. In those cases we can choose for palliative care for various condition. These are listed in Table 6.11.

Table 6.11: Palliative treatment options for end stage COPD		
Symptom	*Advice*	*Caution*
Refractory dyspnoea	1. Opiates (e.g. morphine 5 mg 4th hourly and titrate the dose to achieve relief of dyspnoea).	Opiate can cause respiratory depression, constipation
	2. Cool air, e.g. from a fan can provide comfort.	
	3. Neuromuscular electric stimulation (NMES), chest wall vibration (CWV).	
	4. Pursed-lips breathing	
	5. Positioning	
	6. Targeted inspiratory muscle training	
	7. Short burst O_2 therapy	
	8. Non-invasive ventilation	
	9. Cognitive behavioural therapies (relaxation exercises, biofeedback, social support, hypnosis, music, attention strategies)	
Intractable cough	Morphine 5 mg 4–6 hourly and titrate the dose	Opiate can cause respiratory depression, constipation
Anxiety (high dose of β-agonists can aggravate anxiety)	1. Cognitive behavioural therapy. 2. Benzodiazepines, e.g. alprazolam (start with 0.25 mg daily), zolpidem (5–10 mg daily), diazepam 5–10 mg daily	Avoid over dosage as it may lead to over sedation, affect cognition and respiratory depression
Confusion	Haloperidol 2 mg or levomepromazine 6 mg 12 hourly	Confusion could be a symptom of hypoxia or hypercarbia and hence it must be evaluated prior to pharmacotherapeutic agents

REFERENCES

1. Oroco-Levi M, Garcia- Aymerich J, Villar J, Ramirez-Sarmiento A, Anto JM, Gea J. Wood smoke exposure and risk of chronic obstructive pulmonary disease. Eur Respir J 2006; 27(3): 542–6.

2. Ezzati M. Indoor air pollution and health in developing countries. Lancet 2005; 366 (9480): 104–6.

3. Woodruff PG, Barr RG, Bleecker E, et al. Clinical significance of symptoms in smokers with preserved lung function. N Engl J Med 2016; 374(19): 1811–21.

4. Jones PW, Harding G, berry P, Wiklund I, Chen WH, Kline Leidy N. Development and first validation of the COPD Assessment test. Eur Respir J 2009; 34(3): 648–54.

5. Han MK, Muellerova H, Curran-Everett D, et al. GOLD 2011 disease severity classification in COPD Gene: a prospective cohort study. The Lancet Respiratory medicine 2013; 1(1): 43–50.

6. Jones PW, Tabberer M, Chen WH. Creating scenarios of the impact of COPD and their relationshop to COPD assessment Test (CAT) scores. BMC Pulm Med 2011; 11: 42.

7. Fletcher C, Peto R: The natural history of chronic airflow obstruction. Br Med J 1977; 1(6077): 1645–48.

8. Anthonisen NR, Connett JE, Kiley JP, et al. Effects of smoking intervention and the use of an inhaled anticholinergic bronchodilator on the rate of decline of FEV1. The Lung Health Study. J Am Med Assoc 1994; 272(19): 1497–1505.

9. Continuous or nocturnal oxygen therapy in hypoxemic chronic obstructive lung disease: a clinical trial. Nocturnal Oxygen Therapy Trial Group. Am Intern Med 1980; 93(3): 391–98.

10. Burge PS, Calverley PM, Jones PW, et al. Randomised, double blind, placebo controlled study of fluticasone proprionate in patients with moderate to severe chronic obstructive pulmonary disease: the ISOLDE trial. BMJ 2000; 320(7245): 1297–1303.

11. Group TLHSR: Effect of inhaled triamcinolone on the decline in pulmonary function in chronic obstructive pulmonary disease. N Engl J Med 2000; 343: 1902–09.

12. Cazzola M, Centanni S, Rgolda S, et al. Onset of action of single doses of formoterol admini-stered via Turbuhaler in patients with stable COPD. Pulm Pharmacol Ther 2011; 14: 41–45.

13. Kew KM, Mavergames C, Walters JA. Long acting beta2 agonists for chronic obstructive pulmonary disease. Cochrane Database Syst rev 2013; 10(10): CD010177.

14. Geake JB, Dabscheck EJ, Wood- Baker R, Cates CJ. Indacaterol, a once daily beta2 agonist, versus twice daily beta2 agonists or placebo for chronic obstructive pulmonary disease. Cochrane Database Syst Rev 2015; 1: CD010139.

15. Johnson M, Rennard S. Alternative mech-anisms for long actine beta2 adrenergic agonists in COPD. Chest 2001; 120: 258–70.

16. Gross NJ, Skorodin MS. Anticholinergic, antimuscarinic bronchodilators. Am Rev Respir Dis 1984; 129: 856–70.

17. Karner C, Chong J, Poole P. Tiotropium versus placebo for chronic obstructive pulmonary disease. Cochrane Database Syst Rev 2014; 7: CD009285.

18. Casaburi R, Kukafka D, Cooper CB, Witek TJ, Jr., Kesten S. Improvement in exercise tolerance with the combination of tiotropium and pulmonary rehabilitation in patients with COPD. Chest 2005; 127(3): 809–17.

19. Van Noord JA, Bantje TA, Eland ME, Korducki L, Cornelissen PJ. A randomised controlled comparison of tiotropium and ipratropium in the treatment of chronic obstructive pul-monary disease. The Dutch Tiotropium Study Group. Thorax 2000; 55:289–94.

20. Vogelmeier C, hederer B, Glaab T, et al. Tiotropium versus salmeterol for the pre-vention of exacerbations of COPD. N Engl J Med 2011; 364(12): 1093–103.

21. Cazzola M, Molimard M. The scientific rationale for combining long acting beta2 agonists and muscarinic antagonists in COPD. Pulm Pharmacol Ther 2010; 23(4): 257–67.

22. Gross N, Tashkin D, Miller R, Oren J, Coleman W, Linberg S. Inhalation by nebulisation of albuterol-ipratropium combination (Dey combination) is superior to either agent alone in the treatment of chronic obstructive pulmonary disease. Dey Combination Solution Study Group. Respiration 1998; 65(5): 354–62.

23. Farne HA, Cates CJ. Long acting beta2-agonist in addition to tiotropium versus either tiotropium or long acting beta2-agonist alone for chronic obstructive pulmonary disease. Cochrane Database Syst Rev 2015; 10(10): CD008989.

24. Mahler DA, Kerwin E, Ayers T, et al. FLIGHT1 and FLIGHT2: efficacy and safety of QVA149 (Indacaterol/Glycopyrrolate) versus its monocomponents and placebo in patients with chronic obstructive pulmonary disease. Am J RespirCrit Care Med 2015; 192(9): 1068–79.

25. Wedzicha JA, Decramer M, Ficker JH, et al. Analysis of chronic obstructive pulmonary disease exacerbations with the dual bronchodilator QVA149 comapred with glycopyrronium and tiotropium (SPARK): a randomised, double blind, parallel group study. The Lancet Respiratory Medicine 2013; 1(3): 199–209.

26. Wedzicha JA, Banerji D, Chapman KR, et al. Indacaterol-Glycopyrronium versus Salmeterol-Fluticasone for COPD. N Engl J Med 2016; 374(23): 2222–34.

27. Jones PW, Willits LR, Burge PS, Calverley PM. Disease severity and the effect of fluticasone proprionate on chronic obstructive pulmonary disease exacerbations. Eur Respir J 2003; 21: 68–73.

28. Sin DD, Golmohammadi K, Jacobs P. Cost-effectiveness of inhaled corticosteroids for chronic obstructive pulmonary disease according to disease severity. Am J Med 2004; 116: 325–31.

29. Burge PS, Calverley PM, Jones PW, Spencer S, Anderson JA, Maslen TK. Randomized, double blind, placebo controlled study of fluticasone proprionate in patients with moderate to severe chronic obstructive pulmonary disease: the ISOLDE trial. Br Med J 2000; 320: 1297–1303.

30. Calverley PM, Anderson JA, Celli B, et al. Salmeterol and fluticasone propionate and survival in chronic obstructive pulmonary disease. N Engl J Med 2007; 356(8): 775–89.

31. Nannini LJ, Lasserson TJ, Poole P. Combined corticosteroid and long acting beta2 agonist in one inhaler versus long acting beta2 agonists for chronic obstructive pulmonary disease. Cochrane Database Syst Rev 2012; 9(9): CD006829.

32. Crim C, Dransfield MT, Bourbeau J, et al. Pneumonia risk with inhaled fluticasone furoate and vilanterol compared with vilanterol alone in patients with COPD. Annals of the American Thoracic Society 2015; 12(1): 27–34.

33. Calverley PM, Rabe KF, Goehring UM, et al. Roflumilast in symptomatic chronic obstructive pulmonary disease: two rando-mised clinical trials. Lancet 2009; 374(9691): 685–94.

34. Johnston RN, Mc Neill RS, Smith DH, et al. Five-year winter chemoprophylaxis for chronic bronchitis. BMJ 1969; 4(678): 265–9.

35. Ni W, Shao X, Cai X, et al. Prophylactic use of macrolide antibiotics for the prevention of chronic obstructive pulmonary disease exacerbation: a meta analysis. Plos One 2015; 10(3): e0121257.

36. Uzun S, Djamin RS, Kluytmans JA, et al. Azithromycin maintenance treatment in patients with frequent exacerbations of chronic obstructive pulmonary disease (COLUMBUS): a randomized, double blind, placebo con-trolled trial. The Lancet Respiratory Medicine 2014; 2(5): 361–8.

37. Cazzola M, Calzetta L, Page C, et al. Influence of N-acetylcysteine on chronic bronchitis or COPD exacerbations: a meta analysis. Eur Respir Rev 2015; 24(137): 451–61.

38. Poole P, Chong J, Cates CJ. Mucolytic agents versus placebo for chronic bronchitis or chronic obstructive pulmonary disease. Cochrane Database Syst Rev 2015; (7): CD001287.

39. Rea H, McAuley Sue, Jayaraman L, et al. The clinical utility of long-term humidification therapy in chronic airway disease. Res Med 2010; 104(4): 525–33.

40. Gerard J. Criner MD, John E, et al. Simvastatin for the prevention of exacerbations in moderate to severe COPD. N Engl J Med 2014; 370: 2201–10.

41. Edwards KM, Dupont WD, Westrich MK, Plummer WD, Jr., Palmer PS, Wright PF. A randomised controlled trial of cold-adapted and inactivated vaccines for the prevention of influenza A disease. J Infect Dis 1994; 169(1): 68–76.

42. Bonten MJ, Huijts SM, Bolkenbaas M, et al. Polysaccharide conjugate vaccine against pneumococcal pneumonia in adults. N Engl J Med 2015; 372(12):1114–25.

43. Foulds J, Jarvis MJ. Smoking cessation and prevention. In: Calverley P, Pride N, eds. Chronic Obstructive Pulmonary Disease. London: Chapman & Hall, 1995:373.

44. Lancaster T, Stead L, Silagy C, Sowden A. Effectiveness of interventions to help people stop smoking: findings from the Cochrane Library. BMJ 2000; 321:355–8.

45. Jorenby DE, Leischow SJ, Nides MA, et al. A controlled trial of sustained-release bupropion, a nicotine patch, or both for smoking cessation. N Engl J Med 1999; 340: 685–91.

46. Cranston JM, Crockett AJ, Moss JR, Alpers JH. Domiciliary oxygen for chronic obstructive pulmonary disease. Cochrane Database Syst Rev 2005; (4): CD001744.

47. Long Term Oxygen Treatment Trial Research Group. A randomized trial of long term oxygen for COPD with moderate desaturation. N Engl J Med 2016; 375(17): 1617.

48. Vermeeren M, Creutzberg E, Schols A, et al. Prevalence of nutritional depletion in a large out-patient population of patients with COPD. Respir Med 2006; 100: 1349–55.

49. Fishman A, Martinez F, Naunheim K, et al. A randomized trial comparing lung volume reduction surgery with medical therapy for severe emphysema. N Engl J Med 2003; 348(21): 2059–73.

50. National Emphysema Treatment Trial Research Group. Patients at high risk of death after lung volume reduction surgery. N Engl J Med 2001; 345(15): 1075–83.

51. Marchetti N, Criner GJ. Surgical approaches to treating emphysema: Lung Volume Reduction surgery, Bullectomy and Lung Trans-plantation. Smin Respir Crit Care Med 2015; 36(4): 592–608.

52. Stavem K, Bjortuft O, Borgan O, Geiran O, Boe J. Lung transplantation in patients with chronic obstructive pulmonary disease in a national cohort is without obvious survival benefit. J Heart Lung Transplant 2006; 25(1): 75–84.

53. Klooster K, Ten Hacken NH, Hartman JE, Kerstjens HA, Van Rikxoort EM, Slebos DJ. Endobronchial valves for emphysema without interlobar collateral ventilation. N Engl J Med 2015; 373(24): 2325–35.

54. Davey C, Zoumot Z, Jordon S, et al. Bronchoscopic lung volume reduction with endobronchial valves for patients with heterogenous emphysema and intact interlobar fissures (the BeLieVeR-HIFi trial): study design and rationale. Thorax 2015; 70(3): 288–90.

55. Sciurba FC, Criner GJ, Strange C, et al. Effect of Endobronchial coils vs usual care on exercise tolerance in patients with severe emphysema. The RENEW randomized trial. JAMA 2016; 315(20): 2178–89.

56. Deslee G, Mal H, Dutau H, et al. Lung volume reduction coil treatment vs usual care in patients with severe emphysema. The REVOLENS randomized clinical trial. JAMA 2016; 315(2): 175–84.

Acute Exacerbation of COPD

Arun Sampath, Amit Kumar Verma

Acute exacerbation of COPD (AECOPD) is defined as acute worsening of baseline respiratory symptoms that require change in medications.[1] Exacerbations are usually associated with increased airway inflammation, increased mucus production, dynamic hyperinflation and decline in lung function. COPD exacerbations contribute to disease progression especially when the recovery from AECOPD is slow.[2] AECOPD occurs in more than 20% of patients with severe COPD and exacerbations become more frequent with severe disease (3.43 exacerbation events per year in severe COPD pateints vs 2.68 events/year in moderate COPD).[3] AECOPD usually results in increased dyspnoea (most important symptom) and increased sputum volume with or without sputum purulence. Based on these cardinal symptoms, severity of AECOPD is classified (Table 7.1) into three groups (Anthonisen criteria).[4]

AECOPD are mostly triggered by respiratory viral infections, however, bacterial infections are also responsible either as primary cause or as superimposed secondary infections aggravating the ongoing viral exacerbation. The most common virus isolated is human rhinovirus (common cold virus) and can be isolated even up to a week after AECOPD onset.[5] Viral infections usually cause more severe and prolonged exacerbations. Many patients are sensitive to air pollutants and suffer an exacerbation when ambient levels increase. In about 30% of COPD patients, no cause for

Table 7.1: Classification of acute exacerbation of COPD	
Severity of exacerbations	*Characteristics*
Severe (Type 1)	Increased dyspnoea, sputum volume and sputum purulence
Moderate (Type 2)	Any 2 of the above three cardinal symptoms
Mild (Type 3)	Any 1 of the above three cardinal symptoms and 1 or more of the following minor symptoms or signs: • Cough • Wheezing • Fever without any other obvious source • Upper respiratory tract infection in the past 5 days • Respiratory rate increase >20% over baseline • Heart rate >20% over baseline

AECOPD can be identified. During exacerbations, sputum neutrophilia occurs as a result of heightened inflammation. On contrary, the presence of sputum or blood eosinophilia suggests more vulnerability to viral infections[6] and responsiveness to systemic steroids.[7]

Several studies have shown that inflammatory mediators such as C-reactive protein (CRP), fibrinogen, soluble tumour necrosis factor alpha, inflammatory cytokines are much higher during acute exacerbations. Also, increase in number and activity of neutrophils are noted in the airway lumen during exacerbations. This heightened inflammation may potentially damage lung tissues and lead to an accelerated decline in lung function. About 20% of patients have more decline in lung function and disease severity compared to pre exacerbation state.[8] The mean rate of decline in FEV_1 due to exacerbations was observed to be 36 ml per year and the decline in FEV_1 was greater in patients with frequent exacerbations (40.1 ml/yr vs 32.1 ml/yr, p<0.05).[3] Frequent exacerbations (≥2 exacerbations/year) have been associated with worse outcome, increased dyspnoea, reduced exercise capacity and greater decline in health status. Patients with severe COPD tend to get frequent exacerbations and more severe exacerbations. The median recovery in lung function after an AECOPD is 6 days.[9] However, more severe the exacerbations longer the recovery time (even more than weeks to months). In spite of FEV_1 returning to baseline, about 50% patients perceive their health related quality of life is poor and require assistance for daily activities. Severe AECOPD is associated with increased mortality and studies have reported in-hospital, 6 months, 1 and 2 yrs mortality of 11%, 33% and 49% respectively.[10] However, the severity of the underlying disease may influence the overall patient's outcome.

The predictors of future exacerbations are: Previous exacerbations; worsening FEV_1; severity of emphysema or airway wall thickness as measured by CT scan chest; increase in the ratio of the pulmonary artery to aorta cross sectional dimension (ratio>1);[11] chronic bronchitis. Since COPD patients usually have comorbid conditions, AECOPD must be differentiated from acute coronary syndrome, left ventricular failure, pulmonary embolism. Also, COPD patients are prone to develop other acute pulmonary conditions such as pneumothorax and pneumonia and can mimic as acute exacerbation. Patients with AECOPD are at an increased risk of developing another exacerbation within next 8 weeks and hence close follow-up is needed to promptly detect and treat earlier which can improve treatment outcomes.[12]

MANAGEMENT OF AECOPD

The treatment goals for AECOPD are to minimize the impact of current exacerbation, to minimize loss of lung function, and to prevent future exacerbations. Almost 80% of AECOPD patients can be managed on OPD basis involving bronchodilators, steroid with or without antibiotic. However, certain indicators (Table 7.2) have to be assessed in every COPD patients presenting with exacerbation, based on which the decision for hospitalization has to be made. Early recognition of AECOPD and prompt aggressive intervention is required to prevent further frank respiratory failure.

The decision whether patient with AECOPD could be managed in medical ward or in high dependency unit (HDU)/ Intensive care depends on the severity of respiratory failure (Table 7.3).[13]

Pharmacologic Treatment

Bronchodilators, steroids and antibiotics are the important class of medications commonly used for management of AECOPD.

Table 7.2: Indications for hospitalization

1. Worsening dyspnoea

2. High respiratory rate (> 30 breaths/minute)

3. Increased work of breathing (use of accessory muscles of respiration, paradoxical breathing)

4. Hypoxemia

5. Confusion, drowsiness

6. Hypercarbia

7. Inadequate response to initial medical management for AECOPD

8. Serious cardiovascular conditions (heart failure, arrhythmia, severe hypotension)

9. Inability to tolerate oral medications such as antibiotics or steroids

10. Insufficient home support

11. Older age

12. Frequent exacerbator phenotype

Bronchodilators

Short acting β_2-agonists should be used with or without short acting anticholinergics for initial management for all AECOPD patients. Nebulization therapy is easier than other inhaler devices during an acute exacerbation due to the fact that severely dyspnoeic patients find difficulty in coordinating meter dose inhalers (MDI) and may not generate adequate inspiratory flow required for dry powder inhalers. However, a systematic review[14] found no statistical significant difference in lung function between the MDI and nebulizers during acute exacerbations and hence MDI can be used preferably with spacer if given correctly. It is recommended to give continuous nebulization with short acting bronchodilators initially. If MDI is preferred, then one or two puff to be given every one hour initially and then every 2–4 hours based on the patient's response. There is insufficient data at present for the use of long acting bronchodilators (either LABA or

Table 7.3: Severity classification of respiratory failure in AECOPD

Clinical signs	No respiratory failure	Acute respiratory failure (non-life threatening)	Acute respiratory failure (life threatening)
Respiratory rate	20–30 breaths/minute	>30 breaths/minute	>30 breaths/minute
Use of accessory muscles	No	Yes	Yes
Mental status	Normal	Normal	Acute changes
Hypoxemia	Improved with supplemental oxygen via venturi mask FiO_2<30%	Improved with supplemental oxygen via venturi mask FiO_2<30%	Not improving with supplemental oxygen via venturi mask or requiring high concentration (FiO_2>40%)
Hypercapnia	No rise in $PaCO_2$ levels	Increased compared with patient's baseline or $PaCO_2$ 50–60 mmHg	Increased compared with patient's baseline or $PaCO_2$ >60 mmHg or acidosis pH ≤7.25

LAMA) during exacerbation. Regarding intravenous methylxanthines, such agents are not recommended in AECOPD due to significant side effects.[15]

Glucocorticoids

Systemic steroids use in AECOPD is associated with favourable outcome such as more rapid recovery, improvement in lung function, improve hypoxemia and a reduced risk of early relapse or treatment failure.[16,17] Shorter course (5 days) of systemic corticosteroid was found to be non-inferior to previous recommendation of longer duration (14 days).[18] The present guidelines recommend using 40 mg prednisone per day for 5 days. Oral prednisone is equally effective as intravenous steroids. Glucocorticoids have more effect in eosinophilic phenotype and may be less efficacious in AECOPD patients with lower blood eosinophils levels.[19,6]

Antibiotics

Since AECOPD could be due to viral infections or triggered by environmental causes, the use of antibiotics for all patients still remains controversial. However, systematic review[20] has shown that antibiotics reduce the mortality by 77%, treatment failure by 53% and sputum purulence by 44%. About 50% of AECOPD are associated with *S. pneumoniae*, *H. influenzae* and *M. catarrhalis*.[21] However, it is difficult to differentiate between bacterial respiratory colonization and acute infection. On contrary, even when patients have chronic bacterial colonization, changes in strain may be associated with new exacerbations. Sputum cultures have many demerits like oropharyngeal contamination, lack of differentiation of colonizing bacteria from new one and delay in results. Current guidelines recommend antibiotics to be given for AECOPD patients if they have all

the three cardinal symptoms (increase in dyspnoea, increased sputum volume and purulence); even in moderate severity AECOPD (but sputum purulence should be one of the cardinal symptoms), patients who require ventilation (non-invasive or invasive), and evidence of an infectious process such as fever, leukocytosis, or infiltrates in chest radiograph.[3] The recommended length of antibiotic treatment is 5 to 10 days. The route of administration of antibiotics depends on the patient's ability to eat and the pharmacokinetics of the antibiotic used. The choice of antibiotic should be based on the following factors: Severity of AECOPD, culture reports of previous exacerbations, associated comorbidities, previous pseudomonas colonization and local bacterial resistance pattern. Usual initial empirical antibiotic is an aminopenicillin with clavulanic acid, macrolide or tetracycline (Table 7.4). More resistant pathogens or gram-negative bacteria such as *Pseudomonas aeruginosa* are prevalent in patients with frequent exacerbations/frequent hospitalizations, severe COPD and patients requiring mechanical ventilation.[22] Culture of sputum or samples directly from lower respiratory tract by bronchoscopy should be done for non-responders to initial empirical antibiotics, patients with severe exacerbation or suspicion of pneumonia. Improvement in sputum purulence, fever (if present initially) and dyspnoea indicates antibiotic response.

Respiratory Support

Oxygen Therapy

Supplemental oxygen should be administered if SpO_2 less than 88%, keeping a target to achieve at least 90–92%. After 30–60 minutes, arterial blood gas should be assessed for evidence of carbon dioxide retention. However, carbon dioxide

Table 7.4: Microbial sensitivity profile to commonly used antibiotics

Organism	Antibiotics commonly sensitive	Resistance increasing for
1. *Streptococcus pneumonia*	• Amoxycillin • Amoxycillin-clavulanate • Macrolide (clarithromycin/ azithromycin) • Doxycycline • Second/third generation cephalosporins (cefuroxime/ cefotaxime) • Respiratory fluoroquinolones (levofloxacin/moxifloxacin) • Vancomycin	Penicillins-β-lactamase (with cross resistance to cephalosporins) Macrolides quinolones (due to unnecessary use of this drug)
2. *Haemophilus influenzae*	• β-lactam antibiotics (ampicillin-sulbactum) • Cephalosporins (cefuroxime, cefotaxime, cefixime) • Macrolides • Respiratory fluoroquinolones	Penicillins Cefuroxime Macrolides
3. *Moraxella catarrhalis*	• Macrolides • Second/third cephalosporins • Fluoroquinolones • Trimethoprim-sulfamethaxole	All penicillins
Gram-negative enterics *Klebsiella pneumoniae*	• Third/fourth cephalosporins: Ceftriaxone, cefoperazone, ceftazidime, cefepime • Piperacillin+tazobactum, ticarcillin+ clavulanate • Fluoroquinolnes • Carbapenem (meropenem, imipenem, ertapenem) • Aminoglycosides (as combination therapy)	Penicillins/macrolides (intrinsic resistance) ESBL (extended spectrum beta lactamase) Carbapenamase Fluroquinolones
Pseudomonas aeruginosa Enterobacteriaceae	• Third or fourth generation cephalosporins • Aztreonem • Piperacillin + tazobactum • Fluoroquinolone (levoflox/ciprofloxacin) • Carbapenems • Aminoglycosides (combination therapy)	For ESBL or Carbapenamase organisms: Colistin/ fosfomycin/tigecycline (combined with other agents) Co-trimoxazole for certain of enterobacteriaceae/ strenotrophomonas species

(Contd.)

Table 7.4: Microbial sensitivity profile to commonly used antibiotics *(Contd.)*

Organism	Antibiotics commonly sensitive	Resistance increasing for
Atypical micro-organisms		
Mycoplasma pneumoniae	• Tetracyclines (doxycycline)	Inherent resistance to all
Chlamydia pneumoniae	• Macrolides	β-lactams
Legionella pneumophilia	• Fluoroquinolones	
	• Co-trimoxazole (weekly sensitive)	
Staphylococcus aureus (MSSA)	• Penicillins	Penicillins
	• Penicillinase-resistant	Methicillin or oxacillin
	penicillins (flucloxacillin/	resistance (MRSA)
	dicoloxacillin)	
	• First generation cephalosporins	For MRSA:
	(cefazolin, cephalexin,	Vancomycin, linezolid,
	cephalothin)	telavancin ceftobiprole,
	• Clindamycin	clindamycin (if susceptible)
	• Linezolid	
	• Macrolide	
	• Vancomycin	
	• Others: Rifampicin, co-trimox,	
	doxycycline, quinolone	

retention from depression of hypoxic drive has been overemphasized. Multiple studies in the literature dispute the view that too much oxygen causes significant respiratory depression in COPD patients. With administration of oxygen, $PaCO_2$ rises, but not in proportion to the very minor changes in respiratory drive. Carbon dioxide retention is more likely a consequence of ventilation–perfusion mismatching rather than respiratory center depression. However, this complication is best avoided by titrating oxygen delivery to maintain the SpO_2 ~ 90–92% or PaO_2 at 60–65 mmHg. Controlled oxygen therapy through Venturi masks (high flow with fixed FiO_2) is preferred to other oxygen delivery devices.

Ventilatory Support

AECOPD patients with respiratory failure should be hospitalized immediately for ventilator support, which can be provided either by noninvasive (NIV) or invasive (conventional mechanical ventilation through endotracheal intubation) ventilation. The choice of noninvasive versus invasive ventilation depends upon the severity of respiratory failure, patients' conscious level and ability to protect upper airways and cope with secretions and co-operation and absence of severe cardiovascular compromise (Table 7.5).

Noninvasive Ventilation (NIV)

Wherever feasible, NIV is preferred as initial ventilator support for ACEOPD patients as it has been shown to be successful in about 80–85% cases and can prevent complications of endotracheal intubation such as ventilator associated pneumonia, requirement of prolonged sedation, long hospital stay and inherent complications of mechanical ventilator such as barotrauma.[23-25] NIV alleviates work of breathing by reducing the respiratory muscle load and thus improve respiratory failure. The guidelines recommend that NIV can be safely given for AECOPD patients with mild to moderate respiratory failure with pH not less than 7.25. However, various studies have shown benefit even in lower pH. Also, NIV can be used effectively in respiratory ward settings, provided a trained person is available to monitor the patient carefully.[25] Patients on NIV should be monitored closely initially and ABG has to be obtained after 30 minutes to 1 hour of NIV initiation to assess for the response to therapy. If patient's work of breathing is improving and pH, $PaCO_2$ is improving on NIV, it can be continued with regular monitoring of patients respiratory status. The efficacy of NIV is often made in first hour or two of initiation and if there is no physiologic improvement, NIV is deemed to be failed and patient should be intubated endotracheally and put on invasive ventilation (Fig. 7.1). NIV should be given along with oxygen supplementation, which can be delivered directly through nasal prongs or connected to interface NIV mask. NIV is given through interface mask which can be either nasal, orofacial or whole head (helmet mask). Each interface mask has its own benefits and side effects. Orofacial mask is usually preferred as it is comfortable for patients and provides adequate air seal as compared to nasal mask. Helmet mask is used rarely for some patients who could not tolerate conventional masks. However, claustrophobia is a concern for such mask. Also, NIV can be used as a weaning modality for patients on invasive mechanical ventilation. It has been proved that NIV as a weaning mode allows early weaning and better outcome.[26, 27]

Invasive Ventilation

NIV has revolutionized the respiratory support therapy for AECOPD and replaced invasive ventilation as initial therapy for such respiratory failure cases. However, invasive ventilation is required for the indications as given in Table 7.5. The in-hospital mortality of AECOPD with acute respiratory failure is about 17–49%. However, mortality is lower in AECOPD with respiratory failure as compared to respiratory failure due to other non-COPD conditions. COPD patients with relatively good lung function (FEV_1>30% predicted), no comorbidites, ambulatory before current

Table 7.5: Indications for respiratory support therapy	
Noninvasive ventilation	*Invasive mechanical ventilation*
At least one of the following: • Severe dyspnoea with increased work of breathing such as use of accessory respiratory muscles, paradoxical breathing • Respiratory acidosis ($PaCO_2 \geq 45$ mmHg) and arterial pH ≤ 7.35) • Persistent hypoxemia despite supplemental oxygen therapy AND Absence of all of the following: • Diminished consciousness • Inability to protect airways • Severe hemodynamic instability • Uncooperative	• NIV failure or unable to tolerate NIV • Unconsciousness, extreme agitation • Severe Respiratory acidosis (pH<7.25) • Inability to protect airways/massive aspiration • Severe hemodynamic instability requiring escalating dose of inotropes • Severe ventricular or supraventricular arrhythmias • Status post-cardiac or respiratory arrest • Life-threatening hypoxemia

AECOPD event, not on long term oxygen therapy (LTOT) recovered well with ventilator support. On contrary, very advanced COPD patients with respiratory failure may require prolonged ventilatory therapy with very poor quality of life. Hence the decision to initiate invasive ventilation depends on the likely reversibility of the present exacerbation, patient's wishes, financial status and the availability of intensive care facilities.

Ventilator Settings

NIV: Currently, almost all NIV are given by noninvasive positive pressure ventilation (NIPPV), wherein the positive pressure can be given throughout respiratory cycle either as continuous (CPAP—continuous positive airway pressure) or as biphasic [BiPAP-Bilevel PAP; as IPAP (inspiratory positive airway pressure) and EPAP(expiratory positive Airway Pressure)]. BiPAP is preferred to CPAP for AECOPD patients because it provides support to both phases of respiration and the ability to adjust 'rise time' in BiPAP is very advantageous. COPD patients require longer time for expiration and their inhalations are very quick and short and low rise time settings in BiPAP enables rapid inflow of air during inhalation and prolonged I:E ratio. Various modes and initial settings of BIPAP are listed in Table 7.6 and further explained in Fig. 7.1.

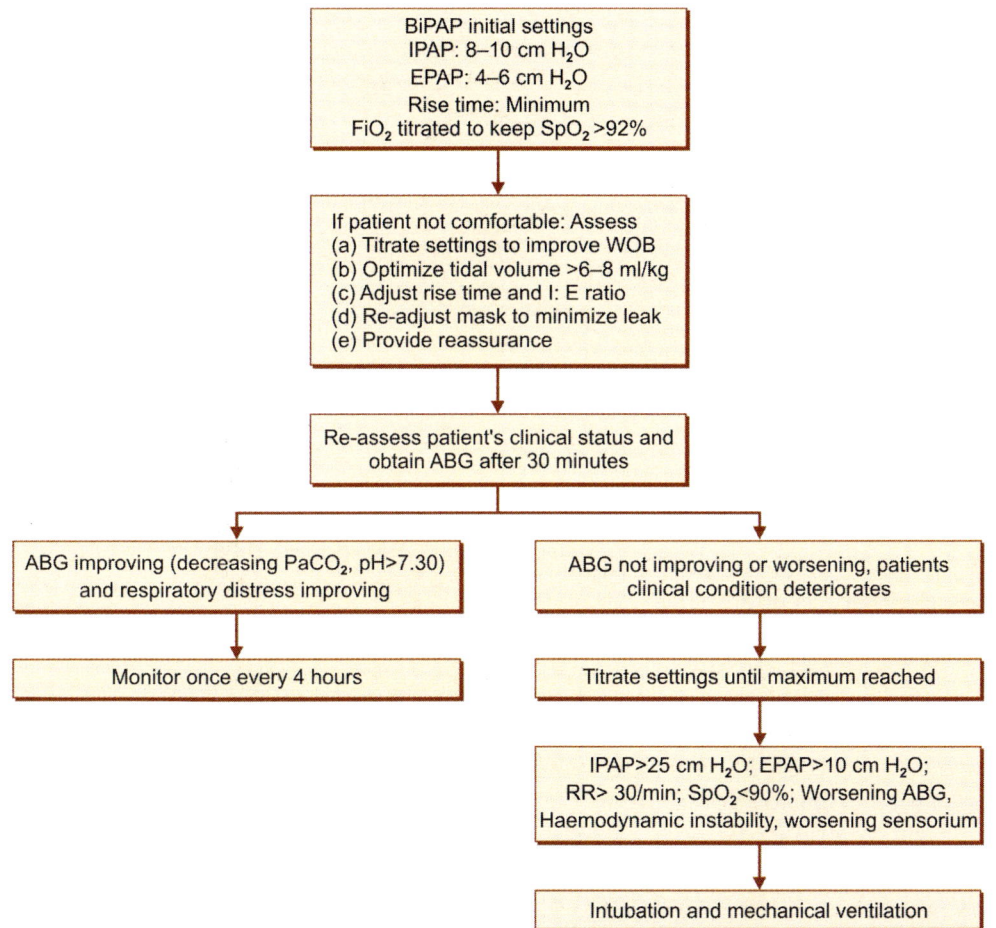

Fig. 7.1: Flow diagram for NIV (BIPAP) for AECOPD

Table 7.6: Modes of NIV and common initial settings

Modes of BiPAP	Initial Settings of BiPAP for AECOPD
• Spontaneous (S mode) • Spontaneous with backup respiratory rate (ST mode). • Time (T) mode (NIV will deliver as per set respiratory frequency). Rarely used as most of the time, apnoeic patient is usually put on IMV • PC mode • AVAPS (average volume assured pressure support)—new advanced technology wherein the machine automatically adjusts with patients' ventilatory requirements (auto-adjusting EPAP), recognizes and compensates for leaks, adjusts variable trigger and cycle thresholds and enables optimum patient/ventilator synchrony	• Start EPAP with 4 to 5 and titrate (in increments of 2 cm H_2O, maximum 25 cm H_2O) according to SpO_2 (target 90–92%). Starting with lower pressures will allow patient tolerance and training. When increasing EPAP, increase IPAP by the same amount to maintain the same level of pressure support. • Start IPAP with 8 to 10 and titrate (in increments of 2–3 cm H_2O, maximum 25 cm H_2O) according to work of breathing/dyspnoea • Keep at least a difference of 4 between IPAP and EPAP • Flow must be synchronized with patient respiratory efforts • Achieve I:E ratio of 1:2 or more • Adjust rise time (the time it takes for the device to change from EPAP to IPAP) according to patient's comfort • Keep RAMP (gradual delivery of pressures according to set time) settings to low so as to initiate delivery of BiPAP pressures quickly • Choose proper interface mask according to patient's acceptance and to minimize air leak (modern NIVs have inherent adjustment to leak of up to 35–40 L) • FiO_2 titrated to achieve SpO_2 >92% • Keep head end of bed raised by 30 degrees or more and explain the therapy to patient and provide reassurance • Closely monitor vitals, work of breathing, sensorium level

Invasive Mechanical Ventilation (IMV)

The pre-requisite to initiate IMV is tubing of the airway either by endotracheal tube or by tracheostomy tube. The parameters of IMV are mostly concerned with inspiration, since expiration is usually passive by elastic recoiling of lung tissue. However, in almost all patients the end expiration is prevented by application of positive pressure through PEEP (positive end expiratory pressure) which prevents complete collapse of each alveoli and maintains functional residual capacity (FRC). The modes of IMV are classi-fied based on 1. Dependency on mechanical breaths (completely controlled by ventilator; partially controlled or spontaneous); 2. Volume targeted (VCV, ACV, VSV) or pressure targeted (PCV, AC-PV, PSV); 3. Limiting factor (inspiratory time or set volume in VCV, inspiratory (i)-time or set pressure in pressure modes) or by 4. Cycling (start of expiration) by i-time or by airflow. Various modes and initial settings of IMV are listed in Table 7.7, these are useful to begin with.

Weaning from mechanical ventilation can be done if following criteria are met: Fully conscious, ability to protect airways,

Table 7.7: Modes of IMV and common initial ventilator settings

Modes of mechanical ventilation	Initial settings of mechanical ventilation for AECOPD
• Controlled modes (VCV, PCV) • Assist control modes (ACV: Volume targeted or pressure targeted) • Intermittent mandatory ventilation (Synchronized intermittent mandatory ventilation: VCV+PS; PCV+PS) • Spontaneous modes (PSV/CPAP) • AVAPS	• Choice of initial mode depends on the treating physician's confidence with a particular ventilator mode • Usually it is advised to start with VCV where tidal volume could be targeted quickly • Pressure modes have advantages such as prevention of barotrauma and patient's own inspiratory flow is allowed which improves patient–ventilator synchrony. However, the delivered tidal volume is variable according to lung compliance and hence it would be difficult to start with PCV • Keep moderately low tidal volume: 6 to 10 ml/kg • Respiratory frequency (f) to match patient's requirement of minute ventilation but avoid hyperventilation as it may affect expiratory time. Start with frequency of 10–14/minute • Inspiratory flow of 80–100 L/minute with square waveform is ideal • Allow longer expiratory time (I:E ratio >1:3 or 1:4) to prevent air trapping • FiO_2 to achieve SpO_2 >92% • Apply external PEEP (less than 75–85% of auto-PEEP) to alleviate respiratory efforts (WOB) • Ventilator trigger setting should be minimal as in the presence of auto-PEEP, patient may not be able to generate enough negative pressure or flow • Target plateau pressure <30 cm H_2O to avoid barotrauma • Closely monitor vitals, work of breathing, ventilator dysynchrony, auto-PEEP, compliance

hemodynamically stable, FiO_2 requirement <50%; rapid shallow breathing index (RSBI: Respiratory rate/tidal volume) <105, and bronchospasm is stabilizing with medications. Weaning can be sometimes difficult and may be a prolonged process in COPD patients, and usually done by either spontaneous breathing trial (T-piece trial) or by pressure support ventilation. However, some patients fail extubation even after careful weaning process. NIV has been found to facilitate weaning, prevent reintubation, reduces risk of respiratory failure post-extubation and lowers 60-day mortality.[26, 27]

HOSPITAL DISCHARGE AND SUBSEQUENT FOLLOW-UP

There is no optimal duration of hospitalization for patients with AECOPD. However, patients can be safely discharged if the following criteria are met: Fully conscious, clinically stable for 24 hrs, ABG parameters stable for 24 hrs, able to take oral diet and medications, able to use inhalers therapy, not significantly dyspnoeic and not requiring frequent SABA's (reliever) therapy, able to sleep without frequent awakenings due to dyspnoea, resting hypoxemia if present can be managed with low flow oxygen supplementation and finally patient/family is educated and confident that patient can manage successfully at home. At the time of discharge, patient has to be educated and explained about drug compliance, inhaler techniques, breathing exercises, domiciliary oxygen/NIV (in selected cases), instructions regarding follow-up visit and when to attend early hospital care (in case of sudden worsening of symptoms/emergency). The usual follow-up visit will be after 4 weeks and patients have to be reassessed about symptoms score, capacity to do daily activities, inhaler technique, spirometry, optimization of medications, assessment and management of comorbidities and reassess need for long term oxygen therapy. Further follow-up can be done once in 3 months and the standard protocol for management of stable COPD can be followed.

Long-term prognosis following hospitalization for AECOPD is poor and 5-year mortality rate of about 50%. Factors associated with poor outcome are given in Table 7.8.

Table 7.8: Factors associated with poor outcome in AECOPD[28,29]

1. Older age
2. Lower BMI
3. Clinical severity of present exacerbation
4. Previous hospitalizations for exacerbations
5. Associated comorbidities (cardiovascular disease, lung cancer)
6. Severity of respiratory symptoms
7. Worse lung function
8. Lower exercise capacity
9. Need for long term oxygen therapy at discharge

SUMMARY

AECOPD is defined as acute worsening of baseline respiratory symptoms that require change in medications. It usually results in increased dyspnoea (most important symptom) and increased sputum volume with or without sputum purulence. The predictors of future exacerbations are: Previous exacerbations, worsening FEV_1, severity of emphysema or airway wall thickness as measured by CT scan chest, increase in the ratio of the pulmonary artery to aorta cross sectional dimension (ratio>1), chronic bronchitis. Up to 80% of AECOPD patients can be managed on OPD basis. Bronchodilators, steroids and antibiotics are the important class of medications commonly used for management of AECOPD. The choice of antibiotic should be based on the following factors: severity of AECOPD, culture reports of previous exacerbations, associated co-morbidities, previous pseudomonas colonization and local bacterial resistance pattern. Respiratory support in the form of oxygen, noninvasive ventilation and invasive ventilation can be decided on case basis.

REFERENCES

1. Wedzicha JA, Seemungal TA. COPD exacerbations: defining their cause and prevention. Lancet 2007; 370(9589): 786–96.
2. Donaldson GC, Law M, Kowlessar B, et al. Impact of prolonged exacerbation recovery in Chronic Obstructive Pulmonary Disease. AM J Respir Crit Care Med 2015; 192(8): 943–50.
3. Donaldson GC, Seemungal TAR, Bhowmik A et al. Relationship between exacerbation frequency and lung function decline in chronic obstructive pulmonary disease. Thorax 2002; 57: 847–52.
4. Anthonisen NR, Manfreda J, Warren Cp, et al. Antibiotic therapy in exacerbations of chronic obstructive pulmonary disease. Ann Intern Med 1987; 106(2): 196–204.

5. White AJ, Gomepertz S, Stockley RA. The aetiology of exacerbations of Chronic Obstructive Pulmonary Disease. Thorax 2003; 58(1): 73–80.

6. Papi A, Bellettato Cm, Braccioni F, et al. Infections and airway inflammation in Chronic Obstructive Pulmonary Disease severe exacerbations. AM J Respir Crit Care Med 2006; 173(10): 1114–21.

7. Bafadhel M, McKenna S, Terry S, et al. Blood eosinophils to direct corticosteroid treatment of exacerbations of Chronic Obstructive Pulmonary Disease: a randomized placebo controlled trial. Am J Respir Crit Care Med 2012; 186(1): 48–55.

8. Seemungal TA, Donaldson GC, Bhowmik A, Jeffries DJ, Wedzicha JA. Time course and recovery of exacerbations in patients with Chronic Obstructive Pulmonary Disease. AM J Respir Crit Care Med 2000; 161(5): 1608–13.

9. Spencer S, Calverley PMA, Burge S, et al. Health status deterioration in patients with chronic obstructive pulmonary disease. Am J Respir Crit Care Med 2001; 163: 122–128.

10. Connors AF Jr, Dawson NV, Thomas C, et al. Outcomes following acute exacerbation of severe chronic obstructive lung disease. The SUPPORT investigators (Study to Understand Prognosis and Preference for Outcomes and Risks of Treatments). Am J Respir Crit Care Med 1996; 154: 959–967.

11. Wells JM, Washko GR, Han MK, et al. Pulmonary arterial enlargement and acute exacerbations of COPD. N Engl J Med 2012; 367(10): 913–21.

12. Hurst JR, Donaldson GC, Quint JK, Goldring JJ, Baghai-Ravary R, Wedzicha JA. Temporal clustering of exacerbations in chronic obstructive pulmonary disease. Am J Respir Crit Care Med 2009; 179(5): 369–74.

13. Celli BR, Barnes PJ. Exacerbations of chronic obstructive pulmonary disease. Eur Respir J 2007; 29(6): 1224–38.

14. Turner MO, Patel A, Ginsburg S, Fitzgerald JM. Bronchodilator delivery in acute airflow obstruction. A meta-analysis. Arch Intern Med 1997; 157(15): 1736–44.

15. Barr RG, Rowe BH, Camargo CA,Jr. Methylxanthines for exacerbations of chronic obstructive pulmonary disease: meta analysis of randomised trials. BMJ 2003; 327(7416): 643.

16. Thompson WH, Nielson CP, Carvalho P, et al, Controlled trial of oral prednisone in outpatients with acute COPD exacerbation. Am J Respir Crit Care Med 1996; 154(2): 407–12.

17. Davies L, Angus RM, Calverley PM. Oral corticosteroids in patients admitted to hospital with exacerbations of chronic obstructive pulmonary disease: a prospective randomised controlled trial. Lancet 1999; 354(9177): 456–60.

18. Leuppi JD, Schuetz P, Bingisser R, et al. Short term vs conventional glucocorticoid therapy in acute exacerbations of chronic obstructive pulmonary disease: the reduce randomised clinical trial. J Am Med Assoc 2013; 309(21): 2223–31.

19. Bafadhel M, McKenna S, Terry S, et al. Acute exacerbations of chronic obstructive pulmonary disease: identification of biologic clusters and their biomarkers. Am J Respir Crit Care Med 2011; 184(6): 662–71.

20. Ram FS, Rodriguez-Roisin R, Granados-Navarrete A, Garcia-Amyerich J, Barnes NC. Antibiotics for exacerbations of chronic obstructive pulmonary disease. Cochrane Database Syst Rev 2006; (2): CD004403.

21. Murphy TF, Sethi S: Bacterial infection in chronic obstructive pulmonary disease. AM Rev Respir Dis 1992; 146(4): 1067–83.

22. Soler N, Torres A, Ewig S, et al. Bronchial microbiological patterns in severe exacerbations of chronic obstructive pulmonary disease (COPD) requiring mechanical ventilation. Am J Respir Crit Care Med 1998; 157(5 Pt1): 1498–505.

23. Brochard L, Mancebo J, Wysocki M, et al. Noninvasive ventilation for acute exacerbation of chronic obstructive pulmonary disease. N Engl J Med 1995; 333(13): 817–22.

24. Kramer N, Meyer TJ, Meharg J, Cece RD, Hill NS. Randomised, prospective trial of noninvasive positive pressure ventilation in acute respiratory failure. Am J Respire Crit Care Med 1995; 151(6): 1799–806.

25. Plant PK, Owen JL, Elliott MW. Early use of non-invasive ventilation for acute exacerbations of chronic obstructive pulmonary disease on general respiratory wards: a multicenter randamoised controlled trial. Lancet 2000; 355(9219): 1931–5.

26. Nava S, Ambrosino N, Clini E, at el. Noninvasive mechanical ventilation in the

weaning of patients with respiratory failure due to chronic obstructive pulmonary disease. A randomized, controlled trial. Ann Med 1998; 128:721–8.

27. Ferrer M, Sellares J, Valencia M, et al. Non-invasive ventilation after extubation in hypercapnic patients with chronic respiratory disorders: randomized controlled trial. Lancet 2009; 374: 1082–88.

28. Singanayagam A, Schembri S, Chalmers JD. Predictors of mortality in hospitalized adults with acute exacerbation of chronic obstructive pulmonary disease. Annals of the American Thoracic Society 2013; 10(2): 81–9.

29. Garcia-Aymerich J, Serra Pons I, Mannino DM, Maas AK, Miller DP, Davis KJ. Lung function impairment, COPD hospitalizations and subsequent mortality. Thorax 2011; 66(7): 585–90.

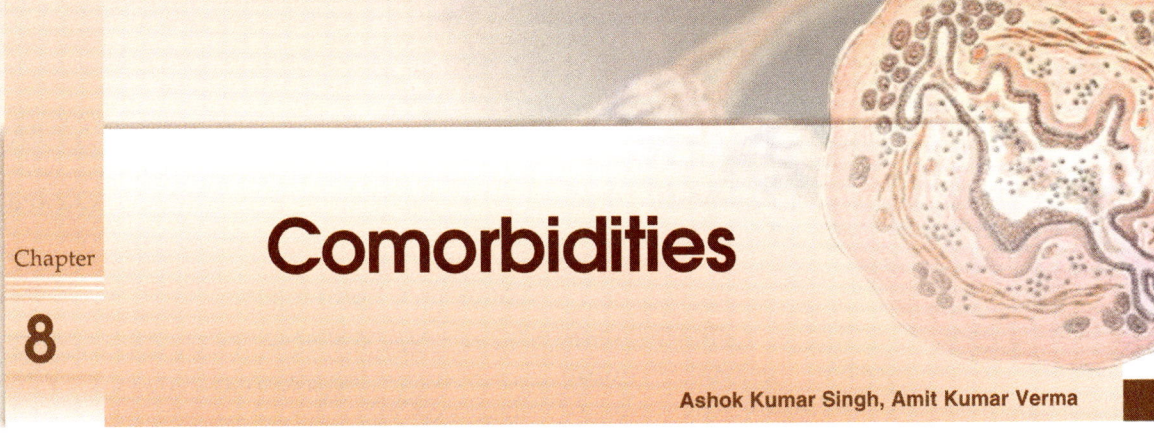

Ashok Kumar Singh, Amit Kumar Verma

Comorbidities

Chapter 8

Management implies investigations, diagnosis, treatment and timely referral to these co-morbid conditions in COPD patients.

Hypertension

Diagnosis of essential hypertension does not require any investigation for confirmation; but measurement of BP on regular basis suspected patient.

BP > 140 mmHg systolic and > 90 mmHg diastolic for persons of COPD age (>40 years), on most of the occasion without any identifiable cause of hypertension suggests the presence of essential hypertension to the COPD patients.

Investigations required when secondary hypertensions are suspected.

Identifiable causes of secondary hypertension are with their diagnostics are listed as follows.

Treatment of Hypertensions

- In the general population, pharmacologic treatment should be initiated when blood pressure is 150/90 mmHg or higher in adults 60 years and older, or 140/90 mmHg or higher in adults younger than 60 years.

- In patients with hypertension and diabetes, pharmacologic treatment should be initiated when blood pressure is 140/90 mmHg or higher, regardless of age.

- Initial antihypertensive treatment should include a thiazide diuretic, calcium channel blocker, ACE inhibitor, or ARB in the general nonblack population or a thiazide diuretic or calcium channel blocker in the general black population.

Sl. No.	Cause	Diagnostics
1.	Sleep apnoea	Polysomnography with split study
2.	Chronic kidney disease (CKD)	S. creatinine, blood urea and GFR
3.	Cushing syndrome	i. 11 am cortisol level in blood ii. 24-hour urine free cortisol iii. Dexamethasone suppression test
4.	Thyroid abnormality	T_3, T_4, TSH in blood
5.	Primary hyperaldosteronism	i. S. adolsterontos and renin ratio (Conn's syndrome) ii. S. K^+, S. Ca^{++}
6.	Pheochromocytoma	Catecholamine metabolites in blood and urine
7.	Hyperparathyoridism	S. paratharmone level
8.	Coarctation of aorta	2D Echocardiography with MRI or CT scan of thorax

- If the target blood pressure is not reached within one month after initiating therapy, the dosage of the initial medication should be increased, or a second medication should be added.

Thiazides with calcium channel blocker or ARB (angiotensine II receptor blocker) are preferred medication in COPD (joint national committee report-7).

ACE-I should be avoided in view of dry cough it causes on long-term use.

One very important point I would like to emphasize here is that cardiovascular literatures and guidelines do not discourage the use of beta-blocker to control the heart rate in hypertensive COPD patients, but literatures support preferably the use of cardioselective beta-blocker, e.g. metoprolol, nabivolol, bisoprolol to control heart rate in hypertensive COPD patients.

Ischaemic Heart Diseases

ECG, stress-echocardiography, myocardial perfusion scan are some of the noninvasive modalities for the diagnosis of IHD in COPD.

Coronary angiography is diagnostic test for ischaemic heart diseases.

Treatment

Always better to refer to cardiac specialist for control of IHD in COPD patients (Fig. 8.1).

It is worth mentioning here that cardioselective beta-blocker can be used to control stress over the heart.

Conversely there are studies which signals use of long acting beta agonist (LABA) and long acting muscrinic receptor antagonist (LAMA) inhalation for COPD with IHD has a cardiovascular risk shortly after introduction of LABA, LAMA medications, but there is no evidence of long-term cardiac risk to these patients on LABA or LAMA therapy.

It is advisable to introduce LAMA, LABA inhalation therapy to COPD patients with IHD in supervision of cardiologists for the first few days.

Congestive Heart failure

Chest X-Ray PA view, ECG, 2D echo, NT pro-BNP are the investigation required to diagnose CHF.

TREATMENT (Fig. 8.2)

1. Cardioselective beta-blocker
2. Diuretics-thiazides, spironolactone preferred in COPD
3. BP monitoring
4. Fluid restriction

Osteoporosis

CT-bone densitometry required to establish the diagnosis.

Treatment

1. Calcium carbonate/citrate tablets
2. Cholecalciferol sachets once a week for 6 to 12 weeks.
3. Bis-phosphonates: Daily dose tablets or weekly dose tablets can be started.
4. Zyludronic acid injection once a year can be given with orthopedician opinion and supervision.

Gastroesophageal Reflux Disease (GERD)

Diagnosis can be made clinically.

If required oesophageal manometry can be done or oesophageal pH monitoring can be done. These tests are used only when symptoms are not typical of acid reflux, but there are frequent exacerbations of COPD.

Treatment

Treated with PPI twice daily and GI motility stimulator like mosapride, levosulpride, itopride, etc.

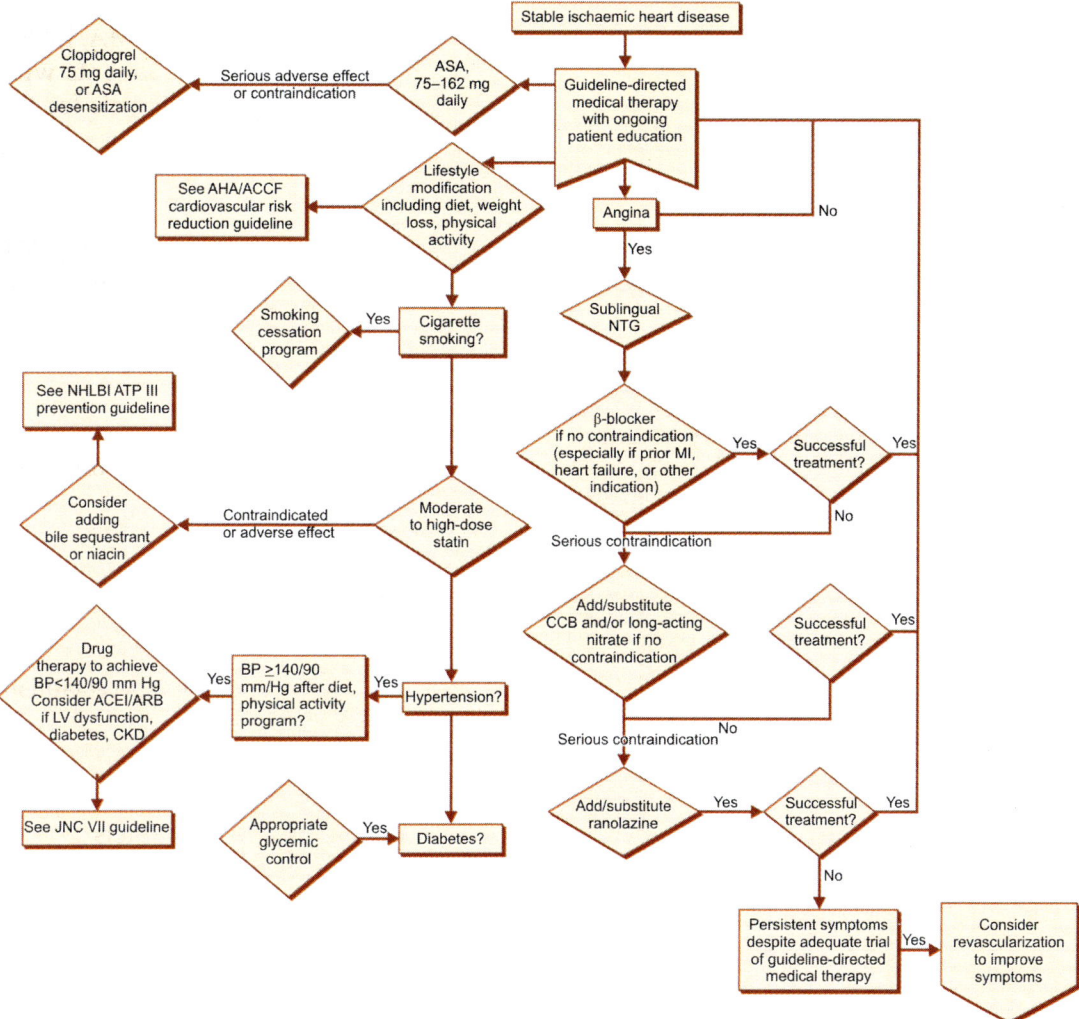

Fig. 8.1: Management of stable Ischemic heart disease

Skeletal–Muscle Dysfunction

Diagnosis of this condition does not require any technical investigation, but Low BMI <18.5, fat free muscle wasting.

These conditions specially found in emphysematous type of COPD.

So, emphysema with low BMI (<18.5) and presence of fat free muscle wasting is diagnostic of this condition.

Treatment

i. Pulmonary rehabilitation: Breathing exercise, physiotherapy.

ii. Improvement of nutrition with high protein diet.
iii. Smoking cessation.
iv. Strict control of COPD.
v. Ventilatory support: Bi-PAP, C-PAP, support.
vi. Anabolic steroid: If required duraboline, deca-duraboline can be given to control any serious muscle wasting taking place.

Depression

Diagnosed by PHQ-9 score as already explained in earlier chapter.

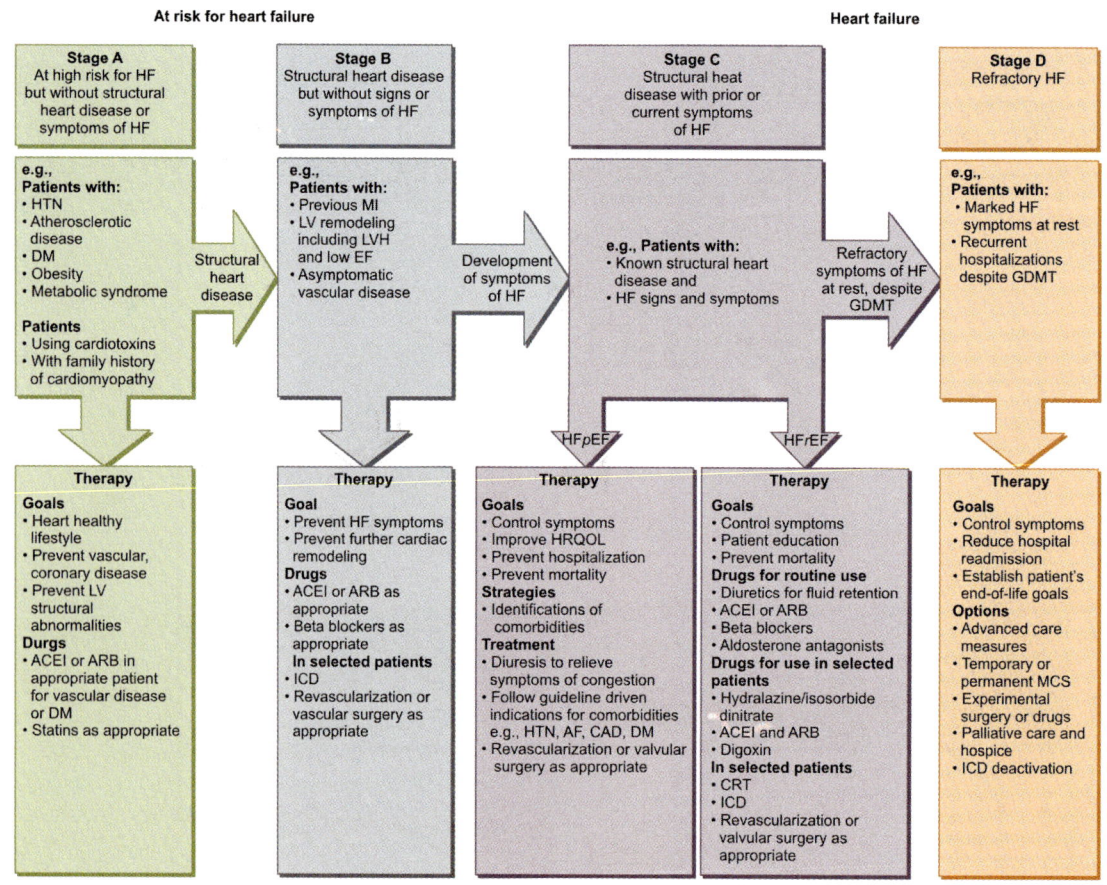

Fig 8.2: Congestive heart failure management

Treatment

1. Counselling and behavioral therapy with the help of psychologist.
2. Good COPD control.
3. Anti-depressant medication only with the guidance of psychologist.

Anaemia

Hemogram with peripheral blood simear.

Serum iron profile, kidney function test required to establish the actual cause of anaemia.

Treatment

1. Antihelminthic—stat dose

2. Iron tablets with folic acid: If microcytic hypochromic anaemia detected in PBS.
3. Vitamin β_{12} supplementation if megaloblastic anaemia detected in PBS.
4. Reference to nephrologist if renal function is grossly abnormal along with anemia and electrolyte disbalance seen. This can be a case of anaemia due to chronic kidney disease.

Diabetes Mellitus

If suspected diagnosis can be confirmed with:

- Fasting plasma sugar
- Post-parandial plasma sugar
- HbA1c percentage in blood

RSSDI (Research Society for Study of Diabetes in India) recommended presence of any of the following for the diagnosis of diabetes mellitus—type II.

1. Fasting plasma sugar (FPG), more than or equal to 126 mg/dl

   OR

2. Oral glucose tolerance test (OGTT) with 75 gm of anhydrous glucose with

   • FPG more than or equal to 126 gm/dl

   • 2-hour plasma glucose more than or equal to 200 gm/dl

   OR

3. HbA1c more than or equal to 6.5%.

   OR

4. Random plasma sugar more than or equal to 200 gm/dl

5. Asymptomatics with single abnormal report should be repeated unless all reports unequivocally abnormal.

Treatment

To start with metformine sustained release tablets in 500 mg twice daily dose can be started with or without glimiperide 1 mg or 2 mg tablets depending upon blood sugar level. Dose of metformine and glimiperide can be titrated with every week fasting blood sugar level and every 12 week HbA1c percentage.

Target to achieve is: Fasting plasma sugar less than 100 mg/dl

Post-parandial plasma sugar less than 140 mg/dl.

HbA1c less than 5.7%.

Minor co-morbidities: Two minor co-morbid conditions that worth discussion here are pneumothorax and oral candidiasis.

OSAS is very big topic itself, hence it should be refered to specialist for diagnosis and treatment. All COPD patients with history of snoring, daytime sleepiness, inability to concentrate on work, and high BMI (>25) should be suspected of OSAS and metabolic syndrome and should be managed by specialist.

Pneumothorax

Most of the time diagnosis is made by obvious clinical history and examination findings with help of urgent expiratory CXR PA view. If confusion is there with big bulla or bullous area or Macleod syndrome (Swyer James syndrome) CXR Lateral view with affected side up can be helpful, or CT-chest can be done to rule out these confusing conditions.

Treatment

Pneumothorax in COPD patients is mostly primary spontaneous.

1. **Wait and watch with moist oxygen inhalation**: If the patient is not symptomatic and pneumothorax is small, i.e. less than 2 cm rim of air in CXR.

2. **Pleurocentesis**: For symptomatic small pneumothorax, i.e. less than 2 cm rim of air in CXR with no free air leak (bronchopleural fistula).

3. **Intercostal drainage tube**: For

   a. Symptomatic bigger pneumothorax, i.e. more than 2 cm rim of air

   b. Any pneumothorax (any size) with FAL

   c. Tension pneumothorax

4. **Plaeurodesis:** If there is history suggestive of recurrent pneumothorax.

Oral Candidiasis

The following steps have to be taken:

i. Stop inhaled or oral Corticosteroid for 1 week.

ii. Regular mouthwash with warm water.

iii. Antifungal mouth paint.

iv. Encourage patients to do mouthwash with lukewarm water everytime after use of inhaled medication.

BIBLIOGRAPHY

1. AntonelliIncalzi R, Fuso L, De Rosa M at al. Co-morbidity contributes to predict mortality of patients with chronic obstructive pulmonary disease. Eur. Respire. J. 10(12), 2794–2800 (1997).
2. Barr RG, Celli BR, Mannino DM et al. Comorbidities, patient knowledge, and disease management in national sample of patients with COPD. Am. J. Med. 122 (4), 348–55 (2009).
3. BTS Guidelines 2003 for management of primary spontaneous pneumothorax.
4. Calverley PM, Anderson JA, Celli B, at al. Salmeterol and fluticasone proportionate and survival in chronic obstructive pulmonary disease. New Engl. J. Med. 2007; 365(8):775–89.
5. Curkendall SM, DeLuise C, Jones JK et al. Cardiovascular disease in patients with chronic obstructive pulmonary disease, Saskatchewan Canada cardiovascular disease in COPD patients. Ann. Epidemiol. 16(1), 63–70 (2006).
6. Feary JR, Rodrigues LC, Smith CJ, Hubbard RB, Gibson JE. Prevalence of major comorbidities in subjects with COPD and incidence of myo-cardial infarction and stroke, a comprehensive analysis using data from primary care. Thorax 65(11), 956–62 (2010).
7. Feldman G, Siler T, Prasad N, at al. Efficacy and safety of indacaterol 150 microg once-daily in COPD: a double-blind, randomized, 12-week study. BMC Pulm. Med. 2010; 10:11. Doi: 10.1186/1471-2466-10-11.
8. Gershon A, Croxford R, Calzavara A, et al. Cardiovascular safety of inhaled long-acting bronchodilators in individuals with chronic obstructive pulmonary disease. JAMA Intern Med. 2013; 173(13): 1175–85.
9. Gottlieb SS, McCarter RJ, Vogel RA, Effect of beta-blocker on mortality among high-risk and low-risk patients after myocardial infarction. New. Engl. J. Med. 339(8), 489-97(1998).
10. Joint National Committee report 2007 for management of hypertension.
11. Kessler R, Faller M, Weitzenblum E, et al. Resp. crit. care. Med. 164(2), 219–24 (2001). "Natural history" of pulm. Hypertension 131 patients with COPD.
12. Mannino DM, Thorn D, Swensen A, Holguin F. Prevalence and outcomes of diabetes, hypertension and cardiovascular disease in COPD. Eur. Respir. J. 32(4), 962–9 (2008).
13. McGarvey LP, John M, Anderson JA, Zvarich M, Wise RA. Ascertainment of cause specific mortality in COPD, operations of the TORCH Clinical Endpoint Committee. Thorax 62 (5), 411–5 (2007).
14. Mills NL, Miller JJ, Anand, et al, Thorax 63 (4), 306–11 (2008). Increased arterial stiffness in COPD for increased cardiovascular risk.
15. RSSDI Guidelines for diagnosis and management of diabetes mellitus 2.
16. Rutten FH, Zuithoff NPA, Hake E, Hoes AW. Beta-blocker may reduce mortality and risk of exacerbation in patients with COPD. Arch. Intern. Med.
17. Rutten FH, β-blocker and their mortality benefit, underprescribed in heart failure and COPD. Future cardiol. 7(1), 43–53 (2011).
18. Salpeter S & E, Ormiston T, Cardiovascular beta-blockers for chronic obstructive pulmonary disease. Cochrane Database Syst Rev. 2005; (4): CD003566.
19. Salpeter S, Ormiston T, Salpeter E, Cardioselective Beta-blockers for chronic obstructive pulmonary disease. Cochrane Database Syst. Rev. (4), CD003566(2005).
20. Sin DD, Man SFP. Why are patients with chronic obstructive pulmonary disease at increased risk of cardiovascular diseases? The potential role of systemic inflammation in chronic obstructive pulmonary disease. Circulation 107(11), 1514–9 (2003).
21. Soriano JB, Visick GT, Mulellerova H, Payvandi N, Hansell AL. Patterns of comorbidities in newly diagnosed COPD and asthma in primary care. Chest 128 (4), 2099-2107 (2005).

Discharge

Ajay Kumar Verma, Anubhuti Singh, Arpita Singh

INTRODUCTION

Chronic obstructive pulmonary Disease (COPD) affects almost 30 crore people throughout the world and is one of the leading causes of morbidity and mortality worldwide.[1] This disease is chronic and progressive in nature, and its course is punctuated by recurrent exacerbations. Exacerbations are any increase in symptoms from the normal day to day variation which requires a change in medication. With each exacerbation, there is significant fall in FEV_1, leading to deterioration of symptoms, poorer prognosis and reduction in life expectancy. Depending on the patient's baseline functional status and severity of exacerbation, patient may be managed at home with stepping up of treatment or may require hospitalization and intensive care unit (ICU) admission. COPD exacerbation is one of the commonest causes of hospitalization in these patients. Frequent exacerbation leading to hospitalization is associated with increased risk of death.[2] Management of a patient with COPD entails all aspects, right from smoking cessation to management of hospitalized patient. Decision regarding discharge of these patients is an important aspect of COPD management. Early discharge is imperative as longer duration of hospitalization is associated with increased chances of nosocomial pneumonias, ventilator dependency and muscle deconditioning. This chapter covers these questions: When and how to discharge a patient with COPD, both from a general ward as well as from ICU, along with advice at discharge, home management and when to have a follow-up visit.

CRITERIA FOR DISCHARGE

An exacerbation is more often than not secondary to an infection of the respiratory tract (viral and bacterial pathogens commonly). It leads to increased inflammatory response in the airways and can decompensate a stable COPD patient. There is deterioration in symptoms, reduction in exercise capacity and quality of life and increased morbidity and mortality. The aim of hospitalization in such patients is to bring them back to their baseline functional status. This is achieved through controlled oxygenation, inhaled bronchodilators (such as long acting muscarinic antagonists (LAMA), long acting beta-agonists (LABA), inhaled corticosteroids (ICS) and short acting beta-agonists (SABA)), antibiotics, systemic corticosteroids, circulatory and ventilatory support. Management of COPD exacerbation has been discussed elsewhere in this book.

Prior to discharge, a patient should be assessed for haemodynamic stability (stable blood pressure and heart rate without vasopressor support) and the ability to maintain adequate saturation through arterial blood gas (ABG) analysis. Inability to do so or marked fluctuations in parameters such as heart rate, blood pressure, oxygen saturation and partial pressures of oxygen or carbon dioxide in blood indicates that hospitalization has to be continued. A normal mental status is also mandatory for discharge. With aggressive treatment, the patient should be able to resume his/her activities of daily living such as walking across the room, eating, sitting up and talking and having an uninterrupted sleep. All the comorbidities need to be addressed and the patient should not have any uncorrected cardiac, haematologic or endocrine status. Hospitalization is an important opportunity to assess the inhalational technique and train the patient accordingly. Lastly, before discharging a patient, it should be ensured that there are adequate facilities for management at home and there are concerned care-takers who understand medication use and can bring the patient back if the need arise. Many guidelines have established the criteria for discharge of COPD patients. We are giving an adapted version of the criteria provided by global initiative for chronic obstructive pulmonary disease (GOLD) (Table 9.1).

Table 9.1: Discharge criteria (adapted from GOLD 2016)[1]

1. Medication use:	Able to use inhaled LABA or LAMA. Use of SABA <6 times a day. Understand correct use of inhalational medication.
2. Clinical status:	Able to walk across room. Able to eat and sleep normally. Haemodynamically stable for 1 day prior to discharge.
3. ABG:	Stable for 1 day prior to discharge
4. Social aspects:	Adequate facilities for management at home (such as oxygen and nursing staff/ family caregiver).

DEVICE ADVICE AT DISCHARGE

The various modes of inhalational drug therapy include pressurized metered dose inhaler (pMDI), dry powder inhaler (DPI), and nebulisation. The potential benefits and disadvantages of these have already been discussed. Here we will discuss their utility in a hospitalized patient and which device to prefer after the patient has been discharged.

All major authorities in the field of respiratory medicine suggest that the use of pMDI with spacer is equivalent to nebulization in relation to efficacy for patients with COPD exacerbations. But, in clinical practice, nebulization is the commonly practiced mode of inhalational therapy in hospitalized patients. It can be used in patients who have poor coordination or suboptimal effort due to poor general condition. It can be administered by health care personnel in a correct way and at correct timings. But at discharge, patient should be prescribed either a pMDI with spacer or a dry powder inhaler (DPI). The decision regarding which device to use is based on patient preferences; compatibility with device and affordability since both has been found to be equally effective. The use of spacer has to be emphasized upon as its use increases drug deposition in the lungs and minimizes oral deposition. The training for correct inhalation technique has to be given to the patient during admission as well as on discharge and during each follow-up visit. Nebulizer therapy use should not be advised on discharge for home therapy as it is expensive and cumbersome, thus giving rise to poor compliance. It should be reserved for management of acute events at home or for patients who are unable to put adequate effort to inhale the medications. The dosage and technique of inhaling should be explained properly to both the patient and an attendant (in case of elderly patients who require assistance for the same). Advice to regularly clean the spacer device with water and detergent should also be provided. The patient should know the maximum doses of reliever medicine which can be taken safely and should know when he/she needs to contact a doctor.

PULMONARY REHABILITATION AT DISCHARGE

The role of pulmonary rehabilitation cannot be over-stated. Multiple studies over the past few decades have established its role in patients with COPD. Exercise capacity and physical activity levels are impaired during and after an exacerbation, particularly of the lower limbs. If pulmonary rehabilitation is commenced within one month of discharge, it is termed 'early' and termed 'late' if commenced thereafter. Participation in pulmonary rehabilitation delivered within one month of hospital discharge reduces short-term risk of future hospital admissions.[3] Rehabilitation has shown multiple benefits, such as, improvement in symptoms, increase in exercise capacity, improved muscle strength (quadriceps), reduction in anxiety and depression and social autonomy.

Rehabilitation is a multi-disciplinary approach of care which encompasses patient education, smoking cessation, nutritional advice and exercise training. Both resistive (strength) and endurance training exercises are undertaken in twice weekly settings under supervision, and continued for 6 to 12 weeks for optimum benefits. Also, breathing exercises such as pursed lip breathing and diaphragmatic breathing and chest physiotherapy in the form of chest percussion should be taught to the patient and the care givers. All these exercises reduce the work of breathing and relieve respiratory muscle fatigue, leading to reduction in dyspnoea and improving quality of life.

In addition to these exercises, all patients with COPD should be advised to lead an active life, with a 30-minute walking schedule (at own place) for at least 5 days a week. At the time of discharge, patients should be advised to continue with their daily routine activities. This builds up the confidence of the patient, as well as prevents peripheral muscle wasting and weakness. It is important for the patients to realize that they can lead a normal life with the medications advised.

NUTRITIONAL ADVICE AT DISCHARGE

COPD exacerbation is a state of increased metabolic demand by the body, because of ongoing inflammation, increased respiratory muscle work and increased cardiac work.

The energy requirements are elevated and have to be met by adequate calorie intake. Thus, at discharge, these patients need to be advised about a healthy diet chart, the importance of timely and adequate meals and a detailed list of do's and don'ts regarding eating habits.

The energy demands of respiratory muscles increase almost 10 times in patients with COPD. Being a chronic inflammatory disorder, there is increased levels of certain inflammatory mediators in patients with

COPD. These mediators are responsible for a number of co-morbidities associated with the disease, including anaemia, osteoporosis, peripheral muscle wasting and cachexia. These issues have to be assessed during hospitalization and managed accordingly at discharge. Also, lower body mass index (BMI) is associated with poorer prognosis. Malnutrition causes decline in pulmonary function, increases susceptibility to infections and decreases exercise capacity. Therefore, it is important to emphasize adequate calorie and protein intake.

Patients with long standing disease usually develop cor pulmonale, which is right-sided heart enlargement secondary to chronic hypoxia. These patients can decompensate into frank heart failure after insults such as lower respiratory tract infection, fluid overload or respiratory failure. A number of COPD exacerbations are a result of right-sided heart failure. In this subgroup of patients, fluid and salt restriction should be advised at discharge to prevent de-compensation.

COPD is frequently associated with osteoporosis as a systemic manifestation of chronic inflammation. If identified, these patients should be prescribed calcium and vitamin D supplements. It is a popular misconception in our country that milk and milk products (which are important sources of calcium) aggravate cough and sputum production, so are usually avoided by COPD patients. This further leads to nutritional deficiency.

Some other general measures which the patients should be advised at discharge include small frequent meals to prevent bloating and distension (which cause upward movement of an already dysfunctional diaphragm) and avoiding caffeine, carbonated drinks and alcohol. They should be encouraged to have an early dinner and have regular exercise.

FOLLOW-UP VISIT

There is no standard guideline for follow-up visits in patients with stable COPD, but according to GOLD, after discharge of a patient with COPD exacerbation, the usual follow-up visit is after 4–6 weeks. But in Indian scenario where no support system is available between treating physician and patients, it is a good practice to call patient after one week of discharge and progressively increase the time interval between visits to 4–6 weeks as recommended. A number of variables have to be assessed at subsequent visits after discharge. These have been enumerated as follows:

1. **Clinical assessment:** All the patients have to be evaluated for improvement or deterioration of symptoms, including breathlessness, cough and expectoration. Dyspnoea can be assessed using modified Medical Research Council (mMRC) scale. Sputum purulence or increase in amount of sputum denotes an infective episode. Any evidence of right-sided heart failure, such as pedal oedema, raised jugular venous pressure (JVP) or tender hepatomegaly should be looked for. Signs of respiratory distress including use of accessory muscles of respiration should be evaluated. Patient's BMI should be measured. Resting oxygen saturation by pulse oximetry (SpO_2) will provide information about need for supplemental oxygenation. ABG analysis should be performed in addition to SpO_2 and if there is persistent hypoxemia (in comparison to ABG and SpO_2 during hospitalization), domiciliary oxygen therapy is indicated.[1]

2. **Assessment of lung function:** If feasible, spirometry should be repeated during follow-up visits to evaluate functional status of the lungs. 6-minute walk test also provides important information regarding overall functional status of the patient and response to treatment. An

increase in walk distance in six minutes during follow-up visit indicates favourable response to treatment.

3. **Assessment of medication use:** Follow-up visits provide an important opportunity for the clinician to assess the patient's inhalational technique. Incorrect inhaler technique is a common cause of frequent exacerbations in patients with COPD. It should be checked at each follow-up visit, along with other aspects such as correct dose, use of spacer device and rinsing of mouth following inhaler use. The patient should be inquired about the common adverse effects of inhaler use such as dry mouth, oral thrush and hoarseness of voice.

4. **Assessment of comorbidities:** The co-morbidities associated with COPD include anaemia, systemic hypertension, congestive heart failure, diabetes mellitus, osteoporosis, sarcopenia, depression and lung cancer among others. One of the most common causes of death in COPD patients is lung cancer. So, evaluation should be done for these factors during follow-up. Any patient with haemoptysis or new nodule on chest radiograph should be evaluated for lung cancer. Long-term use of ICS may pre-dispose to pulmonary tuberculosis, so a patient having persistent purulent cough for >2 weeks duration should undergo a sputum smear examination for detection of acid fast bacilli (AFB). Evaluation of cardiac status and blood pressure monitoring should be done regularly. Hospitalization leads to cognitive disturbances too, including anxiety and depression and continues after discharge.[4] This aspect should also be addressed and a psychiatry consult taken, if required

5. **Smoking cessation counselling:** Follow-up visits provide important opportunity to assess the patient's smoking status. If the patient has not quit smoking since discharge, counselling for cessation should be done and if willing, pharmacotherapy should be considered. If the patient has already quit, then he/she should be encouraged to maintain cessation through counselling.

DISCHARGE FROM ICU

Around 5–10% patients with acute respiratory failure secondary to COPD require ICU/HDU admission.[5] The long term mortality of COPD patients after ICU care is high. Breen et al studied the mortality in invasively ventilated patients and showed a one year and three-year mortality rates of 48.6% and 64.5% respectively.[6] Although no standard guidelines exist for discharge criteria for patients from ICU/HDU, the basic parameters to be assessed remain the same. The patient should be haemodynamically stable, should be able to maintain saturation at room air and should understand medication use. Longer duration of hospitalization is associated with a number of complications, such as nosocomial pneumonia including hospital acquired pneumonia (HAP) and ventilator associated pneumonia (VAP), deep vein thrombosis and pulmonary thromboembolism. Also, patients who are on mechanical ventilation for prolonged duration develop diaphragmatic dysfunction and critical care myopathy, which makes weaning and discharge difficult. So, it is imperative to plan discharge as soon as the patient comes off mechanical ventilation.

If the patient meets the criteria for long-term oxygen therapy as per GOLD,[1] then discharge should be done only after arrangement for oxygen, either in the form of concentrator or oxygen cylinders, has been made by the caretakers. For patients who require prolonged ventilator support (>2 weeks), tracheostomy is performed. In such patients, wound care should be taught to the patient and caregivers. If there is no evidence of infection or pneumonia, antibiotics are prescribed for 5–7 days, but if patient develops HAP/VAP, antibiotics can be given for longer duration. The importance of proper inhalational technique cannot be stressed upon. Patients, who have very poor effort and are not able to take inhalational medications, can be advised home nebulisation until general condition improves. Proper nebulisation technique needs to be trained, with advice regarding which medications can be mixed together during nebulisation and which drugs cannot. Rehabilitation is particularly important for patients who have been discharged from ICU/HDU to overcome diaphragmatic and other respiratory muscle dysfunction which occur during mechanical ventilation. Pursed lip breathing and diaphragmatic breathing techniques help in re-conditioning of these muscles. Patients should be encouraged to remain ambulatory and resume his or her activities of daily living after discharge. This advice is also applicable to even those patients who are on domiciliary oxygen therapy.

SAMPLE CASE

A 55-year-old smoker male presented to the emergency department with the complaints of:

- Progressive breathlessness × 6 years (symptoms increased for past 5 days). Insidious in onset, progressive, no orthopnea/paroxysmal nocturnal dyspnoea, aggravated during winters.
- Cough occasionally with expectoration × 6 years, which is occasionally yellow colour and aggravated during winters.

On examination: Conscious, oriented, with:

- Tachypneic
- Tachycardic

- On auscultation—bilateral rhonchi present.
- No pedal oedema

At admission ABG:

- pCO_2: 62;
- pO_2: 54;
- pH: 7.305;
- SO_2: 82%;
- HCO_3: 35

Vitals at admission: BP—124/74 mmHg; PR—108/min; RR—22/min; SpO_2—82%.

He was managed with:

- Intravenous antibiotics
- Bronchodilators and inhalational steroids through nebulisation.
- Oxygen therapy (controlled to maintain SpO_2 between 88% and 92%)
- Intravenous steroids

Patient improved after 2 to 3 days and discharge was planned after 5 days when:

- Vitals became stable
- SpO_2>90%
- ABG—normal
- The patient was shifted to inhalers and was trained to use them.
- Intravenous steroids were changed to oral steroids.

ADVICE AT DISCHARGE

The following advice was given:

- Correct inhaler technique taught to both patient and attendant.
- The use, dosage and timings of medications properly explained to the patient.
- The oral steroids and oral antibiotics must be stopped after prescribed timing (i.e., after 5 or 7 days).
- Smoking cessation was advised with proper counselling and if required must be therapeutically intervened.

- Rehabilitation exercises were explained to the patient and the patient was encouraged to get registered in the rehabilitation program in the next follow-up visit.
- Nutritional advice including high protein diet, low salt diet and low fluid intake.
- Monthly or two monthly follow-up advised initially and the frequency can be reduced thereafter.
- Red flag signs were explained, i.e. when to come for emergency consultation (severe/sudden onset breathlessness, pedal oedema, chest pain, increased sputum purulence).
- In patients who are discharged on long term oxygen therapy (LTOT), advised to use inhaled oxygen for >15 hours/day, at low flow (2–3 litres/ minute). They must be advised not to smoke while on inhaled oxygen.

SUMMARY

The management of a patient with COPD ranges from preventive measures such as smoking cessation up to end-of-life and palliative care of the terminally ill patient. The decision regarding discharge of a hospitalized COPD patient is an important, although often overlooked aspect of the management strategy. This chapter has covered the assessment of hospitalized COPD patients for discharge planning, including discharge criteria, advise at discharge, with respect to medication use, oxygen and ventilator support, smoking cessation, nutrition and pulmonary rehabilitation and timings and indications for follow-up visits.

KEY POINTS

1. It is important to recognize the importance of early discharge in a hospitalized COPD patient.
2. To be fit for discharge, a patient should be haemodynamically stable, should have normal blood gases, should know correct use of medications and should have concerned caretakers at home.
3. At the time of discharge, the patient should be taught correct inhalational medication use.
4. Also, emphasis on nutrition and pulmonary rehabilitation needs to be given.
5. All efforts should be made to encourage the patient to quit smoking and maintain cessation if already quit.
6. Home management strategies and red flag signs for immediate medical consultation have to be explained.
7. Finally, the patient should know when to come for follow-up visits.

REFERENCES

1. Global strategy for the diagnosis, management, and prevention of chronic obstructive pulmonary disease-updated 2016.
2. Soler-Cataluria JJ, Martinez Garcia MA, Salcedo E, Navarro M, Ochando R. Severe acute exacerbations and mortality in patients with COPD. Thorax 2005; 60: 925–31.
3. Bolton CE, Bevan-Smith EF, Blakey JD, et al. British Thoracic Guideline on pulmonary rehabilitation in adults. Thorax 2013; 68: ii1–ii30.
4. Escarrabil J. Discharge planning and home care for end stage COPD patients. Eur Respir J 2009; 34: 507–12.
5. Davidson AC. The pulmonary physiology in intensive care: critical care management of respiratory failure resulting from COPD. Thorax 2002; 57: 1079–84.
6. Breen D, Churches T, Hawker F, Torzillo PJ. Acute respiratory failure secondary to chronic obstructive pulmonary disease treated in the intensive care unit: a long term follow up study. Thorax 2002; 57: 29–33.

Guidelines and their Deficiencies

Adesh Kumar, Aditya Kumar Gautam, Ashish Kumar Gupta, Prashant Yadav, Harender Singh

Chronic Obstructive Pulmonary Disease (COPD) is a common, preventable and treatable disease that is characterized by persistent respiratory symptoms and airflow limitation that is usually caused by significant exposure to noxious particles or gases.

Management of COPD includes pharmacological and non-pharmacological aspects. Global community has created many guidelines for the management of COPD and GOLD guidelines are most referred in India, although Indian guidelines are also available.

In the management of COPD the treating physician has to deal also with other diseases which are oftenly present in these patients, called comorbidities. These diseases have significant impact on the prognosis. Some of these arise independently of COPD, whereas others may be causally related. Either with shared risk factors or by one disease actually increasing the risk of another. Whether or not COPD and comorbid diseases are related, management of the COPD patient must include identification and treatment of its comorbidities. The recommendations in GOLD guideline of COPD are insufficient for the management of comorbidities and cannot substitute for the use of guidelines for the management of each comorbidity. There is no recommendation for comorbidity management in Indian guideline.

This chapter also highlights other available guidelines. The later part of this chapter compares and details the deficiencies, which in the opinion of authors are present. However, the aim is not to undermine the great efforts put while making these guidelines but stress out the Indian patients and health care system is different from the other parts of the world. The reasons are:

1. Health care system is not well organised.
2. Patients feel that his doctor must be able to treat all conditions.
3. Patients are often not willing to continue long term medications especially for respiratory diseases.
4. Most patients are not covered with any type of insurance and they are not able to afford multidisciplinary care.
5. Government institutions are not uniformly available.
6. PFT is often said to be best test for diagnosis and monitoring of COPD patients, but its results are also dependent on the skill of operator and ability of patient to understand procedure. Hence in spite of availability, PFT results may not be acceptable.

Many COPD patients already on treatment and return with persistent symptoms after initial therapy or less commonly with resolution of some symptoms that subsequently require less therapy. Therefore, recommendation of escalation and de-escalation strategy.

GOLD GUIDELINE

The lowest estimates of prevalence are those based on self-reporting of a doctor diagnosis of COPD or equivalent condition. For example, most national data show that less than 6% of the adult population has been told that they have COPD.[1] This likely reflects the widespread under-recognition and underdiagnosis of COPD.[2]

The burden of obstructive lung diseases (BOLD) program has carried out surveys in several parts of the world and has documented more severe disease than previously found with a prevalence of COPD grade 2 or higher of 10.1% (SE 4.8) overall, 11.8% (SE 7.8) for men and 8.5% (SE 5.8) for women[3] and a substantial prevalence (3–11%) of COPD among never smokers.[3]

Based on BOLD and other large-scale epidemiological studies, it is estimated that the number of COPD cases was 384 million in 2010, with a global prevalence of 11.7% (8.4–15%).[4] Globally, there are around three million deaths annually.[5]

The Global Burden of Disease Study projected that COPD, which ranked sixth as a cause of death in 1990, will become the third leading cause of death worldwide by 2020; a newer projection estimated COPD will be the fourth leading cause of death in 2030.

In the European Union, the total direct costs of respiratory disease are estimated to be about 6% of the total health care budget, with COPD accounting for 56% (3860 crore Euros) of this cost of respiratory disease.[6] In the United States the estimated direct costs

of COPD are 3200 crore dollar and the indirect costs $2040 crores.[7] In 2005, COPD was the eighth leading cause of DALYs lost in the world but by 2013 COPD was ranked as the fifth leading cause of DALY lost.[8]

Diagnosis and Initial Assessment

COPD should be considered in any patient who has dyspnoea, chronic cough or sputum production and/or a history of exposure to risk factors for disease. Spirometry requires to make the diagnosis in the clinical context.[9] The presence of a post-bronchodilator $FEV_1/FVC < 0.70$ confirms the presence of persistent airflow limitation and thus of COPD in patients with appropriate symptoms and significant exposures to noxious stimuli.

Symptoms

Dyspnoea: Dyspnoea, a cardinal symptom of COPD, is a major cause of the disability and anxiety that is associated with the disease.[10] Typical COPD patients describe their dyspnoea as a sense of increased effort to breathe, chest heaviness, air hunger or gasping.

Cough: Chronic cough is often the first symptom of COPD and is frequently discounted by the patient as an expected consequence of smoking and/or environmental exposures. Initially, the cough may be intermittent, but subsequently may be present every day, often throughout the day. Chronic cough in COPD may be productive or unproductive.[11] In some cases, significant airflow limitation may develop without the presence of cough.

Sputum production: COPD patients commonly raise small quantities of tenacious sputum with coughing. Sputum production can be intermittent with periods of flare-up interspersed with periods of remission.[12] The presence of purulent sputum reflects an increase in inflammatory mediators.

Wheezing and chest tightness: Wheezing and chest tightness are symptoms that may vary between days, and over the course of a single day. Audible wheeze may arise at laryngeal level and need not be accompanied by abnormalities heard on auscultation. Alternatively, widespread inspiratory or expiratory wheezes can be present on auscultation. Chest tightness often follows exertion is poorly localised and muscular in character and may arise from isometric contraction of the intercostal muscles.

Additional features in severe disease: Fatigue, weight loss and anorexia are common problems in patients with severe and very severe COPD.

Spirometry

Spirometry is the most reproducible and objective measurement of airflow limitation. The spirometric criterion for airflow limitation remains a post-bronchodilator fixed ratio of $FEV_1/FVC<0.70$. It should be noted that the use of the fixed FEV_1/FVC ratio to define airflow limitation may result in more frequent diagnosis of COPD in the elderly and less frequent diagnosis in adults <45 years, especially in mild disease, comparing to using a cut-off based on the lower limit of normal (LLN) values for FEV_1/FVC.[13] The LLN values are based on the normal distribution and classify the bottom 5% of the healthy population as abnormal.

Assessment

The goals of COPD assessment are to determine the level of airflow limitation, its impact on the patient's health status and the risk of future events (such as exacerbations, hospital admissions or death), in order to eventually guide therapy.

Classification of Severity of Airflow Limitation

Classification of severity of airflow limitation in COPD (based on post-bronchodilator FEV_1) in patients with FEV_1/FVC < 0.70 (Table 10.1).

Table 10.1: Classification of severity of airflow limitation		
GOLD 1	Mild	$FEV_1 \geq 80\%$ predicted
GOLD 2	Moderate	$50\% > FEV_1 <$ 80% predicted
GOLD 3	Severe	$30\% > FEV_1 <$ 50% predicted
GOLD 4	Very severe	< 30% predicted

It should be noted that there is only a weak correlation between FEV_1, symptoms and impairment of a patient's health status.[14] For this reason, formal symptomatic assessment is required.

Assessment of Symptoms

In the past, COPD was viewed as a disease largely characterised by breathlessness. A simple measure of breathlessness such as Modified British Medical Research Council (mMRC) Questionnaire was considered adequate for assessment of symptoms as mMRC relates well to other measures of health status and predict future mortality risk.

However, it is now recognised that COPD impacts patients beyond just dyspnoea.[15] For this reason, a comprehensive assessment of symptoms is recommended rather than just a measure of breathlessness. The most comprehensive disease specific health status questionnaires such as the Chronic Respiratory Questionnaire (CRQ) and St. Georges Respiratory Questionnaire (SGRQ) are too complex to use in routine practice, but shorter comprehensive measures, e.g. COPD Assessment Test (CAT) (Table 10.2) and the COPD Control Questionnaire (The CCQ) have been developed and are suitable.

Table 10.2: Revised combined COPD assessment

Patient category	Exacerbations per year	CAT	mMRC
A	≤1	<10	0–1
B	≤1	≥10	≥2
C	≥2	<10	0–1
D	≥2	≥10	≥2

Effective management should be based on an individualized assessment of disease in order to reduce both current symptoms and future risks (Fig. 10.1).

Treatment of Stable COPD

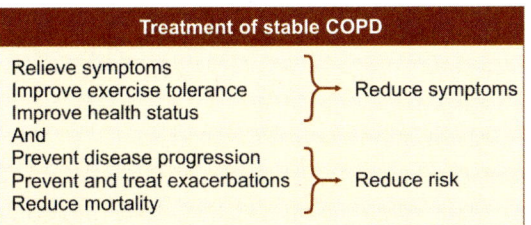

Fig. 10.1: Goals for treatment of stable COPD

Identify and Reduce Exposure To Risk Factors

1. **Tobacco smoke:** Smoking cessation is the key intervention for all COPD patients who continue to smoke. Healthcare providers are important to the delivery of smoking cessation messages and interventions and should encourage all patients who smoke to quit, even when patients visit a healthcare provider for reasons unrelated to COPD or breathing problems.

2. **Occupational:** Although studies as yet have not been done to demonstrate whether interventions to reduce occupational exposures also reduce the burden of COPD, it seems common sense to advise patients to avoid continued exposures.

3. **Indoor and outdoor air pollution:** Reduction of exposure to smoke from biomass fuel, particularly among women and children, is a crucial goal to reduce the prevalence of COPD worldwide. Efficient ventilation, non-polluting cooking stove and similar interventions are feasible and should be recommended.

This is in keeping with the fact that most of the clinical trial evidence about treatment efficacy in COPD is oriented around baseline FEV_1. However, FEV_1 alone is a poor descriptor of disease status. Hence the treatment strategy for stable COPD should also consider an individual patient's symptoms and future risk of exacerbations.

Non-pharmacologic Treatment (Table 10.3)

1. **Smoking cessation:** Smoking cessation should be considered the most important intervention for all COPD patients who smoke regardless of the level of disease severity.

2. **Physical activity:** Physical activity is recommended for all patients with COPD. There is very little COPD-specific evidence to support recommendations for physical activity other than studies of pulmonary rehabilitation.

3. **Rehabilitation:** All COPD patients appear to benefit from rehabilitation and maintenance of physical activity, improving their exercise tolerance and experiencing decreased dyspnoea and fatigue.

4. **Vaccination:** Influenza vaccination is recommended for all patients with COPD. Pneumococcal vaccination, PCV_{13} and $PPSV_{23}$ are recommended for all patients >65 years of age. The $PPSV_{23}$ is also recom-

Table 10.3: Non-pharmacologic management of COPD			
Patient Group	*Essential*	*Recommended*	*Depending on local guidelines*
A	Smoking cessation (can include pharmacologic treatment)	Physical activity	Flu vaccination Pneumococcal vaccination
B–D	Smoking cessation (can include pharmacologic treatment) Pulmonary rehabilitation	Physical activity	Flu vaccination Pneumococcal vaccination

mended for younger COPD patients with significant comorbid conditions including chronic heart or lung disease.[16]

Pharmacological Treatment

Pharmacologic therapy in COPD is used to reduce symptoms, reduce the frequency and severity of exacerbations, and improve health status and exercise tolerance.

Group A

- All Group A patients should be offered bronchodilator treatment based on its effect on breathlessness. This can be either a short or a long acting bronchodilator.

- This should be continued if symptomatic benefit is documented.

Group B

- Initial therapy should consist of a long-acting bronchodilator. Long-acting inhaled bronchodilators are superior to short-acting bronchodilators taken as needed.

- There is no evidence to recommend one class of long-acting bronchodilators over another for initial relief of symptoms in this group of patients. In the individual patient the choice should depend on the patient's perception of symptom relief.

- For patients with persistent breathlessness on monotherapy[17] the use of two bronchodilators is recommended.

- For patients with severe breathlessness initial therapy with two bronchodilators may be considered.

- If the addition of a second bronchodilator did not improve symptoms, we suggest the treatment could be stepped down again to single bronchodilator.

- Group B patients are likely to have comorbidities that may add to their symptomatology and impact their prognosis and these possibilities should be investigated.

Group C

- Initial therapy should consist of a single long-acting bronchodilator. In two head to head comparisons[18] the tested LAMA was superior to the LABA regarding exacerbation prevention, therefore starting therapy with LAMA is recommended in this group.

- Patients with persistent exacerbations may benefit from adding a second long acting bronchodilator (LABA/LAMA) or using combination of a long-acting β_2 agonist and an inhaled corticosteroid (LABA/ICS). As ICS increases the risk for developing pneumonia in some patients, so primary choice is LABA/LAMA.

Group D

- GOLD guideline recommend starting therapy with a LABA/LAMA combination because:

  o In studies with patient reported outcomes as the primary endpoint LABA/LAMA combination showed superior results compared to single substances. If a single bronchodilator is chosen as initial treatment, a LAMA is preferred to exacerbation prevention based on comparison to LABA.

o A LABA/LAMA combination was superior to a LABA/ICS combination in preventing exacerbations and other patient reported outcomes in group D patients.

o Group D patients are at higher risk of developing pneumonia when receiving treatment with ICS.[19]

- In some patients initial therapy with LABA/ICS may be the first choice. These patients may have a history and/or findings suggestive of asthma-COPD overlap. High blood eosinophil counts may also be considered as a parameter to support the use of ICS.

- In patients who develop further exacerbations on LABA/LAMA therapy GOLD guideline suggests two alternate pathways:

o Escalation to LABA/LAMA/ICS.

o Switch to LABA/ICS. However, there is no evidence that switching from LABA/LAMA to LABA/ICS results in better exacerbation prevention. If LABA/ICS therapy does not positively impact exacerbation, a LAMA can be added.

- If patients treated with LABA/LAMA/ICS still have exacerbations, the following options may be considered:

o Add roflumilast. This may be considered in patients with an FEV_1 <50% predicted and chronic bronchitis,[20] particularly if they have experienced at least one hospitalisation for an exacerbation in the previous year.

o Add macrolide. The best available evidence exists for the use of azithromycin.[21]

o Stopping ICS. A reported lack of efficacy, an elevated risk of adverse effects (including pneumonia) and evidence showing no significant harm from withdrawl support this recommendation.

Bronchodilators—Recommendations

- For both β_2-agonists and anticholinergics, long-acting formulations are preferred to short-acting formulations.

- Patients may be started on single long acting bronchodilator therapy or dual long acting bronchodilator therapy. In patients with persistent dyspnoea on one bronchodilator, treatment should be escalated to two.

- Based on efficacy and side effects inhale bronchodilators are preferred over oral bronchodilators.

- Based on evidence of relatively low efficacy and more side effects, treatment with theophylline is not recommended unless other long-term treatment bronchodilators are unavailable or unaffordable.

Anti-Inflammatory Agents—Recommendations

- Long-term monotherapy with ICS is not recommended.

- Long-term treatment with inhaled corticosteroids may be considered in association with LABA for patients with a history of exacerbations despite appropriate treatment with long-acting bronchodilators.

- Long-term monotherapy with oral corticosteroids is not recommended in COPD.

- Long-term treatment containing inhaled corticosteroids should not be prescribed outside their indications, due to the risk of pneumonia and the possibility of an increased risk of fractures following long-term exposure.

- The phosphodiesterase-4 inhibitor, roflumilast, may also be used to reduce exacerbations for patients with chronic bronchitis, severe and very severe COPD, and frequent exacerbations that are not adequately controlled by long-acting bronchodilators.

- In former smokers with exacerbations despite appropriate therapy, macrolide can be considered.

- Antioxidant mucolytics are recommended in selected patients.

- Statin therapy is not recommended for prevention of exacerbations.

Monitoring and Follow-up

Monitor disease progression and development of complications.

Measurements

Decline in lung function is best tracked by spirometry performed at least once a year to identify patients whose lung function is declining quickly. Functional capacity as measured by a timed walking test (6-minute walking distance) provides additional information regarding prognosis.[22] Measurement of oxygenation at rest in an arterial blood gas sample may help identify patients who will benefit from supplemental oxygen to improve both symptoms and survival in those with severe resting hypoxaemia.

Symptoms

At each visit, inquire about changes in symptoms since the last visit, including cough and sputum, breathlessness, fatigue, activity limitation, and sleep disturbances.

Smoking Status

At each visit, determine current smoking status and smoke exposure; strongly encourage participation in programs to reduce and eliminate wherever possible exposure to COPD risk factors.

Monitor Pharmacotherapy and other Medical Treatment

In order to adjust therapy appropriately as the disease progresses, each follow-up visit should include a discussion of the current therapeutic regimen. Dosages of various medications, adherence to the regimen, inhaler technique, effectiveness of the current regime at controlling symptoms, and side effects of treatment should be monitored. Treatment modifications should be recommended as appropriate with a focus on avoiding unnecessary polypharmacy.

Monitor Exacerbation History

Evaluate the frequency, severity, and likely causes of any exacerbations. Increased sputum volume, acutely worsening dyspnoea, and the presence of purulent sputum should be noted.

Severity of exacerbations can be estimated by the increased need for bronchodilator medication or corticosteroids and by the need for antibiotic treatment.

Monitor Comorbidities

Comorbidities are common in COPD, amplify the disability associated with COPD, and can potentially complicate its management. Until more integrated guidance about disease management for specific comorbid problems becomes available, the focus should be on identification and management of these individual problems in line with local treatment guidance.

INDIAN GUIDELINE

COPD is a common, preventable lung disorder characterized by progressive, poorly reversible airflow limitation often with systemic manifestations, in response to tobacco smoke and/or other harmful inhalational exposures.

A diagnosis of COPD should be considered in persons having chronic symptoms of cough, sputum production, shortness of breath, and/or wheezing; especially among those with prolonged exposure to risk factors for the disease.

A postbronchodilator FEV_1/FVC below the LLN (lower fifth percentile of values from a reference population) should be used as the criterion for diagnosis of airflow obstruction.

DIAGNOSIS

FEV_1/FVC 0.7 criterion leads to over-diagnosis of the disease as compared to a more statistically sound lower limit of normal (LLN) criterion. Moreover, studies have also shown that 0.7 also potentially 'underdiagnoses' younger patients with airflow obstruction.[23] Young subjects, especially below the age of 40 years, might have a FEV_1/FVC below the LLN for their

age, but might get misclassified as normal as the ratio may be greater than the fixed cut off of 0.7.[24]

For simplicity and ease of use, mMRC questionnaire (Table 10.4) rather than CAT has been incorporated into classification as a measure of patient symptoms.

Recommendations *(Table 10.5)*

- ICS have a beneficial effect in subgroup of COPD patients with $FEV_1 < 50\%$.
- ICS have a beneficial effect in subgroup of COPD patients with frequent exacerbations (≥ 2 exacerbations/ year).
- The risk benefit profile favours use of ICS in patients with severe COPD.
- LAMA is superior to LABA monotherapy.
- ICS monotherapy should not be used.
- SABA and SAMA are equally effective when used for COPD.
- LAMA plus LABA may be used in patients who continue to have symptoms on monotherapy, except for those with frequent exacerbations.

Table 10.4: Classification of severity of COPD

Severity	Post-bronchodilator FEV_1 % predicted	MMRC grade	Exacerbation Frequency per year	Complications Haematocrit>55% cor pulmonale pO_2 <60 pCO_2 >50
Mild	≥80	<2	<2	No
Moderate	50–79	≥2	<2	No
Severe	<50	≥2	≥2	Yes

Table 10.5: Management of stable COPD

Category	First choice	Alternative choice	Add-on therapy (if patient continues to have symptoms)
Mild	SABA or SAMA	Methylxanthines	
Moderate	LAMA	LABA	Methylxanthines to LAMA/ LABA
Severe	ICS plus LABA	LAMA	Methylxanthines to LAMA or ICS plus LABA

- LABA plus ICS should be preferred to LABA alone in patients with $FEV_1 < 50\%$ or those having frequent exacerbations.
- In patients of severe COPD ($FEV_1 < 50\%$), triple therapy may be used in those who are symptomatic despite single or dual bronchodilator therapy.
- There is a lack of sufficient data to recommend ICS LABA or ICS LAMA combination over LAMA monotherapy.

Comparison of GOLD and Indian guideline of COPD is given in Table 10.6.

American College of Physicians, American College of Chest Physicians, American Thoracic Society, and European Respiratory Society

A diagnosis of COPD is confirmed when a patient who has symptoms of COPD is found to have airflow obstruction generally defined as a postbronchodilator FEV_1/FVC ratio less than 0.70.

This guideline does not address all components of management of a patient with COPD and is limited to pharmacologic management, pulmonary rehabilitation, and oxygen therapy. It does not cover smoking cessation, surgical options, palliative care, end-of-life care, or nocturnal ventilation.

There is no evidence to support the use of routine periodic spirometry after initiation of therapy to monitor disease status or to modify therapy in symptomatic patients. Improvements in clinical symptoms do not necessarily correlate with spirometric responses to therapy or reduction of long-term decline in FEV_1. Because of the wide intra-individual variation, the spirometric decline of lung function cannot be used to measure individual long-term response to treatment.

Monotherapy with a long acting inhaled agent (long-acting anticholinergic, long-acting β_2-agonist, or corticosteroid) was superior to placebo or short-acting anticholinergic therapy in reducing exacerbations.

BTS GUIDELINE

COPD is a chronic, slowly progressive disorder characterised by airways obstruction ($FEV_1 < 80\%$ predicted and FEV_1/FVC ratio $< 70\%$) which does not change markedly over several months (Table 10.7). The impairment of lung function is largely fixed but is partially reversible by bronchodilator therapy.

A positive spirometric response to bronchodilators or corticosteroids is considered to be present when the FEV_1 increases by 200 ml and 15% of the baseline value.

Deficiency of Guidelines

Health Education

Health education is an integral component of a COPD management program. Special importance should be given to inhaler technique, which should be demonstrated to the patient and accompanying attendants and reinforced at every visit. This is particularly true for elderly patients.

For COPD patients who are not active smokers, potential environmental exposures (environmental tobacco smoke, biomass fuel smoke, and others) should be asked for and avoided. Reassure patient that inhaler medication will not lead to addiction, minimise side effect of oral/parenteral medication.

Inhaler Training Technique

Correct technique for using inhaler should be mentioned. Wrong inhalation technique would not benefit patient's symptom and lead to poor compliance to inhaler medication.

Table 10.6 : Comparison of GOLD and Indian guideline of COPD

GOLD guideline	Indian guideline
1. Chronic Obstructive Pulmonary Disease (COPD) is a common, preventable and treatable disease that is characterized by persistent respiratory symptoms and airflow limitation that is due to airway and/or alveolar abnormalities usually caused by significant exposure to noxious particles or gases.	Chronic obstructive pulmonary disease is a common, preventable lung disorder characterised by progressive, poorly reversible airflow limitation often with systemic manifestations, in response to tobacco smoke and/or other harmful inhalational exposures.
2. The spirometric criterion for airflow limitation remains a post-bronchodilator fixed ratio of $FEV_1/FVC < 0.70$.	A postbronchodilator FEV_1/FVC below the LLN (lower fifth percentile of values from a reference population) should be used as the criterion for diagnosis of airflow obstruction.
3. Classification includes four grades.	Classification includes three grades.
4. Complications like haematocrit>55%, cor pulmonale, pO_2 <60 pCO_2 >50 not included for classification criteria.	Complications like haematocrit>55%, cor pulmonale, pO_2 <60 pCO_2 >50 included for classification criteria.
5. Recommend a comprehensive assessment of symptom (CAT score) rather than just a measure of breathlessness (mMRC).	Indian guideline assess only breathlessness (mMRC) for grading COPD. CAT score is not recommended in Indian guideline.
6. Nebulised budesonide alone may be an alternative to oral corticosteroids in the treatment of exacerbations.	ICS are not routinely recommended in management of AECOPD.
7. Antibiotics should be given to patients with exacerbations of COPD who have 1. Three cardinal symptoms—increase in dyspnoea, sputum volume, and sputum purulence. 2. Two of the cardinal symptoms, if increased purulence of sputum is one of the two symptoms. 3. Or require mechanical ventilation (invasive or noninvasive)	Antibiotics should be prescribed for all exacerbations of COPD.
8. Prophylactic antibiotic for prevention of exacerbation is recommended.	Prophylactic antibiotic for prevention of exacerbation is not recommended.
9. Mucolytic agent is recommended for prevention of exacerbation.	Mucolytic agent is not recommended.
10. Escalation and de-escalation strategy for management of stable COPD is given.	Escalation and de-escalation strategy for management of stable COPD is not given.
11. Management of co-morbidities is given.	Management of co-morbidities is not given.

	Table 10.7: Classification of COPD (BTS guidelines)	
Category of COPD	*FEV_1 (% predicted)*	*Symptoms and signs*
Mild	60–80	No abnormal signs, smoker's cough, little or no breathlessness
Moderate	40–59	Breathlessness (±wheeze) on moderate exertion. Cough (±sputum). Variable abnormal signs (general reduction in breath sounds, presence of wheezes)
Severe	<40	Breathlessness on any exertion/at rest. Wheeze and cough often prominent. Lung overinflation usual; cyanosis, peripheral oedema and polycythemia in advanced disease, especially during exacerbations.

Comorbidity Management

COPD often coexists with other diseases (comorbidities) that may have a significant impact on prognosis. Some of these arise independently of COPD, whereas others may be causally related, either with shared risk factors or by one disease actually increasing the risk of another. Whether or not COPD and comorbid diseases are related, management of the COPD patient must include identification and treatment of its comorbidities. The recommendations in **GOLD** guideline are insufficient for the management of comorbidities and cannot substitute for the use of guidelines for the management of each comorbidity. There is no recommendation for comorbidity management in **Indian guideline**. Ideally patient should refer to concerned specialist for comorbidity management where no available guideline should include management of comorbidity. To formulate the guideline for coexisting comorbidity the treatment should be added with concession of concerned physician.

Escalation and de-escalation Strategy

Many COPD patients already on treatment and return with persistent symptoms after initial therapy or less commonly with resolution of some symptoms that subsequently require less therapy. Therefore, recommendation of escalation and de-escalation strategy.

Easy Way of Monitoring of COPD

- **Pulmonary lung function testing:** Spirometry is the most reproducible and objective measurement of airflow limitation. The spirometric criterion for airflow limitation remains a post-bronchodilator fixed ratio of $FEV_1/FVC<0.70$. Decline in FEV_1 can be tracked by spirometry performed at least once in a year to identify those patients who are declining quickly.

- **Six minutes walk test (6MWT):** The 6-minute walk test has historically been used to characterise the functional status of COPD patients. The 6MWT is a practical simple test that requires a 100-ft hallway but no exercise equipment or advanced training for technicians. Walking is an activity performed daily by all but the most severely impaired patients. This test measures the distance that a patient can quickly walk on a flat, hard surface in a period of 6 minutes (the 6MWD). It evaluates the global and integrated responses of all the systems involved during exercise, including the pulmonary and cardiovascular systems, systemic circulation, peripheral circulation, blood, neuromuscular units, and muscle metabolism. The strongest indication for the 6MWT is for measuring the response to medical interventions in patients with moderate to severe heart or lung disease. The 6MWT has also been used as a one-time measure of functional status of patients, as well as predictor of morbidity and mortality.

- DLCO should be routinely recommended for severe COPD at tertiary care centre.

Sequelae Management

- **Cor pulmonale:** Pulmonary hypertension and consequent right ventricular failure, cor pulmonale, are usually the consequence of chronic alveolar hypoxia, with secondary contributions from destruction of the alveolar capillary bed, lung hyperinflation, and increased blood viscosity.[25] Diagnosis of pulmonary hypertension and right ventricular failure can be difficult, as physical findings of venous engorgement, and right ventricular hypertrophy and dilatation are late signs. Peripheral edema is poorly correlated with resting right atrial pressure and may reflect fluid retention from activation of the renin–angiotensin–aldosterone system. Functional imaging studies including echocardiography or radionuclide ventriculography are more probative for evaluation of right ventricular function. Doppler echocardiographic measures of pulmonary artery systolic pressure correlate weakly with severity of pulmonary hypertension by right heart catheterization.[26]

    The primary treatment of cor pulmonale consists of continuous oxygen to overcome hypoxemia and diuretic to optimize volume status. Calcium channel blockers and other vasodilators can dilate the pulmonary circulation, but they worsen hypoxemia and their benefit is not established. Phlebotomy increases exercise capacity when the haematocrit exceeds 55%, but persistent erythrocytosis suggests inadequate oxygen supplementation or another cause. Anticoagulation, which is considered beneficial in severe pulmonary vascular hypertension of other causes, is of uncertain benefit in patients with pulmonary hypertension caused by COPD.

- **Pulmonary arterial hypertension:** Pulmonary arterial hypertension (PAH) is a progressive disease of the pulmonary vasculature in which an ever increasing resistance to circulatory flow imposes a mounting afterload for the right heart to overcome. Without therapy, and frequently despite it, patients with PAH suffer progressive and inexorable right heart failure, functional decline, and ultimately die.

    PAH is one of several possible causes of pulmonary hypertension. Pulmonary hypertension is defined as a mean pulmonary artery pressure greater than or equal to 25 mmHg at rest. It can be due to diseases primarily isolated to the pulmonary vasculature itself, as in PAH, or can be a complication of other diseases, including hypoxemic lung disorders (e.g., chronic obstructive pulmonary disease [COPD]), left heart disease (e.g., systolic, diastolic, or valvular dysfunctions), or thromboembolism. Identification of its cause is essential, as appropriate therapy for pulmonary hypertension is aimed at its underlying cause—be that repair of a stenotic mitral valve, bronchodilators for obstructive lung disease or, in the case of PAH, the use of advanced therapies targeted at the pulmonary vasculature.

General measures include exercise and the avoidance of deconditioning, oxygen therapy, immunizations, fluid management and diuretics, digitalis, anticoagulation, contraception for pregnancy.

PAH-specific pharmacotherapy includes calcium channel antagonists, endothelin receptor antagonists, phosphodiesterase inhibitors, prostenoid therapies.

- **Hypertension:** Blood pressure should be regularly monitored and managed.
- **Osteoporosis:** Osteoporosis is a disease characterised by low bone mass and density. The National Osteoporosis Foundation, the American Medical Association, and other major medical organizations recommend a dual-energy X-ray absorptiometry scan (DXA, formerly known as DEXA) be used for the diagnosis of osteoporosis. DXA typically measures bone density in the hip, the spine, and the forearm. The test takes only five to 15 minutes to perform, exposes patients to very little radiation (less than one-tenth to one-hundredth of the amount used on a standard chest X-ray), and is quite precise. Lifestyle changes, including quitting cigarette smoking, curtailing excessive alcohol intake, exercising regularly, and consuming a balanced diet with adequate calcium and vitamin D can prevent osteoporosis. Medications that stop bone loss and increase bone strength, such as alendronate, risedronate, raloxifene, ibandronate, calcitonin, zoledronate.

Indian Mind Setup When to Stop Medicines

Education and counselling for continue medication. Many COPD patients already on treatment and return with persistent symptoms after initial therapy or less commonly with resolution of some symptoms that subsequently require less therapy, treatment can be modified by regular visit but not stopped completely. Patient should follow schedule for influenza and pneumococcal vaccination.

How Much Practical is to Implement Guideline in Daily Practice

It is possible to implement guideline in daily practice with some modification as per clinical observation of the respiratory physician.

SUMMARY

Chronic obstructive pulmonary disease (COPD) is a common, preventable and treatable disease that is characterized by persistent respiratory symptoms and airflow limitation that is usually caused by significant exposure to noxious particles or gases.

Comorbidities have significant impact on the prognosis. Some of these arise independently of COPD, whereas others may be causally related. Indian patients and healthcare system is different from the other parts of the world. In spite of this GOLD guidelines are cornerstone in the management of COPD, the available Indian guideline tries to deal with local issues but it has not provided satisfactory remarks as to adjust management as per Indian mindset. Detailed guidelines are not available how to select among spectrum of devices available, inhaler technique standards, co-morbidity management, escalation or de-escalation of therapy, easy way to monitor disease in follow-up period.

REFERENCES

1. Halbert RJ, Natoli JL, Gano A, Badamgarav E, Buist AS, Mannino DM. Global burden of COPD: systematic review and meta analysis. Eur Respir J 2006; 28(3): 523–32.

2. Quach A, Giovannelli J, Cherot-Kornobis N, et al. Prevalence and underdiagnosis of airway obstruction among middle-aged adults in northern France: The ELISABET study 2011–2013. Respir Med 2015; **109**(12): 1553–61.

3. Lamprecpt B, McBurnie MA, Vollmer WM et al. COPD in never smokers; results from the population based burden of obstructive lung diseases study, Chest 2011; 139(4): 752–63.

4. Adeloye D, Chua S, Lee C, et al. Global and regional estimates of COPD prevalence. Systemic review and meta-analysis. Journal of global health 2015; 5(2): 020415.

5. Global Burden of Disease Study Collaborators. Global, regional and national age-sex specific all-cause and cause-specific mortality for 240 causes of death, 1990–2013: a systematic analysis for the Global Burden of Disease study 2013. Lancet 2015; 385 (9963): 117–71.

6. Stein BD, Bautista A, Schumock GT, et al. The validity of International Classification of Diseases, Ninth Revision, Clinical Modification diagnosis codes for identifying patients hospitalised for COPD exacerbations. Chest 2012; 141(1): 87–93.

7. Guarascio AJ, Ray SM, Finch CK, Self TH. The Clinical and economic burden of chronic obstructive pulmonary disease in the USA. Clinico Economics and outcomes research: CEOR 2013; 5: 235–45.

8. DALYs GBD, Collaborators H, Murray CJ, et al. Global, regional, and national disability-adjusted life years (DALYs) for 306 diseases and injuries and healthy life expectancy (HALE) for 188 countries, 1990–2013: quantifying the epidemiological transition. Lancet 2015; 386 (10009): 2145–91.

9. Buist AS, McBurnie MA, Vollmer WM, et al. International variation in the prevalence of COPD (the BOLD study): A population-based prevalence study. Lancet 2007; 370(9589): 741–50.

10. Miravitilies M, Worth H, Soler Cataluna JJ, et al. Obsevational study and their relationship with patient—reported outcomes: results from the ASSESS study. Respir RES2014; 15: 122.

11. Cho SH, Lin HC, Ghosal AG, et al. Respiratory Disease in the Asia-pacific region: Cough as a key symptom. Allergy Asthma Proc 2016; 37(2): 131–40.

12. Allinson JP, Hardy, Donaldson GC, Shaheen SO, Kuh D, Wedzicha JA. The presence of chronic mucus hypersecretion across adult life in Relation to Chronic Obstructive Pulmonary Disease Development. Am J Respir Crit Care Med 2016; 193(4): 662–72.

13. Gudur G, Brenner S, Angermann CE, et al. GOLD or lower limit of normal definition? A comparison with expert-based diagnosis of chronic obstructive pulmonary disease in a prospective cohort-study. Respir Res 2012; 13(1): 13.

14. US Preventive services Task Force, Siu AL, Bibbins-Domingo K, et al. Screening for Chronic Obstuctive Pulmonary Disease: US Preventive Services Task Force Recommendation Statement. JAMA 2016; 315(13): 1372–7.

15. Jones PW. Health status measurement in chronic obstructive pulmonary disease. Thorax 2001; 56(11): 880–7.

16. Tomczyk S, Bennett NM, Stoecker C, et al. Use of 13 valent pneumococcal conjugate vaccine and 23 valent pneumococcal polysaccharide vaccine among adults aged>/=65 years: recommendations of the advisory committee on immunization practices (ACIP). MMWR Morb Mortal Wkly Resp 2014; 63(37): 822–5.

17. Karner C, Cates CJ. Long-acting beta$_2$ agonist in addition totiotropium versus either tiotropium or long acting beta 2 agonist alone for chronic obstructive pulmonary disease. Cochrane Data base Syst Rev 2012; (4): Cd008989.

18. Vogelmeir C, Hederer B, Glaab T, et al. Tiotropium versus salmeterol for the prevention of exacerbations of COPD. N Engl J Med 2011; 364(12): 1093–103.

19. Crim C, Dransfield MT, Bourbeau J, et al. Pneumonia risk with inhaled fluticasone fuorate and vilanterol compared with vilanterol alone in patients with COPD. Annals of American Thoracic Society 2015; 12(1): 27–34.

20. Martinez FJ, Calverley PM, Gooehring UM, Brose M, Fabbri LM, Rabe KF. Effect of roflumilast on exacerbation in patients with severe chronic obstructive pulmonary disease uncontrolled by combination therapy (REACT): a multicentre randomised controlled trial. Lancet 2015; 385(9971): 857–56.

21. Albert RK, Connett J, Bailey WC, et al. Azithromycin for prevention of exacerbations of COPD. N Engl J Med 2011; 365(8): 689–98.

22. Jones PW, Harding G, Berry P, Wiklund I, Chen Wh, Kline Leidy N. Development and first

validation of the COPD assessment Test. EurRespir J 2009; 34(3): 648–54.

23. Cerveri I, Corsico AG, Accordini S, Niniano R, Ansaldo E, Anto JM, et al. Underestimation of airflow obstruction among young adults using $FEV_1/FVC < 70\%$ as a fixed cutoff: A longitudinal evaluation of clinical and functional outcomes. Thorax 2008; 63: 10405.

24. Aggarwal AN, Gupta D, Agarwal R, Jindal SK. Comparison of the lower confidence limit to the fixed percentage method for assessing airway obstruction in routine clinical practice. Respir Care 2011; 56: 177884.

25. Naeije R. Pulmonary hypertension and right heart failure in chronic obstructive pulmonary disease. Proc Am Thorac Soc. 2005; 2(1): 20–22.

26. Fisher MR, Criner GJ, Fishman AP, et al. Estimating pulmonary artery pressures by echocardiography in patients with emphysema. Eur Respir J. 2007; 30(5): 914–21.

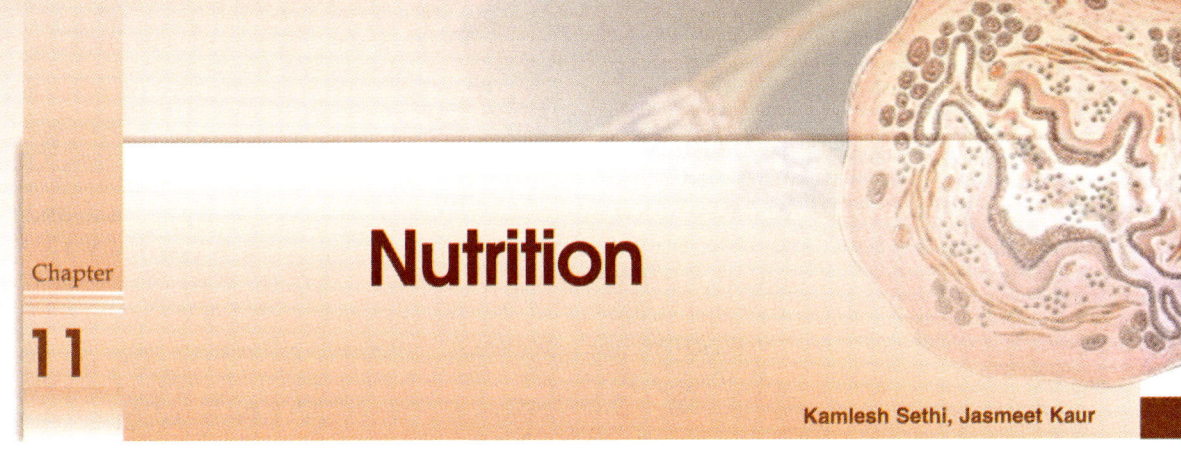

Chapter

11

Kamlesh Sethi, Jasmeet Kaur

Nutrition

INTRODUCTION

Nutritional and respiratory status are related in a variety of ways. Malnutrition, either in isolation or as the result of acute or chronic illness, impairs respiratory function directly by weakening diaphragmatic contractions (Table 11.1). Malnutrition impacts the respiratory system indirectly by causing relative immunosuppression.

The link between diet and the pulmonary system is especially clear in patients with limited respiratory reserve and carbon monoxide retention. Evidence that manipulation of diet to reduce the respiratory quotient will modify long-term outcomes in patients with chronic obstructive pulmonary disease (COPD) is lacking, although the practice is supported by short-term studies.

Table 11.1: Adverse effects of lung disease on nutrition status	
Adverse effects of lung disease on nutrition status	
Increased energy expenditure	Increased work of breathing
	Chronic infection
	Medical treatments (e.g. bronchodilators, chest physical therapy)
Reduced intake	Fluid restriction
	Shortness of breath
	Decreased oxygen saturation when eating
	Anorexia resulting from chronic disease
	Gastrointestinal distress and vomiting
Additional limitations	Difficulty in preparing food because of fatigue
	Lack of financial resources
	Impaired feeding skills (for infants and children)
	Altered metabolism

Source: Mahan K and Escott-Stump S. *Krause's Food and Nutrition Therapy*, 12th ed. Saunders Elsevier, 2008, 903.

Dietary triggers of asthma and exacerbations of COPD are under investigation. Dietary intake may influence the production of surfactant. Whereas conclusive evidence supports a role for adequate nutritional status in obstructive pulmonary disease, evidence for a protective or provocative role of specific micronutrients is mostly preliminary to date.

OBESITY, ADIPOKINASE AND RESPIRATORY DISEASES

Overnutrition and resulting obesity are clearly linked with asthma, though the mechanisms involved are still under investigation. COPD is characterized not only by pulmonary deficits but also by chronic systemic inflammation and co-morbidities which may develop in response to the metabolic deregulation that occurs with excess adipose tissue.[42] A recent meta-analysis of leptin levels in COPD reported a correlation with body mass index (BMI) and fat mass per cent in stable COPD though absolute levels were not different to healthy controls.[51]

Undernutrition and Respiratory Disease

Amongst the obstructive lung diseases, Undernutrition is most commonly recognized in COPD. Itoh et al[44] present a review on undernutrition in COPD and the evidence for nutritional therapy in management of the disease. Weight loss, low body weight and muscle wasting are common in COPD patients with advanced disease and are associated with reduced survival time and an increased risk of exacerbation.[45] The causes of under-nutrition in COPD are multifactorial and include reduced energy intake due to decreased appetite, depression, lower physical activity and dyspnoea while eating.[46] In addition, resting energy expenditure is increased in COPD, likely due to higher energy demands from increased work of breathing.[47] Also systemic inflammation which is a hallmark of COPD may influence energy intake and expenditure.[48] Cigarette smoke may also have deleterious effects on body composition in addition to the systemic effects of COPD. Smoking causes muscle fibre atrophy and decreased muscle oxidative capacity shown in cohort of non-COPD smokers.[49, 50]

Reduced Dietary Intake

Dietary intake in weight losing patients is lower than in weight stable patient both in absolute terms as well as in relation to measured REE (resting energy expenditure). The reason for the relatively low dietary intake seen in COPD is not completely understood. Patient with COPD may eat suboptimal due to the changes in breathing pattern and low oxygen saturations (SaO) seen with chewing and swallowing. Indeed in hypoxemic patients a rapid decrease in SaO (% saturation of Hb with oxygen in arterial blood) is seen, which slowly recovers after completion of the meal. The decrease in SaO is related to increased dyspnoea sensation. The severity of the drop may differ, depending on the composition of the meal. Gastric emptying time of a meal may also affect dietary intake since gastric filling in COPD patients reduces the functional residual capacity and leads to an increase in dyspnoea. Simple dietary practices may help to overcome these problems are listed in Table 11.2.

Systemic factors may also affect dietary intake. Recent studies suggest that appetite regulation may be adversely affected by systemic inflammation. The adipocyte-derived hormone leptin represents the afferent hormonal signal to brain in a feedback mechanism regulating fat mass, circulating leptin levels are increased in some patients. This increased plasma leptin level is positively related to an increase in

Table 11.2: Simple dietary practices for COPD patients

S.No.	Respiratory symptom	Dietary Modification
1.	Dyspnoea	• Small frequent meals and snacks • Soft meals to reduce work of chewing and swallowing. • Sit up for meals and of bed if possible
2.	Oxygen therapy	Wear nasal prongs instead of oxygen mask when eating
3.	Dry mouth	Moist meals
4.	Constipation	Increased fluid and fibre intake
5.	Dysphagia	Speech and language therapy
6.	Taste alterations	Provide meals and drinks with strong flavours
7.	CPAP/BiPAP	Nasogastric feeding
8.	Regurgitation of meals	Post-pyloric enteral feeding
9.	Immobility	Social review regarding home help and help with shopping and meal preparation

some of the markers of systemic inflammation and inversely related to dietary intake adjusted for REE.

AN OVERVIEW ON DIET

Malnutrition has been shown to be common among patients with clinically significant obstructive airway disease, ranging from 20% to 70%[6–8]. Mortality rates among patients with COPD rise substantially with the advent of malnutrition.

Cytokines associated with the disease state may contribute to catabolism and attenuate appetite. Negative energy balance during acute exacerbations of COPD apparently is due to both reduced energy intake relative to baseline and an increase in resting energy expenditure.[9, 10]

In COPD, energy intake of 1.4 to 1.6 times the resting energy expenditure is indicated during periods when lean body mass is being recovered; energy then should be maintained at 1 to 1.2 times resting energy expenditure to avoid increased CO generation.[11]

Protein supplementation at approximately 1.5 g/kg/day is advocated by some in the aftermath of COPD exacerbation to facilitate the reconstitution of lean body mass.[9]

The energy requirements of patients with COPD and malnutrition are estimated at 45 kcal/kg/day, approximately 80% to 90% higher than predicted resting energy expenditure. In such a patient, expert opinion favours a diet relatively high in total fat (45% to 55% of total calories), with low intake of saturated fat to avoid cardiovascular sequel.[12]

Although nutritional support with high-fat rather than high carbohydrate preparations offers the theoretical advantage of a lower respiratory quotient, in most cases the actual clinical significance appears to be small.[11]

Oxidative injury by free radicals is thought to be a key factor in acute lung injury. Preliminary evidence suggests that antioxidant supplementation in the form of vitamins E and C, retinol, and β carotene may have protective effects. Dietary addition of n-3 fatty acids may also be beneficial in patients with acute lung injury.[15]

A recent area of active investigation is the potential associations between both dietary antioxidants and n-3 fatty acids and the rising incidence of asthma. Although epidemiological and observational studies suggest benefits from higher intake of these nutrients, clinical intervention trials have, for the most part, been less encouraging.[16] Evidence that a variety of dietary antioxidants may protect against COPD is preliminary but provocative.[17]

Smoking

Population based survey data suggest an inverse association between dietary fish intake and the development of smoking related COPD.[13] Apart from cigarettes, people from India smoke tobacco using bidis, hookahs and chillums among several other forms of smoking. It is important to note that the harmful effects of each of these are different. Bidis are more harmful than cigarettes (although they contain only one fourth the amount of nicotine, they produce four to five times more tar than cigarettes, making one bidi as harmful as one cigarette), hookahs are more harmful than bidis and the chillum is the most harmful of the lot[52] suggesting that other factors also are important; Diet probably is one of these factors, but data on the diet–COPD association remain scare, particularly when compared with the enormous literature on the role of diet in other chronic diseases.

Dietary Intake

Various dietary patterns have been linked to the risk of respiratory diseases.[27] The Mediterranean diet has been found to have protective effects for allergic respiratory diseases in epidemiological studies.[28] This dietary pattern consists of a high intake of minimally processed plant foods, namely fruit, vegetables, breads, cereals, beans, nuts and seeds, low to moderate intake of dairy foods, fish, poultry and wine and low intake of red meat.

The "western" dietary pattern, prevalent in developed countries, is characterized by high consumption of refined grains, cured and red meats, desserts and sweets, French fries, and high fat dairy products.[26, 29] In adults, a western diet has been shown to be positively associated with increased frequency of asthma exacerbation,[30] but not related to asthma risk. In addition, an acute challenge with a high fat fast food meal has been shown to worsen airway inflammation.[31] Cross sectional studies have also found that the "western" diet is associated with an increased risk of COPD.[26]

IMPORTANT NUTRIENTS

Phosphorus

Hypophosphatemia is known to impair diaphragmatic contractility and exacerbates CO retention. Phosphorus depletion commonly occurs due to intracellular shifts following the correction of respiratory acidosis.[6, 18] Impaired skeletal muscle function, attributable to loss of lean body mass, is associated with functional deterioration in COPD.[14]

Antioxidant and Oxidative Stress

Dietary antioxidants are an important dietary factor in protecting against the damaging effects of oxidative stress in the airways, a characteristic of respiratory diseases.[32] Oxidative stress caused by reactive oxygen species (ROS), is generated in the lungs due to various exposures, such as air pollution, airborne irritants and typical airways inflammatory cell responses.[33] Antioxidants including vitamin C, vitamin E, flavonoids and carotenoids are abundantly present in fruits and vegetables, as well as nuts, vegetable oils, cocoa, red wine and green tea (Table 11.3). Inverse association between dietary antioxidant and asthma and COPD have been reported in

Table 11.3: Various sources of antioxidant in diet

	Sources of antioxidants
Vitamin A	Liver, sweet potatoes, carrots, milk, egg yolk
Vitamin C	Oranges, kiwi, mangoes, broccoli, spinach, capsicum and strawberries
Vitamin E	Vegetable oil, avocados, nuts, seeds and whole grains
Lycopene	Tomatoes, grapefruit, watermelon
Flavanoids	Tea, green tea, citrus fruits, onion, apples
Catechins	Tea, sesamol
Anthocyanins	Egg plant, grapes berries
β-carotene	Pumpkin, mangoes, apricots, carrots, spinach, parsley
Zeaxanthin	Spinach and all green vegetables
Manganese	Whole grains, pulses and legumes, cereal products, tea, fruits, vegetables, nuts
Zinc	Whole grains, legumes, leafy vegetables, nuts and oil seeds, milk, eggs, cheese, nuts
Selenium	Whole grains, pulses and legumes, cereal products, tea, fruits, vegetables, nuts.
Copper	Seafood, lean meat and milk, nuts
Polyphenols	Tea, thyme and oregano
Cryptoxanthins	Red capsicum, pumpkin and mangoes
Allium sulphur compounds	Leeks, onion and garlic

epidemiological and observational studies. A case control study note diverse association with zinc, magnesium, and manganese, as well as vitamin C.[19] Theoretical support is strongest for vitamin C, which is found abundantly in pulmonary secretions;[20] however, interventional studies have not shown significant clinical benefit.[21, 22]

Flavonoids

Flavonoids are potent antioxidants and have anti-inflammatory as well as anti-allergic actions due in part, to their ability to neutralize reactive oxygen species (ROS).[34] There are 6 classes of flavonoids flavonols, flavanones, isoflavones and flavanols,[35] which are widely distributed throughout the diet and found in fruit, vegetables, nuts, seeds, stems, flowers, roots, bark, dark chocolate, tea, wine and coffee.[35]

Magnesium

Magnesium relaxes bronchial and vascular smooth muscle. It has been studied for the treatment of acute, reversible bronconstriction, and early studies have shown mixed results in mild to moderate asthma. Recent randomized control trials have demonstrated safety and efficacy of both intravenous[23] and nebulized[24] magnesium sulphate as adjuvant treatment of severe asthma exacerbations.

Omega-3 Fatty Acids and Fish

Consumption of oily fish or supplementation with omega-3 PUFA's may have positive effects in asthma and COPD, through strong evidence to support the experimental and epidemiological data is not yet available. There is considerable interest in the potential benefits of n-3 fatty acid on inflammatory conditions in general and pulmonary diseases in particular. Evidence in support of this interest is limited to date, and interventional trials thus far have yielding conflicting results.[25]

Vitamin D

Only one intervention trial has been conducted using vitamin D in adults with asthma, which found that rate of first exacerbation was reduced in subjects who demonstrated an increase in circulating vitamin D_3 following supplementation.[36] Data for the role of vitamin D in COPD onset is limited, though several cross-sectional studies have reported an association between low vitamin D levels, or deficiency, with COPD incidence.[37] Blood vitamin D levels have also been correlated with lung function in COPD patients.[38, 39]

The extra-skeletal effect of vitamin D is associated with documented in both asthma and COPD, and deficiency is associated with negative respiratory and immune outcomes. At this stage however, more evidence from supplementation intervention is needed before widespread adoption of supplementation can be recommended.

Minerals

Some minerals have also been found to be protective in respiratory conditions. Dietary magnesium may have beneficial bronchodilator effects in asthma.[40] Studies on dietary intake of minerals and associations with COPD are sparse. A small study in Sweden found that in older subjects with severe COPD, intakes of folic acid and selenium were below recommended levels, and although intake of calcium was adequate, serum calcium levels were low, likely related to their vitamin D status as intake was lower than recommended.[41] Mineral intake may be important in respiratory diseases, yet evidence for supplementation is weak. It is

likely that adequate intake of these nutrients in a whole diet approach is sufficient.

FORMULATION OF DIET

Ideal COPD diet includes small frequent meals of nutrients dense foodstuff like fruits, vegetables, milk, dairy products, lean protein sources and unrefined grain or complex carbohydrates that are high in dietary fibre. Nutrition education is an excellent impetus for changing poor food habits through nutritional counselling.

Balanced Diet

A balanced diet is one which provides all the nutrients in the required amounts and proper proportion. It can be easily achieved through a blend of Food Group Systems.

Balanced diet can be defined as one which contains different types of foods in such quantities and proportions that the needs for all the nutrients are adequately met and a small extra allowance is made as a margin of safety (Tables 11.4–11.6).

Why a healthy diet with COPD is important to maintain body weight?

- People with chronic bronchitis have a tendency to be obese, while those with emphysema have a tendency to be underweight. This makes diet and nutrition assessment a vital part of COPD treatment.

- Some symptoms of COPD, like lack of appetite, depression, or feeling unwell in general, can cause to be become underweight. Because COPD requires using more energy when breathing, it may need up to 10 times more calories per day than a person without the condition.

- If person is underweight, it is advised to include healthy, high calorie snacks in the diet. In overweight person heart and lungs have to work harder, making breathing more difficult. Excess body

Food groups	Representative foods	Nutritional significance
Grains	Wheat, rice, corn, oat, and other grain-based foods	Major source of energy (due to their sheer size in an average diet), carbohydrates, protein, minerals and fibre. Some are also fortified with vitamins.
Vegetables	Carrots, potato, onion, green beans, green peas, spinach, tomatoes, sweet potatoes, pumpkin, bitter gourd, bottle gourd, and others.	Rich source of vitamins, minerals, and fibre. The vitamin and mineral content varies between different vegetables.
Fruits	Apple, apricot, banana, dates, grapes, orange, melon, peaches, pears, mango, pineapple, raisins, grapefruit, strawberries and others.	Important sources of vitamins, minerals and fibre. The vitamin and mineral content varies between different fruits
Milk and dairy products	Fat-free (skim) or low fat (1%) milk or buttermilk, low fat, or reduced-fat cheese, fat-free or low fat regular or frozen yogurt.	Major sources of calcium, protein, vitamin B_1 and B_2, often also fortified with vitamin A and D.
Legumes	Lentils, kidney beans, dry beans, chickpea, and other pulses.	Good sources of protein, carbohydrates, vitamins, minerals (particularly magnesium) and fibre.
Meats, fish and eggs	Lean meats, fish, poultry and eggs	Rich sources of protein, zinc, iron, vitamins B_1, B_2, B_6, B_{12}, folate and niacin.
Oils and fats	Vegetable oils, viz. groundnut, mustard, olive, corn, safflower, and sunflower oil; butter, and ghee	Rich sources of energy, essential fatty acids, vitamins A and E.
Sweets and added sugars	Low fat sweets and added sugars	Calories with no other nutritive value.

Table 11.4: Representative foods and nutritional significance of various food groups

* *Source:* Srivastava RK, Tiwari BK, Agarwal Y. Current Nutritional Therapy Guidelines in Clinical Practice. Directorate General of Health Services, Government of India, 2008.

weight may also increase the demand for oxygen. So losing weight may be recommended.

- However, some people with COPD lose weight, which they do not need to lose and which can also make symptoms worse. They may need help to gain weight again and maintain a healthy weight, such as dietary advice about eating enough protein and calories.

- COPD can be a challenging condition to live with, so it is important to make food preparation a straightforward and stress-free process. Make meal time easier encourage underweight people to eat and stick to a healthy eating plans.

ESSENTIAL GUIDELINES FOR A DIETETICS ADVICE

- Many patients require dietary modification as a part of the therapeutic demand. Some imagination and creativity are essential when planning meals acceptable for a varied population.

Table 11.5: Comprehensive food exchange list

Food exchange	Raw food		Protein (g)	Carbo-hydrates (g)	Fat (g)	Energy (kcal)
	Amount (g)	Measure				
Milk (cow)	250 ml	1 C	8	12	10	170
Skim milk	320	13 C	8	14.7	–	93
Meat	40	2 pcs./1egg	7	neg.	6	80
Lean meat	35	2 pcs.	7	–	0.5	35
Pulses	30	3 T	7	17	neg.	100
Cereal/starch	20/variable	3 T	2	15	neg.	70
Vegetable A*	100	½ C	1	3.5	neg.	20
Vegetable B*	Variable	–	2	7	neg.	40
Fruit	Variable	1 portion	neg.	10	neg.	45
Fat	5	lt	–	–	5	45
Sugar	5	lt	–	5	–	20

* Two exchanges of vegetable A are calculated as one exchange of vegetable B. neg.—negligible, C—cup, T—tablespoon, lt—leveled teaspoon.
* *Source:* Khanna Kumud, Gupta Sharda. *Textbook of Nutrition and Dietetics,* 2nd ed., Department of Food and Nutrition, Institute of Home Economics, University of Delhi, 2016.

Alteration must be given to the colour, texture, composition and temperature of the foods, care also should be taken to supply the nutrients in a manner that the body can use them. A diet may need to be altered and adjusted in many ways before it meets the needs of individual patients.

- Changes in consistency—some patients may require fully liquid diet, soft diet, and normal diet.
- Changes in calorie contents—Some patients may require a high calorie diet, other a weight reduction diet.
- Restriction, elimination or increase in amount of a specific dietary nutrient.

    Dictated by their clinical condition, some patients may require a sodium restricted diet, while others may need a lactose restricted diet, gluten free diet, etc. This requires a thorough knowledge of nutrients contents of different foods.

- Changes in protein, fats and carbohydrates contents

    Patients with hyperlipidemia require a low fat diet, while patients of renal failure and advanced liver disease, a low protein diet and malnourished patients, a high protein high calorie diet.

- Changes in frequency of meals
- Dietary counseling.
- Failure of the patients to follow the prescribed drug regimen leads to great increase in recurrence and repeated hospitalization. Good nutrition is likewise important in preventing recurrence. The characteristics of normal diet, with special emphasis on a liberal milk intake, protein rich foods, fruits and vegetables, must be pointed out. To increase the calcium and protein intake 3–5 tablespoons of non-fat dry milk may be added to 250 ml milk (one glass).

Table 11.6: One serving portion of various foodstuffs for an adult (average)

Foodstuffs	Preparation	Household measures	Amount of raw foods (edible portion)
Cereals			
• Wheat flour	Chapatti/Prantha/Poori.	4–5	80–120 g
• Rice	Boiled rice, pulao	1 full plate	80–120 g
Breakfast cereals			
• Dalia/cornflakes/puffed	Porridge	1 bowl	20 g
• Wheat bread	Toast with butter	2 slices	60 g
Pulses			
• Washed pulses (moong, lentil, arhar, urad, chana dal)	Dal preparation	1 katori	30 g
• Whole pulses (soya bean, rajma, lobia, chana)	Whole pulse preparation	1 katori	30–35 g
Milk and milk products			
• Milk	Milk as such	1 glass	250 ml
• Curd	Curd as such	1 katori	100 g
	As raita	1 katori	75 g
• Paneer	As paneer curry	1 katori	60–80 g
	With peas or some other vegetables	1 katori	30–40 g
Vegetables			
• Green leafy vegetables	Vegetable preparation, e.g. Saag	1 katori	100–150 g
• Roots and tubers (potato, sweet potato, arbi)		1 katori	90–120 g
• Other vegetables	As vegetable preparation	1 katori	100–125 g
	As vegetable preparation		
Fruits			
• Guava, apple, pear, etc.	Fruit as such	1 med. size	100 g
	Added to puddings	1 bowl	40–50 g
• Melon, watermelon	Fruit as such	1 small plate	200–300 g
Meat, fish and poultry			
• Egg	As breakfast preparation	One	40–50 g
• Mutton	As curry	1 katori	80–100 g
• Fish	As curry	1 bowl	80–100 g
• Chicken	As fried	1 fillet	100 g
	As curry	1 bowl	80–100 g
• Keema	As roasted	1 piece	200 g
	As kababs	2 kababs	50 g
	As kofta curry	1 bowl	60–70 g
	As curry with peas	1 bowl	40 g

* To be served with approximately 150 ml. of milk and sugar to taste.
* *Source:* Khanna Kumud, Gupta Sharda. *Textbook of Nutrition and Dietetics*, 2nd ed., Department of Food and Nutrition, Institute of Home Economics, University of Delhi.

DIETARY MANAGEMENT

I. **Eat balanced diet:** A healthy diet includes a variety of foods. Try to include these food items in the diet.

- Low fat protein foods such as low fat milk, fresh paneer, tofu, lean meat, poultry and fish.
- Complex carbohydrate such as whole cereal, whole wheat product, Dal (whole/split), beans; these foods are also high in fiber.
- Fresh fruits and vegetables: These contain essential vitamins, minerals and fiber, which will help to keep body healthy and improve the function of the digestive system.
- Food contains high level of potassium such as banana, oranges, dark green leafy vegetables, tomatoes, beets and potatoes.

II. **Fluid intake:**

- Try to drink plenty of fluids throughout the day. Around six to eight glasses of non-caffeinated beverages are recommended per day. Adequate hydration keeps mucus thin and makes it easier to cough up.
- Limit or avoid caffeine altogether, as it could interfere with the medication. Caffeinated drinks include coffee, tea, sodas and energy drinks.

III. **Alcohol:** It is advised to avoid or limit alcohol beverages as they can interest with medications. Alcohol may also slow down breathing rate and make it more difficult to cough up mucus.

IV. **Supplements:** Certain supplements, such as omega-3-fatty acids, may, but have not been proven to help reduce inflammation and lung function.

V. **Reduce salt:** Salt intake makes body retain water, which increases swelling.

This makes breathing more difficult. To reduce salt intake read food nutritional label. Try using no-salt spices and avoid adding salt while cooking.

VI. **Avoid food that causes wind or bloating:** If wind or bloating is a problem, consider reducing consumption of foods and drinks such as: Apple, peaches, melons, beans, cauliflower, turnip, cabbage, sprouts; broccoli, peas, onions, and soya bean may also cause gas. Fizzy drinks, fried, spicy or greasy foods.

VII. **Dairy products:** Some people find that dairy products, such as milk and cheese, make phlegm thicker. If dairy products do not seem to make phlegm worse, so can be continued to eat them.

VIII. **Chocolate:** Chocolate contains caffeine which may interfere with medication.

IX. **Fried foods:** Foods that are fried, deep dried or greasy can cause gas and indigestion. Heavily spiced foods can also cause discomforts and may affect breathing.

X. Avoid empty foods, junk foods such as crisps and sweets, do not provide any nutritional value.

MAKE EATING EASIER WITH COPD

Try these tips for easier eating:

- Keep healthy foods visible and within easy reach.
- Eat variety of healthy foods, especially favourite foods.
- Use colourful place settings or play background music while eating.
- Eat with other people as often as you can.
- Drink fluids at the end of the meal so avoid feeling of fullness.
- Take small bites, chew slowly, and breathe deeply while chewing.

- Try to eat main meal early in the day this will boast energy levels for the whole day.
- Choose foods that are quick and easy to prepare to avoid wasting of energy.
- Sit down when preparing meals or ask family and friends to assist you with meal preparation.
- Sit up comfortably in a high backed chair when eating to avoid putting too much pressure on lungs.
- Freeze extra portions and take them out when you are too tired to cook.
- Choose easy to chew foods.
- Eat smaller more frequent meals.

SPECIAL CONSIDERATION

- Small frequent nutrients dense and easy to digest meals should be given.
- During the acute phase, a semi-soft or soft diet is recommended (khichri, kheer, boiled/mashed/pureed vegetables and/or fruits, custard, yoghurt, etc.). A regular diet is suggested during the recovery phase. Indoor patients suffering from severe form/COPD may need to be given a full fluid diet which can be supplemented with high energy, high protein eternal feeds.
- Meal pattern should be adjusted according to work schedule of the patients. It has generally been observed that several ambulatory patients (particularly sweepers, carpenters, construction workers) follow a two or maximum three meal pattern. They should be encouraged to consume meal more frequently and advised regarding the concept of carrying easy to digest, nutrient dense, non-perishable food items, such as sweet dalia, sujikheer, stuff roti/paranthas/missi roti/besan laddoo, upma, etc.
- Many of the patients suffering from COPD have limited purchasing power.

They should therefore be counseled effectively regarding the low cost nutritious foods available in their region such as guava, dates, jiggery, jowar, bajra, chirwa, milk and milk products ready to eat foodstuff or prepared at home.

- The patient should be convinced and encouraged to consume drugs as per the schedule. Avoid residing in area with poor hygiene/sanitation conditions and avoid smoking.

STABLE COPD PATIENTS IN OPD

Step 1. Check the weight and height of the patient.

Step 2. Categories the patient on the basis of BMI or the weight for height chart.

Step 3. Calculate the daily menu on the basis of the calories allowances of the patients (Table 11.7).

Step 4. Draw the daily menu on the basis of the calories allowances of the patients.

Body Mass Index (BMI)

This is the measure of the relative body fatness to evaluate risk factors associated with obesity. It is based on weight (in kg) with minimal clothing and height (in meters) without shoes.

BMI is expressed as W/H^2 where W is weight in kg and H is height in metres.

The WHO classification based on BMI is given in Table 11.8. However, lower BMI cut offs have been given for Asians as they have a greater risk of no communicable diseases (Misra 2009) (Table 11.8).

Diet for Patients who are Elderly and Living Alone

Many of the COPD patients are in Geriatrics age group. As per WHO guidelines people aged 60–74 years are

Table 11.7: *Calculating the daily calories requirements**		
BMI ≥25.0 kg/m²	*BMI 18.50 – 24.99 kg/m²*	*BMI<18.5 kg/m²*
Overweight patients 20 × body wt (in kg) = kcal	Ideal body weight patient 30 × body wt (in kg) = kcal	Underweight patient 35 × body wt (in kg) = kcal
For example, a patient of 95 kg will need = 20 × 95 = 1900 kcal	For example, a patient of 75 kg will need = 30 × 75 = 2250 kcal	For example, a patient of 46 kg will need = 35 × 46 = 1610 kcal
Pick a 1900 kcal menu	Pick a 2250 kcal menu	Pick a 1600 kcal menu

* (Daily calorie requirements worked out on the basis of Association of Physicians of India. API-ICP Guidelines on Diabetes 2007. JAPI 2007; 55:1-50(www.japi.org).)

Table 11.8: Classification of BMI (kg/m²)		
Category	*WHO (2004)*	*Asians*
Underweight	<18.5	<18
Normal	18.5–24.9	18.0–22.9
Overweight	25.0–29.9	23.0–24.9
Obesity	≥30	>25

Source: WHO (2004), Misra (2009)

called elderly. Influence of ageing on nutritional requirement also changes because of the ageing process that may affect their physiological, psychological and functional status.

The aged or the elderly (more than 60 years of age) belong to postmature adult group of population. The physiological and pathological changes that inevitably accompany ageing result in degenerative process and lower functional capacity.

Dietary Tips for the Elderly

The diet of the elderly may be modified according to physical activity of an individual and general health condition (Table 11.9).

Table 11.9: Nutritional modification in elderly	
Problem	*Nutritional modification*
Decline in the relative mass of immune tissue and an associate decline in immune function.	Increased vitamin intake and multivitamin as a supplement.
Decreased bone density and skin synthesis of vitamin D.	Regular exercise, adequate calcium intake.
Dysphasia, weaking of gas reflux, causes swallowing difficulties.	Modified food consistency (chopped, ground pureed or soft). Seasoning and flavouring to promote better intake. The consistency of liquid can be modified to thin nectar, honey or budding consistency using thickening agents. Appropriate body position (sit in upright position) also helps to reduce the risk of choking.
Constipation	Provide sufficient fibre and fluids. Encourage consumption of fruits, vegetables and whole grain bread and cereals.

- Take simple but nutritious diet.
- Improve the quality of diet by adding liberal amount of fruits, green leafy vegetables, seasonal vegetables and whole cereals.
- Take frequent but small meals.
- Take plenty of fluids and semi-solids. Avoid fried foods. Reduce total fats, salts and refined carbohydrates.
- Avoid fasting.

RECIPES FOR THE ELDERLY

As the age advances, old people have some problems of chewing foods and digestion, sometime the elderly people are forced to live on their own and cook their own food, hence they need some simple but nutritious recipes to maintain good health, the recipes have been formulates as they should be a nutrition supplement on a minimal, easy to cook, involve minimal time for cooking or no cooking, ready to eat as and when necessary (Table 11.10).

NORMAL DIET

A normal diet is used for most of the patients who are permitted to eat without any restriction in respect of the type and amount of food. Such a diet is known by various names—regular, general or full diet. However, for most acute illnesses, the consistency of the diet is modified to either soft or liquid, depending upon the tolerance of the patient (Tables 11.11, 11.12).

SOFT DIET

This diet is soft in texture, low in residue, easily digested, and well tolerated. It provides the essential nutrients in the form

Table 11.10: Recipes for the elderly	
Easy to cook foods	*Ready to store foods*
Sweet dalia	Besan ladoo/barfi
Sevian	Coconut ladoo
Curd chirwa	Chirwa
Savianupma	Paushtic barfi (atta + besan + peanuts + gur + ghee)
Sujiupma	Panjiri (atta + besan + drynuts)
Poha	Chikki (til + peanut)
Stuffed Prantha	Biscuits
Curd salad (with boiled vegetables)	Cakes
Dalia pulao	Roasted dalia, suji, chidwa to make porridge.
Sujikheer	
Rice kheer/phirni	
Khichri	
Cheela (veg)	
Suji/atta/Besan halwa	
Dalia khichri	
Bajra khichri	
Pongal sweet	

Table 11.11: Menu for normal diet	
Food items	*Amount (gm)*
Atta/rice	300 gm
Bread	60 gm
Dal	50 gm
Vegetable	300 gm
Potatoes	100 gm
Fruit	One portion (100 gm)
Milk	650 ml
Fat	20
Sugar	30
Butter	10
Approx nutritive value	
Calories	2279 kcal
Protein	72 gm
Fat	49 gm
Carbohydrate	384 gm

Table 11.12: Detailed menu

Meal	Menu	Amount (gm)
Early morning	Tea	1 cup
Breakfast	Milk	250 ml (1 glass)
	Bread omllete/butter	2 slice
	Fruit	One
Lunch	Chapatti	100 gm (4 chapatti)
	Rice	50 gm
	Dal	25 gm
	Curd	75 gm
	Seasonal vegetable	150 gm
	Potato	50 gm
Evening Tea	Tea	1 cup
Dinner	Chapatti	100 gm (4 chapatti)
	Rice	50 gm
	Dal	25 gm
	Curd	75 gm
	Seasonal vegetable	150 gm
	Potato	50 gm

of liquids and semisolid foods, such as milk, fruit, juices, eggs, cheese, custards and puddings, strained soups and vegetables, rice, boiled or baked potatoes, wheat, corn, or rice cereals, and breads.

Omitted are raw fruits and vegetables, coarse breads and cereals, rich desserts, strong spices, all fried foods, nuts, and raisins. It is commonly recommended for people who have GI disturbances or acute infections and those unable to tolerate a normal diet.

This diet is modified in consistency only to facilitate chewing, swallowing and/or digestion. Foods used may be modified variedly depending on your condition (Tables 11.13. to 11.15).

Liquid Diet for COPD Patients

Liquid diet or fluid diets are used in febrile states, or whenever the patient is unable to

Table 11.13: Menu for semi-solid diet

Food items	Amount (gm)
Rice/dalia	200 gm
Bread	120 gm
Dal	100 gm
Vegetable	300 gm
Potatoes	100 gm
Fruit	One portion (100 gm)
Milk	625 ml
Fat	20
Sugar	30
Butter	10
Butter	10
Approx nutritive value	
Calories	2290 kcal
Protein	69 gm
Fat	49 gm
Carbohydrate	388 gm

Table 11.14: Detailed menu

Meal	Menu	Amount (gm)
Early morning	Tea	1 cup
Breakfast	Milk	250 ml (1 glass)
	Bread omllete/butter	2 slice
	Fruit	One
Lunch	Rice	100 gm
	Dal	50 gm
	Curd	75 gm
	Seasonal vegetable	150 gm
	Potato	50 gm
Evening tea	Tea	1 cup
	Bread	60 gm (2 slice)
Dinner	Rice	100 gm
	Dal	50 gm
	Curd	75 gm
	Seasonal vegetable	150 gm
	Potato	50 gm

Table 11.15: Options for semi-liquid/soft diet in COPD

Khichri (plain)	Sheera (besan/atta)	Khichri kanji	Idli
Veg khichri	Milk shakes (Banana/mango)	Raita (boondi/ vegetable/bathua)	Cornflakes with milk
Sweet dalia with milk	Sweet sago	Semia	Oats with milk
Rice kheer	Milk with supplements	Lassi	Bread with milk
Phirni	Badam milk	Sujisheera	Fresh paneer
Sabudana kheer	Mashed vegetable	Sharbat milk	Custard
Suji kheer	Mashed potato	Sweet sattu	Poha with curd
Custard with milk	Dal soup	Upma	

tolerate solid food. These diets are used for patients requiring easily digested foods which are free from mechanical and chemical irritants. The degree of nutritional adequacy of these diets will depend upon the type of liquids permitted (Table 11.16).

- Quantity to be khichri feed (200 ml)
  1. Cooked khichri—2 tbsp (30 gm)
  2. Cooked soft dal—2 tbsp (30 gm)
  3. Soft vegetables—2 tbsp (30 gm) (ghiya, tori, tinda, pumpkin)
  4. Oil—1 tsp.

Table 11.16: Menu for liquid diet

Timing	Feeds
6 am	Lukewarm water + Supplement
8 am	Milk/high protein feed
10 am	Soup
12 noon	Coconut water/lassi/roohafza water/rice kanji
2 pm	Khichri feed (dal + veg + rice + salt + 1 tsp.oil)
4 pm	Milk—thin custard/milk shake/fruit shake
6 pm	Soup
8 pm	Khichri feed
10 pm	Milk/high protein feed

- Quantity to be high protein feed (1 Lt)
  1. Milk—1 L
  2. Sugar—50 gm
  3. Arrowroot powder—25 gm
  4. Egg—1 no.

Instructions for Feed

- All feeds should be mashed and strained properly.
- No spices should be added, only salt and turmeric can be used.
- Quantity of feeds should be measured.
- Feeds are to be given at lukewarm temperature.
- Consistency of the feed should be checked it should not be thick as it may clog the tube.
- Timings specified for the feeds should be followed accurately.
- All feeds should be hygienically made.

CONCLUSION

Dietary intake appears to be important in both the development and management of respiratory diseases, shown through epidemiological and cross-sectional studies and supported by mechanistic studies in animal models. Although more evidence is needed from intervention studies in humans, there is a clear link for some nutrients and dietary patterns.

The dietary patterns associated with benefits in respiratory diseases include high fruit and vegetable intake, Mediterranean style diet, fish and omega-3 intake, while fast food intake and westernized dietary patterns have adverse associations.

Dietary counselling for COPD patients is still at the beginning as compared to other chronic degenerative diseases like diabetes, cardiac, hypertensive to comply information from various texts is also minimum. Special efforts has to take for planning a diet for different stages of COPD and further research is required in nutritional and dietary management for COPD patients.

REFERENCES

1. Michael J, Gibney, Marinos Elia, Olle L. jungqvist and Julie Dowsell. Clinical Nutrition 2nd edition. The Nutrition Society Textbook series. Blackwell Publishing, 2005; 239–42.
2. Srivastava RK, Tiwari BK, Agarwal Y. Current Nutritional Therapy Guidelines in Clinical Practice. Directorate General of Health Services, Government of India, 2008; 215.
3. Mahan K and Escott-Stump S. Krause's Food and Nutrition Therapy. 12th Edition. Saunders Elsevier, 2008; 903.
4. Khanna Kumud, Gupta Sharda. Textbook of Nutrition and Dietetics 2nd ed. Department of Food and Nutrition. Institute of Home Economics. University of Delhi, 2016; 28, 202, 168–70.
5. David L, Katz Rachel SC. Friedman. Nutrition in Clinical Practice. A comprehensive, evidence-based manual for the practitioner. 2nd ed. 2010; 214–17.
6. Chin R Jr, Haponik EF. Nutrition, respiratory function, and disease. In: Shils ME, Olson JA, Shike M, eds. Modern nutrition in health and disease, 8th ed. Philadelphia: Lea & Febiger 1994.

7. Cano NJ, Roth H, Court-Ortune I, et al. Nutritional depletion in patients on long-term oxygen therapy and/or home mechanical ventilation. Eur Respir J 2002; 20: 30–7.

8. Cote CG. Surrogates of mortality in chronic obstructive pulmonary disease. Am J Med 2006; 119: 54–62.

9. Vermeeren MAP, Schols AMWJ, Wouters EFM. Effects of an acute exacerbation on nutritional and metabolic profile of patients with COPD. Eur Respir J 1997; 10: 2264.

10. Agusti A, Morla M, Sauleda J, et al. NF-kappa β activation and iNO Supregulation in skeletal muscle of patients with COPD and low body weight. Thorax 2004; 59: 483–87 .

11. Pezza M, Iermano C, Tufano R . Nutritional support for the patient with chronic obstructive pulmonary disease. Monaldi Arch Chest Dis 1994; 49: 33.

12. Goldstein – shapes SA. Nutritional treatment in chronic respiratory failure: the effect of macronutrient on metabolism and ventilation. Monaldi Arch Chest Dis 1993; 48: 535.

13. Silverman EK, Speizer FE. Risk factors for the development of chronic obstructive pulmonary disease. Med Clin North Am 1996; 80: 501.

14. Schols AMWJ. Nutrition and outcome in chronic respiratory disease. Nutrition 1997; 150: 1569–74.

15. Nathens AB. Neff MJ, Jurkovich GJ, et al. Randomized, prospective trial of antioxidant supplementation in critically ill surgical patients. Ann Surg 2002; 236: 814–22.

16. McKeever TM, Britton J. Diet and asthma. Am J Respire Crit Care Med 2004; 170: 725–29.

17. Burney P. The origins of obstructive airway disease. A role for diet ? Am J Respire Crit Care Med 1995; 151: 1292.

18. Fiaccadori E, Coffrini E, Fracchia C, et al. Hyphophasphatemia and phosphorus deletion in respiratory and peripheral muscles of protein with respiratory failure due to COPD. Chest 1994; 105: 1392–8.

19. Soutar A, Seaton A, Brown K. Brochinal reactivity and dietary antioxidants. Thorax 1997; 52: 166.

20. Hatch GE. Asthma, inhaled oxidants, and dietary antioxidant. Am J Clin Nutr 1995; 61: 625s.

21. Fogarty A, Lewis SA, Scrivener SL, et al. Oral magnesium and vitamin C supplement in asthma: a parallel group randomized placebo-controlled trial. Clin Exp Allergy 2003; 33: 1355–59.

22. Ram FS, Rower BH, Kaur B. Vitamin C supplementation for asthma. Cochrane Database Syst Rev 2004; 3: CD000993.

23. Silverman RA, Osborn H, Runge J, et al. IV magnesium sulfate in the treatment of acute severe asthma: a multicentre, randomized controlled trial. Chest 2002; 122: 1870.

24. Hughes R, Goldkorn A, Masoli M, et al. Use of isotonic nebulized magnesium sulphate as an adjuvant to salbutamol in treatment of severe asthma in adults: randamozed placebo-controlled trial. Lancet 2003; 361: 2114–7.

25. Woods RK, Thein FC, Abramson MJ, Dietary marine fatty acids (fish oil) for asthma in adults and children. Cochrane Database Syst Rev 2002; 3: CD001283.

26. Varraso R, Fung TT, Barr RG, Hu FB, Willett, W. Camargo, CAJ Prospectivctive study of dietary patterns and chronic obstructive pulmonary disease among US women. Am. J. Clin. Nutr. 2007, 86, 488–95.

27. Saadeh D, Salameh P, Baldi I, Raherison C. Diet and allergic disease among population aged 0 to 18 years: Myth or reality? Nutrients 2013, 5, 3399–423.

28. Willett WC Sacks F, Trichopoulou, A, Drescher G, Ferro-Luzzi, A, Helsing, E, Trichopolulos, D. Mediterranean diet pyramind: A cultural model for healthy eating. Am. J. Clin. Nutr. 1995, 61, 1402S–1406S.

29. Wood LG, Gibson PG, Dietary factors leads to innate immune activation in asthma. Pharmacol. Ther. 2009, 123, 37–53.

30. Varraso R, Kauffmann F, Leynaert B, Le Moual N, Boutron–Ruault, M.C, Clavel-Chapelon, F, Romieu, I. Dietary patterns and asthma. In the E3N study. Eur. Respir. J. 2009, 33, 33–41.

31. Wood LG, Gibson, PG A high fat challenge increase airway inflammation and impairs bronchodilator recovery in asthma. J. Allergy Clin. Immunol. 2011, 127, 1133–40.

32. Wood LG, Gibson, PG, Garg, ML Biomarkers of lipid peroxidation, airway inflammation and asthma. Eur. Respir. J. 2003, 21, 177–86.

33. Kelly FJ. Vitamins and respiratory disease: Antioxidant micronutrient in pulmonary health and disease. Proc. Nutr. Soc. 2005, 64, 510–26.

34. Tanaka T, Takahashi R, Flavonoids and asthma. Nutrient 2013, 5, 2128–43.

35. Manach C, Scalbert A, Morand C, Remesy C, Jimenez L. Polyphenols: Food sources and bioavailability. Am. J. Clin.2004, 79, 727–747.

36. Castro M, King TS, Kunselman SJ, Cabana MD, Denlinger L, Holguin F, Kazani SD, Moore, WC, Moy, J, Sorkness, CA, et al. Effect of vitamin D_3 On asthma treatment failures in adults with symptomatic asthma and lower vitamin D levels: The VIDA randomized clinical trial. JAMA 2014, 311, 2083–91.

37. Janssens W, Bouillon R, Claes B, Carremas C, Lehouck A, Buysschaert I, Coolen J, Mathieu C, Decramer M, Lambrechts, D. Vitamin D deficiency is highly prevalent in COPD and correlates with variants in the vitamin D–binding gene. Thorax 2010, 65, 215–20.

38. Black PN, Scragg R. Relationship between serum 25-hydroxyvitamin D and pulmonary function survey. Chest 2005, 128, 3792–8.

39. Persson LJ, Aanerud M, Hiemstra PS, Hardie JA, Bakke PS, Eagan, t.m. Chronic obstructive pulmonary disease is associated with low levels of vitamin D. PloS One 2012, 7, e389334.

40. Mathew R, Altura B. The role of magnesium in lung disease: Asthma, allergy, and pulmonary hypertension. Magnes.Trace Elem. 1991, 10, 220–8.

41. Andersson I, Gronberg A, Slinde F, Bosaeus I, Larsson S. Vitamin and mineral status in elderly patients with chronic obstructive pulmonary disease. Clin. Respir. J. 2007, 1, 23–9.

42. Franseen FM, O"Donnell DE, Goossens, GH, Bllaak, EE, Schols AM. obesity and the lung: 5. obesity and COPD. Thorax 2008, 63, 1110–17.

43. Bianco A, Mazzarella G, Turchiarelli V, Nigro, E, Corbi, G, Scudiero, O, Sofia, M, Daniele, A. Adiponectin: An attractive marker for metabolic disorders in chronic obstructive pulmonary disease (COPD). Nutrient 2013, 5, 4115–522.

44. Itoh M, Tsuji T, Nemoto K, Nakamura H, Aoshiba K. Undernutrition in patients with COPD and its treatment. Nutrients 2013, 5, 1316–35.

45. Hallin R, Koivisto-Hursti, UK, Linberg E, Janson C. Nutritional status, dietary energy intake and the risk of exacerbations in patients with chronic obstructive pulmonary disease (COPD). Respire. Med. 2006, 100, 561–7.

46. Gronberg AM, Slinde F, Engstrom CP, Hulthen L, Larsson S. Dietary problems in patients with severe chronic obstructive disease. J. Hum. Nutr. Diet. 2005, 18, 445–52.

47. Wilson DO, Donahoe M, Rogers RM, Pennock BE. Metabolic rate and weight loss in chronic obstructive lung disease. J. Parenter. Enter. Nutr. 1990, 14, 7–11.

48. Gan WQ, Man, SF, Senthilselvan A, Sin DD. Association between chronic obstructive pulmonary disease and systemic inflammation: A systematic review and a meta-analysis. Thorax 2004, 59, 574–80.

49. Orlander J, Kiessling KH, Larsson L. Skeletal muscles metabolism, morphology and function in sedentary smokers and nonsmokers, Acta Physical. Scand.1979, 107, 39–46.

50. Kok MO, Hoekstra T, Twisk J.W.R. The Longitudinal Relation between Smoking and Muscles Strength in Healthy Adults. Eur. Addict. Res. 2012, 18, 70–5.

51. Zhou, L, Yuan, C, Zhang, J, Yu, R, Huang, M, Adcock, I.M, Yao, X. Circulating Leptin Concentrations in Patients with Chronic Obstructive Pulmonary Disease: A systematic Review and Meta-Analysis. Respiration 2014, 86, 512–22.

52. Singh S, Soumya M, Saini A, Mittal V, Singh UV, Singh V. Breath carbon monoxide levels in different forms of smoking. *Indian J Chest Dis Allied Sci* 2011; 53: 25–8.

Physiotherapy and Yoga

VG Prabhu Ramnath

INTRODUCTION

COPD is a progressive disease with poor prognosis.[1] At severe stages treatment options are limited and oxygen supplement and bronchodilators, which are the only treatment modality that prolongs survival.[2] With disease advancement, comorbidities and recurrent exacerbations make a patient disabled. Decreased activity is an independent predictor of mortality in COPD.[3]

The aim of physiotherapy is to break this vicious cycle and help the COPD patients to participate in daily activity. Even in normal lungs exercise results in tenfold improvement in performance. Similarly a patient with chronic obstructive pulmonary disease (COPD) who is unable to walk 100 metres can be trained under physiotherapy to walk greater distances and perform tasks which he could not do previously. Exercise training has been shown to reduce disability in many chronic respiratory diseases.[4, 5] Pulmonary rehabilitation is an essential component of care for patients with chronic lung disease. Pulmonary rehabilitation is defined as an evidence based, multidisciplinary, and comprehensive intervention for patients with chronic respiratory diseases who are symptomatic and often have decreased daily activities. Integrated into the individualized treatment of the patient, pulmonary rehabilitation is designed to reduce symptoms,

optimise functional status, increase participation, and reduce healthcare costs through stabilizing or reversing systemic manifestations of the disease. Pulmonary rehabilitation aims to restore patients to an independent, productive and satisfying life and prevent further clinical deterioration to the maximum extent compatible with the stage of the disease. This goal may be accomplished, without materially improving lung function, by helping the patients to become more aware of their disease, more actively involved in their own healthcare and more independent in performing daily care activities, attempting to reverse the disability from disease.

Components of comprehensive pulmonary rehabilitation

Patient assessment

Education

Exercise training

Psychosocial and behavioural support

Nutritional support

Outcome assessment

BREATHING TECHNIQUES

Breathing training techniques means learning techniques that decrease the work of inhalation and exhalation. Pursed lip breathing and diaphragmatic breathing are the two breathing techniques which helps to lessen the breathlessness during exercise and other daily activities.

Pursed Lip Breathing (Fig.12.1)

Inhaling through the nose and exhaling through pursed lips makes breathing easier. First we should relax our neck and shoulder muscles, inhale slowly through our nose for at least 2 counts. Then pucker the lips as if to blow out a candle and then exhale slowly and gently through pursed lips for at least twice as long as we inhaled. Pursed lip breathing involves active expiration against resistance.[6] Resistance may be provided at a level of lips or tongue and a whistling is produced during expiration.[7] Pursed lip breathing improves ventilation, releases trapped air in the lungs, keeps the airways open longer and decreases the work of breathing and prolongs exhalation to slow the breathing rate. This procedure reduces respiratory rate and improves tidal volume.[8] Other theories are alteration in respiratory muscle recruitment,[9] and development of positive pressure in the airways during breathing, thereby preventing dynamic airway collapse.[10]

Diaphragmatic Breathing (Fig. 12.2)

It is known that diaphragmatic dysfunction is an important deleterious consequence of the progression of the severity of COPD. With the increase in airflow resistance, air trapping and hyperinflation in this disease, the inspiratory muscles are passively shortened and placed at a mechanical disadvantage. Therefore, a progressive reduction occurs in the mobility of the diaphragm and in its relative contribution to thoraco-abdominal movements, and as a compensatory mechanism, there is a greater

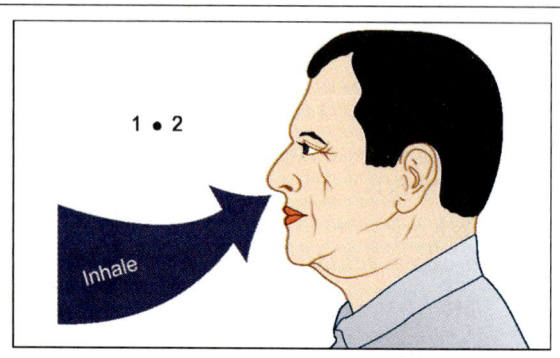

Inhale through nose with slow counting of 1 and 2

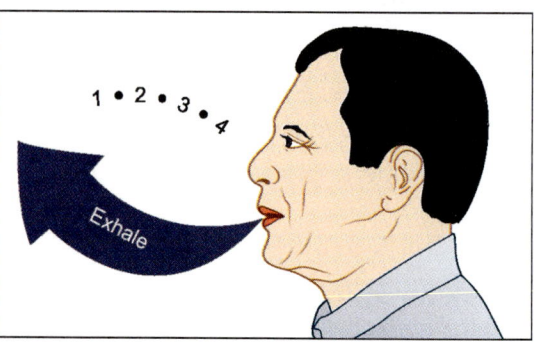

Exhale through mouth with puckered lips with slow counting of 1, 2, 3, 4

Fig. 12.1: Pursed lip breathing

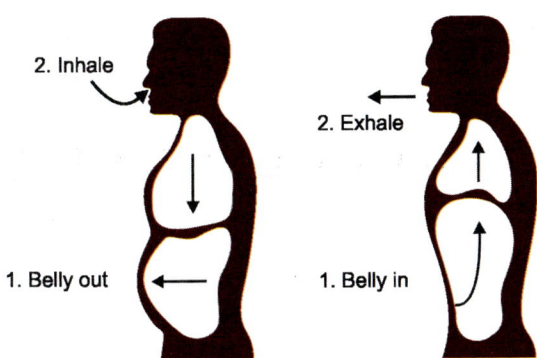

2. Inhale

2. Exhale

1. Belly out

1. Belly in

Fig. 12.2: Diaphragmatic breathing

recruitment of respiratory muscles of the rib cage. In this context, both the reduction in diaphragm mobility and the greater activity of the rib cage respiratory muscles are associated with the increase in dyspnoea and intolerant to physical exercise. To reduce or minimize these alterations, diaphragmatic breathing is found useful for improving diaphragmatic mobility and thereby reducing the deleterious effect of diaphragmatic dysfunction.

We should learn to breathe with diaphragm, because by using only one muscle to breath we will use only less energy. For this we must sit or lie on our back and inhale slowly through our nose. As we inhale our stomach should move out. Breathe out through pursed lips and as we exhale we should feel our stomach move in. The possible mechanism of action of this method is altered respiratory muscle recruitment and reduction in respiratory frequency.[11] Diaphragmatic breathing is most helpful when used for at least 20 minutes two to three times daily.

EXERCISES

It has been observed that around 30% of muscle mass gets wasted in an average COPD patient.[12] Poor muscle mass leads to early fatigue and decrease exercise tolerance. Exercise training replaces type 2 muscle fibres (fast, fatigable, low oxidative) with type 1 fibres (slow, fatigue resistant, high oxidative).[13] Thus exercise training builds up muscle mass and strength. It has been known to improve health related quality of life measures, increases exercise capacity and reduces symptoms of breathlessness. Exercise also has psychosocial benefits with reduced prevalence of depression.[14]

Usually patients of COPD with severe breathlessness interfering with daily activity, decreased tolerance to exercise and patients in pre-operative period are suitable candidate for physiotherapy programme. Some guidelines refer patients with MRC breathlessness scale of more than III.[15] However, one study observed benefit in COPD patients of any GOLD stage.[16]

Patients should work toward a goal of 30–60 minutes of exercise, most days of the week. And make exercise as a part of their daily routine. While doing exercise breathlessness is acceptable as long as they can talk and are in control of their breathing. If they have increased breathlessness, exercise should be slowed down. And if it continues exercise should be stopped immediately. Oxygen if prescribed should be used during exercise.

Contraindications to exercise: Patients with recent myocardial infarction (within past 3 months), unstable angina, uncontrolled hypertension, debilitating arthritis, congestive heart failure and peripheral vascular disease are not suitable for physiotherapy exercise.[17]

Training programmes of longer duration have been known to produce more benefits as compared to shorter duration programmes. Training sessions of at least three sessions per week are followed. Minimum of 6–8 weeks duration of programme is followed. Training of less than 6 weeks duration is of less benefit.[18]

Types of Exercises

Endurance or Aerobic Exercises

Endurance exercises help to condition our muscles and improve the function of our lungs and heart. These are aerobic exercises, meaning they help our body use oxygen better and over time they will help to have more energy and less breathlessness. Riding a stationary bicycle (Fig. 12.3), using a treadmill (Fig. 12.4) and home walking programme are endurance exercises.

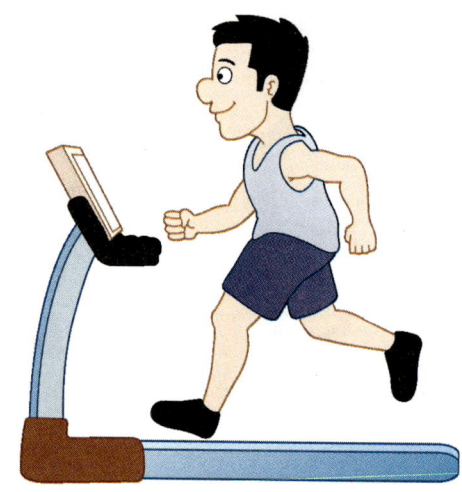

Fig. 12.4: Using a treadmill

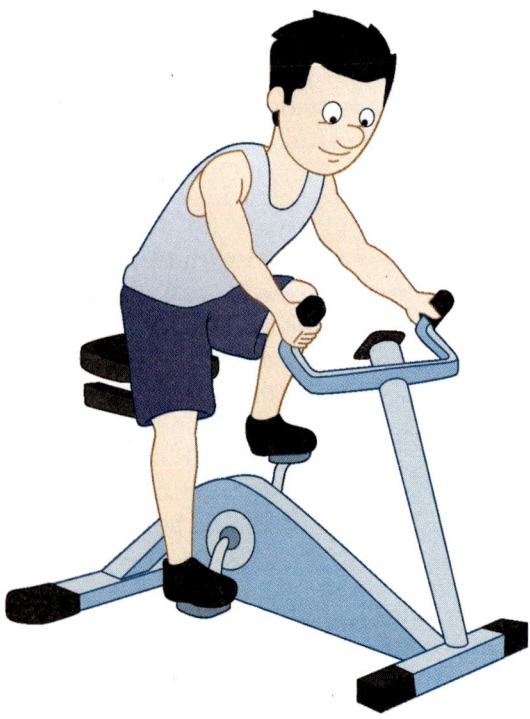

Fig. 12.3: Riding a stationary bicycle

Riding a stationary bicycle, adjust the seat so their knees are only slightly bend when the pedals are at their lowest point. Begin to pedal at a comfortable pace. Do pursed lip breathing while peddling.

Start walking at a comfortable pace. Do pursed lip breathing while walking.

Home walking program: Patient should start walking slowly up to their normal rate.

Then rate should be increased if possible. When they are ready to work harder, begin to walk a small incline or hill. Do pursed lip breathing while walking.

Strengthening or Resistance Exercises

Strengthening or resistance exercise helps build muscles, improves strength and maintain bone health. Building muscle strength will allow us to do many activities with less effort. As a result we may find that we are more active but have less breathlessness. Biceps curl (Fig. 12.5), side lift (Fig. 12.6), leg raise (Fig. 12.7), lifting weights and working with stretchy resistant bands (Fig. 12.8) are good way to increase strength.

Stand or sit with a weight in each hand. Keep the arm very close to the sides, with palm facing forward and inhale. Exhale slowly as bending our arms and lift the weight to shoulder level. Inhale while slowly returning to the starting position.

Stand straight and hold on to the chart with one hand, inhale. Exhale as we lift our foot to the side. We need to lift it a few inches only. Keep the toes pointing forward. Hold the lift until we are finished exhaling. Inhale while bringing our leg back to our side. Then switch sides.

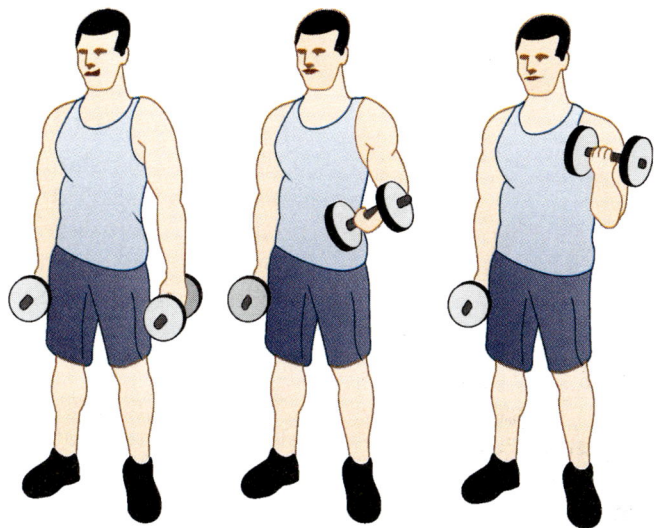

Fig. 12.5: Biceps curl

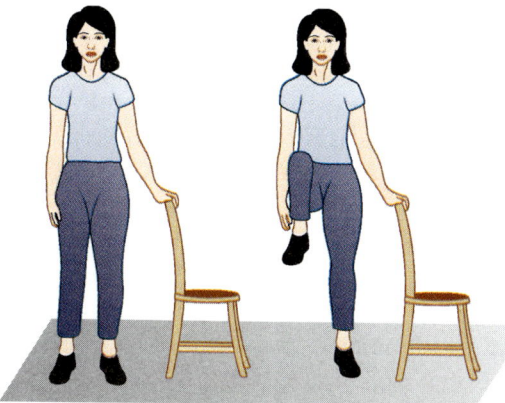

Fig. 12.6: Side lift

We should lie on our back, a mat and pillow may be kept to make comfortable. Bend one knee and keep the other leg straight. Inhale, then while exhaling we should lift our straight leg until our knees are lined up. Inhale while we lower our legs. Then switch legs.

Stand with feet slightly apart. Hold the both ends of the resistant band, and raise our hand to chest height. Exhale through pursed lips as we stretch the band outwards. Stop when we feel tension between our shoulder blades. Inhale, holding this position. Then

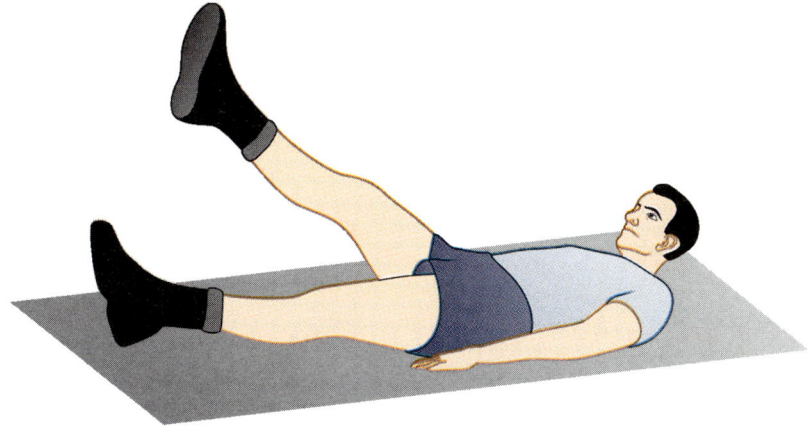

Fig. 12.7: Leg raise

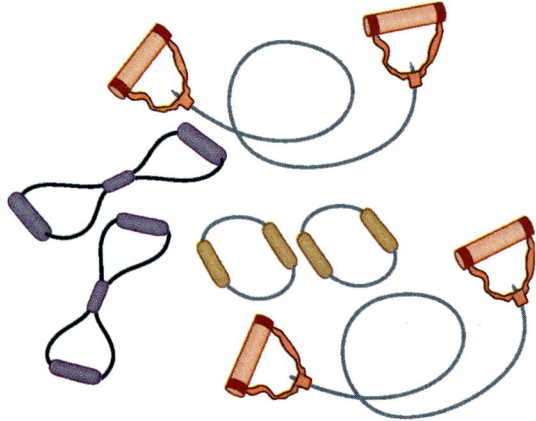

Fig. 12.8: Resistant bands

exhale as we squeeze our shoulder blades together. Inhale as we slowly return to the start position.

Flexibility Exercise or Stretching

Flexibility exercise or stretching help improve range of motion, posture and breathing. Stretching may also reduce muscle soreness cause by endurance or strengthening exercise. Head tilt (Fig. 12.9), shoulder rolls (Fig. 12.10), calf stretch (Fig. 12.11) and quadriceps stretch (Fig. 12.12) are flexibility exercises.

Sit or stand with relaxed shoulder, breath in. Slowly lower chin as we blow out. We will feel a stretch in the back of the neck. While inhaling return to starting position. Then exhale, slowly moving our head right and left as if we are saying no.

Stand with our shoulders relaxed. Put the hands on our shoulder, breath in. Slowly breathe out while rolling our shoulder forward. Continue until we are done exhaling, then relax the shoulder. Repeat the above step while rolling the shoulder backwards.

Stand facing the wall with our feet side by side. Put our arms out at shoulder level. Rest our hands against the wall with our elbow slightly bend, without pushing the wall. Do pursed lip breathing throughout this stretch. Step back with our left foot. Gently lower our heel to the floor. Keep our toes pointing forwards and our right knee slightly bend. We will feel the stretch in the back of our left calf. Hold the stretch for 15–30 seconds while doing pursed lip breathing. Return to the starting position, repeat the stretch using our right leg.

Stand holding on to a study chair for balance, inhale. While exhaling, reach back and grasp the ankle that is farthest from the chair. Pull our leg back until our knees line up. Keep our hips facing forward and our knees pointed towards the floor. We will feel

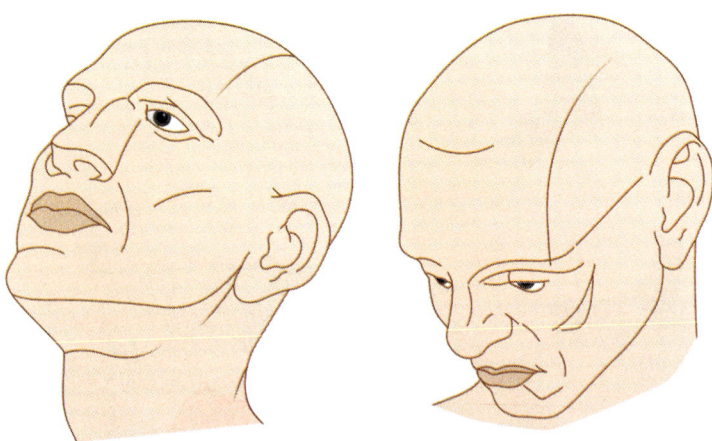

Fig. 12.9: Head tilt

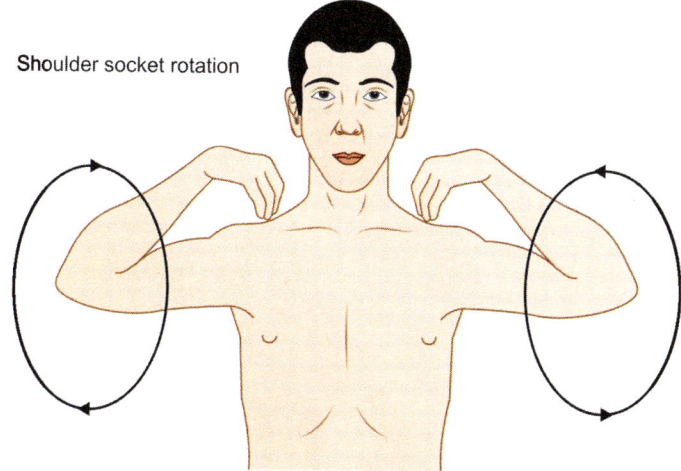

Shoulder socket rotation

Fig. 12.10: Shoulder roll

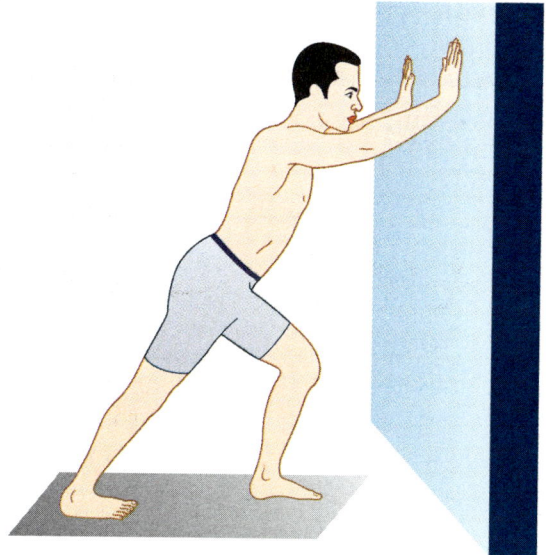

Fig. 12.11: Calf stretch

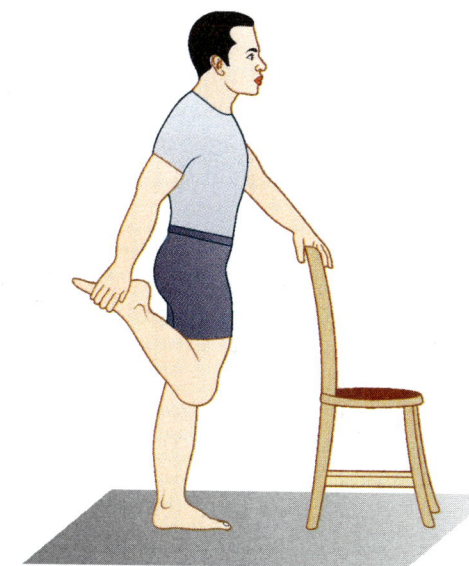

Fig. 12.12: Quadriceps stretch

the stretch in our thigh. Hold until we finish exhaling. Then inhale while slowly lowering our legs. Then turn and grasp the chair with our other hand, repeat the stretch with our other leg.

Inspiratory Muscle Training

Inspiratory muscle training can be used as an adjunct to aerobic and resistant exercises. The rationale behind the use of inspiratory muscle training is that patients with COPD have weak respiratory muscle.[19] There are three types of inspiratory muscle training, namely isocapnic hyperventilation, inspiratory threshold loading and inspiratory resistive loading. The use of inspiratory muscle training has been shown to increase inspiratory muscle strength and endurance, improve exercise capacity, improve quality of life, and decrease breathlessness in patients with stable COPD.[20] Results of various studies with the above three techniques are inconclusive with no distinct advantage of one technique over the other.

Acute Exacerbation

Acute exacerbation of COPD is characterised by increased cough, sputum volume and sputum purulence. Physiotherapy plays an integral role in the treatment of people with exacerbation of COPD, with high level evidence that physiotherapy can aid recovery and prevent recurrences. Physiotherapy frequently used are breathing exercises to relieve dyspnoea, improve thoraco-abdominal coordination and enhance functional capacity. Commonly used technique are pursed lip breathing, diaphragmatic breathing and airway clearance techniques. Airway clearance technique involves application of physical forces to enhance removal of sputum from the airway.[21] Forced expiration technique (huffing), manual chest physiotherapy and positive pressure devices are commonly used airway clearance techniques. Despite their widespread use in clinical practice, evidence for important benefits of breathing exercise in acute exacerbation of COPD is scarce. Recent randomised controlled trials provide some evidence that breathing exercises may provide symptomatic relief in patients who are hospitalised with acute exacerbation of COPD. Patients who undertook twice daily sessions of controlled breathing consisting of relaxation exercises, pursed lip breathing and active expiration, had greater improvements in anxiety, depression and breathlessness than those who undertook usual care.[22]

YOGA IN COPD

Yoga denotes the union between the individual self and the transcendental self. The body's organ and systems are cleansed through asanas (postures) and pranayama (controlling the breath). The yoga training has a positive improvement effect on lung function and exercise capacity and can be used as an adjunct to pulmonary rehabilitation program for COPD patients.[23, 24] Studies have indicated an increase in tidal volume and FVC, reduction in respiratory rate, increase in FEV_1, $FEV_1\%$, maximum voluntary ventilation and breath holding capacity after short-term yoga practice.[25, 26] Further studies suggested that yoga training may improve exercise capacity, prevent lung function decline, improve quality of life, and reduce breathlessness in a patients with COPD.[27, 28] One meta-analysis suggested that yoga training that lasts from 12 weeks to 9 months may have beneficial effect in patients with COPD compared with conventional therapy.[29]

Standing mountain pose (*tadasana*) (Fig. 12.13): This straightforward pose

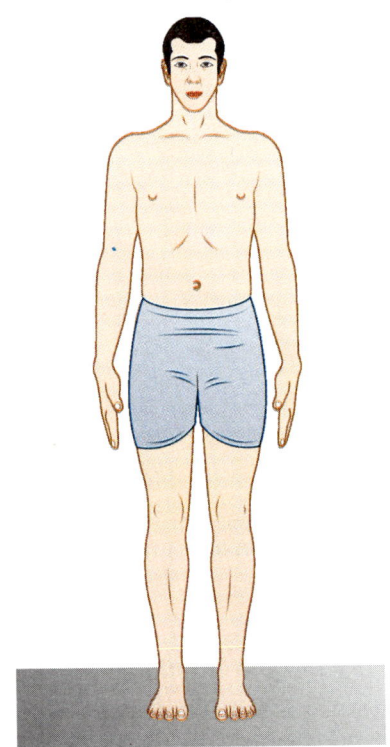

Fig. 12.13: Tadasana

requires us to stand tall to open up our chest. Arms can be raised or left at our sides.

Standing side bends (Chakrasana) (Fig. 12.14): These bends will help strengthen our diaphragm while also improving the flexibility of the rib cage.

Standing back bend (Anuvittasana) (Fig. 12.15): This pose also helps to open up the muscles of our chest but needs to be practised carefully to avoid muscle strain and breathlessness.

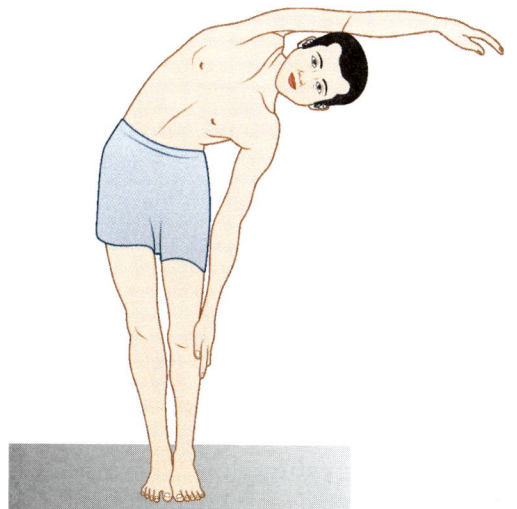

12.14: Chakrasana

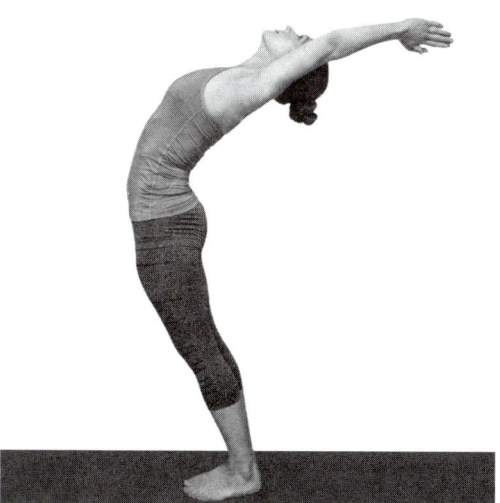

Fig. 12.15: Anuvittasana

Seated forward bends (*Paschimottanasana*) (Fig. 12.16): These pose help strengthen our respiratory system.

KEY POINTS

1. Physiotherapy consists of breathing techniques, exercises and clearing of secretions.
2. Breathing techniques include pursed lip breathing and diaphragmatic breathing.
3. Exercise training includes aerobic exercise, resistant training, flexibility exercise and inspiratory muscle training.
4. Aerobic exercise includes riding a stationary bicycle, using a treadmill and home walking program.
5. Resistant training includes biceps curl, side lift, leg raise and resistant bands.
6. Flexibility exercise includes head tilt, shoulder rolls, calf stretch and quadriceps stretch.
7. The yoga training can be used as an adjunct to pulmonary rehabilitation program for COPD patients.

SAMPLE EXERCISE PLAN FOR COPD PATIENTS

However, there is no sample plan available in literature to be prescribed in COPD patients. In the opinion of the author a simple sequence as suggested below can be prescribed initially in patients of COPD. This is pure arbitrary plan but in practical it works. As a practitioner one can modify according to the need of patient.

1 minute head tilt; 1 minute shoulder rolls; 1 minute calf stretch; 1 minute quadriceps stretch; 2 minutes riding a stationary bicycle; 2 minutes treadmill; 1 minute biceps curl; 1 minute side lift; 1 minute leg raise; 1 minute resistant bands.

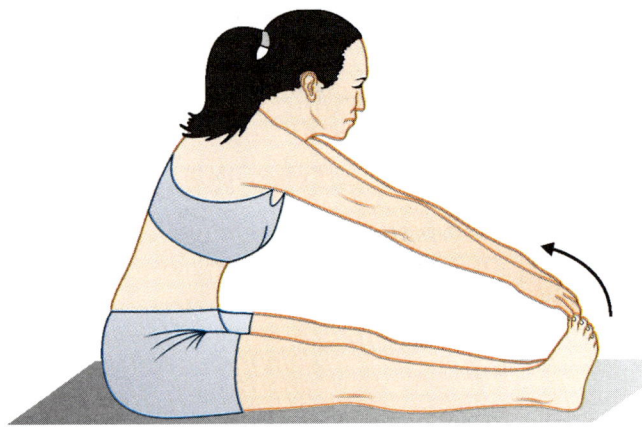

Fig. 12.16: *Paschimottanasana*

Rest for 10 seconds between exercises.

Initially all these exercises are done as one set later it can be done as two sets.

In general, to achieve maximum benefit, we should gradually work up to an exercise session lasting 20 to 30 minutes, at least three to four times a week.

Always breathe slowly to save our breath. Inhale through our nose, keeping our mouth closed. This warms and moisturizes the air we breathe and at the same time filters it. Exhale through pursed lips.

Rated Perceived Exertion (RPE) Scale

The RPE scale is used to measure the intensity of our exercise. The RPE scale runs from 0 to 10.

    0 – Nothing at all
    0.5 – Just noticeable
    1 – Very light
    2 – Light
    3 – Moderate
    4 – Somewhat heavy
    5 – Heavy
    6
    7 – Very heavy
    8
    9
    10 – Very, very heavy

In most cases we should exercise at a level that feels 3 (moderate) to 4 (somewhat heavy).

SUMMARY

Chronic obstructive pulmonary disease (COPD) is characterised by expiratory airflow obstruction, abnormalities in gas exchange, inspiratory muscle dysfunction and cardiac dysfunction. The motion of thorax is restricted due to hyperinflation and thereby capacity to increase tidal volume is limited which leads to activity limitation and breathlessness. Physiotherapy and yoga has been shown to benefit patients with chronic lung disease. Increase in exercise tolerance, reduction in breathlessness, improvement in health related quality of life and reduction of healthcare utilization are the benefits.

Physiotherapy consists of breathing techniques, exercises and clearing of secretions. Breathing techniques include pursed lip breathing and diaphragmatic breathing. Exercise training includes aerobic exercise, resistant training, flexibility exercise and inspiratory muscle training. Clearing of secretions is done by chest physiotherapy, controlled cough and forced expiration.

The current limited evidence suggests that yoga training has a positive effect on improving lung function and exercise capacity and could be used as an adjunct pulmonary rehabilitation programme in COPD patients. Despite the well-known benefits associated with this, physiotherapy is often underutilized. The inclusion of physiotherapy as a routine part of the overall care of a patient with COPD will results in improved patient care.

REFERENCES

1. Global initiative for chronic obstructive airway diseases. Global strategy for the diagnosis, management, and prevention of chronic obstructive pulmonary diseases. Updated 2007. MCR vision inc 2007; 2.
2. Nocturnal Oxygen Therapy Trial Group. Continuous or nocturnal oxygen therapy in hypoxemic chronic obstructive lung diseases: a clinical trial. Ann Intern Med 1980; 93: 391–8.
3. Yohannes AM, Baldwin RC, Connolly MJ. Predictors of 1 year mortality in patients discharged from hospital following acute exacerbation of chronic obstructive pulmonary disease. Age Aging 2005; 34: 491–6.
4. Singh V, Wisniewski A, Britton J, Tattersfield AE. Effect of yoga breathing exercises (pranayama) on airway reactivity in subjects with asthma. Lancet 1990; 335: 1381–83.
5. Singh V. Effect of respiratory exercises on asthma: The Pink City Lung Exerciser. J Asthma 1987; 24: 355–59.
6. Faling LJ. Pulmonary rehabilitation—physical modalities. Clin Chest Med 1986; 7: 599–18.
7. Rodenstein DO, Stanescu DC. Absence of nasal airflow during pursed lip breathing: the soft palate mechanism. Am rev Respir Dis 1983; 128: 716–18.
8. Mueller R, Petty F, Fiflev G. Ventilation and arterial blood gas changes induced by pursed lip breathing. J Appi Physiol 1970; 28: 784–89.
9. Breslin EH. The pattern of respiratory muscle recruitment during pursed lip breathing. Chest 1992; 101: 75–8.
10. Ingram RU, Schilder DP. Effect of pursed lips expiration on the pulmonary pressure flow relationship in obstructive lung disease. Am Rev Respir Dis 1967; 96: 381–88.
11. O Donnell DE, Webb K, Mcguire M. Controlling breathlessness and cough. In: Bourbeau J, Nault D, Borycki E. Chronic obstructive pulmonary disease. London: BC Decker Inc, 2002; 149–70.
12. Bernard S, Leblanc P, whittom F, et al. Peripheral muscle in patients with chronic obstructive airway disease. Am J Respir Crit Care Med 1998; 158: 629–34.
13. Howard H, Hoppeler H, Claasen H, et al. Influences of endurance training on the ultrastructural composition of the different muscle fibre types in human. Pflugers Arch 1985; 403: 369–76.
14. American college of chest physician/Americal association of cardiovascular and pulmonary rehabilitation guidelines panel. Pulmonary rehabilitation. Joint ACCP/AACVPR evidence based guidelines. Chest 1997; 112: 1363–96.
15. Berry MJ, Rejeski WJ, Adair NE, Zaccaro D. exercise rehabilitation and chronic obstructive pulmonary disease stage. Am J Respir Crit Care Med 1999; 160: 1248–53.
16. Maltais F, Hershfield ES, Stubbing D, et al. Exercise training in patients with COPD.In: Bourbeau J, Nault D, Borycki E, editors. Chronic obstructive pulmonary disease. London: BC Decker Inc, 2002; 185–214.
17. Green RH, Singh SJ, Williams J, Morgan MD. A randomised controlled trial of four weeks versus seven weeks of pulmonary rehabilitation in chronic obstructive pulmonary disease. Thorax 2001; 56: 143–45.
18. American Thoracic society/European Respiratory Society. Skeletal muscle dysfunction in chronic obstructive pulmonary disease: a statement of the Americal Thoracic Society and European Respiratory Society. Am J Respir Crit Care Med 1999; 159: S1–S40.
19. O Brien K, Geddes EL, Reid WD, Brooks D, Crowe J. Inspiratory muscle training compared with other rehabilitation interventions in chronic obstructive pulmonary disease. J Cardiopulm Rehabil 2008; 28(2): 128–41.
20. Holland AE, Button BM. Is there a role for airway clearance technique in chronic obstructive pulmnory disease? Chron Respir Dis 2006; 3(2); 83–91.
21. Valenza MC, Valenza-pena G, Torres-Sanchez I, Gonzalez-JimenezE, Conde-Valero A,

Valenza-Demet G. Effectiveness of controlled breathing techniques on anxiety and depression in hospitalized patients with COPD: a randomized clinical trial. Respir Care. 2014; 59(2): 109–15.

22. Tamdon Mk. Adjunct treatment with yoga in chronic severe airway obstruction. Thorax 1978; 33: 514–17.

23. Kulpati DD, Kamath RK, Chauhan MR. The influence of physical conditioning by yogasanas and breathing exercises in patients of chronic obstructive lung disease. J Assoc Physicians India 1982; 30: 865–68.

24. Makwana K, Khirwadkar N, Gupta HC. Effect of short term yoga practice on ventilator function tests. Indian J Physiol Pharmacol 1988; 32: 202–08.

25. Joshi LN, Joshi VD, Gokhale LV. Effect of short term pranayama practice on breathing rate and ventilator functions of lung. Indian J Physiol Pharmacol 1992; 36: 105–08.

26. Behera D. Yoga therapy in chronic bronchitis, J Assoc Physicians India 1998; 46: 207–8.

27. Fulambarker A, Farooki B, Kheir F, et al. Effect of yoga in chronic obstructive pulmonary disease. Am J Ther 2012; 19: 96–100.

28. Xun-Chao Liu, Lei Pan, Qing Hu, Wei-Ping Dong, Jun-Hong Yan, Liang Dong. Effects of yoga training in patients with chronic obstructive pulmonary disease: 1 systamatic review and meta analysis. J Thorac Dis 2014; 6(6): 795–802.

Prevention

Shiva Narang, Apoorva Tomar, Amit Kumar Verma

INTRODUCTION

The Global Initiative for Chronic Obstructive Lung Disease (GOLD) defined COPD as

"Chronic obstructive pulmonary disease (COPD), a common preventable and treatable disease, is characterized by persistent airflow limitation that is usually progressive and associated with an enhanced chronic inflammatory response in the airways and the lung to noxious particles or gases. Exacerbations and comorbidities contribute to the overall severity in individual patients." [1]

According to World Health Organization estimates, 6.5 crore people have moderate to severe COPD. It is estimated to be the third leading cause of death by 2030.[2]

Its prevalence is increasing each year and this rise is much faster in the developing world.

In India, non-communicable diseases accounted for 53% of all deaths and 44% of disability adjusted life years (DALYs) lost in 2005. Out of these chronic respiratory diseases estimated for 7% deaths and 3% DALYs lost.[3] According to crude estimates, 3 crore COPD patients estimated in India.[4] India also contributes a significant and growing percentage of COPD mortality estimated to be amongst the highest in the world, i.e. more than 64.7 estimated age standardized death rate per 100,000 amongst both sexes. This would translate into approximately 556,000 in case of India (>20%) out of a world total of 2,748,000 annually.[5]

An old proverb "Prevention is better than cure" still holds true for most of the chronic illness we encounter. Prevention can be primary, secondary and tertiary.

A. **Primary prevention:** One that strives to prevent the development of the disease and remains the most important step. It promotes the reduction or avoidance of personal exposure to common risk factors.

These risk factors are tobacco smoking, exposure to indoor pollution as well as outdoor pollution and occupation related risk factors.

B. **Secondary prevention:** It includes early detection by spirometry and screening of population, however, the cost effectiveness and implementation of the widespread screening is questionable. It also includes prevention and treatment of exacerbations.

C. **Tertiary prevention:** It involves the pulmonary rehabilitation.

ASSOCIATIONS OF COPD AND THEIR ROLE IN PREVENTION

Smoking Cessation and COPD

Tobacco smoking is associated with chronic obstructive pulmonary disease (COPD) in most of cases and its use should be strongly discouraged. Smoking cessation remains to be the most important intervention to decrease the progression of chronic obstructive pulmonary disease (COPD).[6] There is increased rates of FEV_1 decline in smokers and cessation leads to less steep rates of decline in pulmonary function.[7] Among the various studies conducted, smoking cessation provides numerous benefits to smokers suffering from disease such as improvement in symptoms of coughing and wheezing, decreasing frequency of COPD exacerbation and slows the decline in FEV_1 in COPD cases.

According to a Lung Health Study[8] conducted recruiting 5887 current smokers with mild to moderate COPD smoking cessation was associated with decrease in decline in FEV_1, hospitalisation and total mortality.

Participants in the special intervention group plus a placebo inhaler, who became sustained quitters, experienced a forced expiratory volume in one second (FEV_1) decline of only 34 ml/year. In contrast, those who continued to smoke experienced an FEV_1 decline of 63 ml/year[7]. Thus, smoking cessation nearly halved the rate of descent in FEV_1 in patients with mild to moderate COPD, female smokers experienced larger gains in lung function when they stopped smoking compared with male quitters (Fig. 13.1).

According to curve showing relation between lung age and smoking (Fig. 13.2) which has been plotted in between lung function FEV_1 (% of value at age 25) and age (years) conclusions drawn are that in chronic smokers rate of decline in FEV_1 with age is greater than in non-smokers and smokers at age of 52 years has FEV_1 equivalent to that of a 75 years old who has never smoked[9] (Fig. 13.2).

There have been several approaches towards smoking cessation to elaborate a few we have:

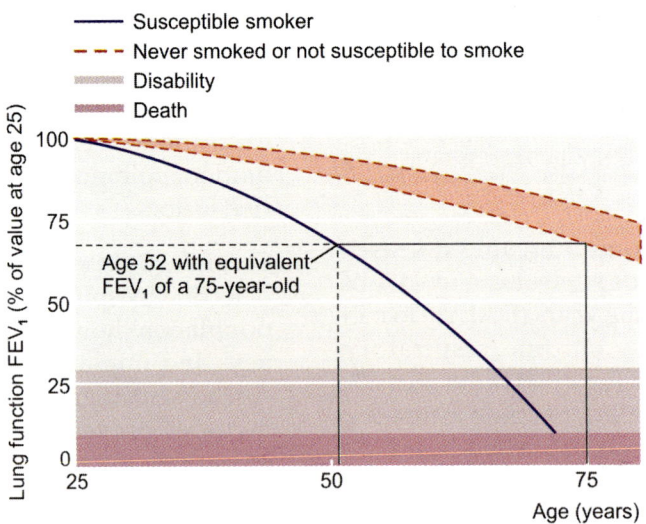

Fig. 13.1: Lung function against age graph (adapted from Fletcher and Peto)

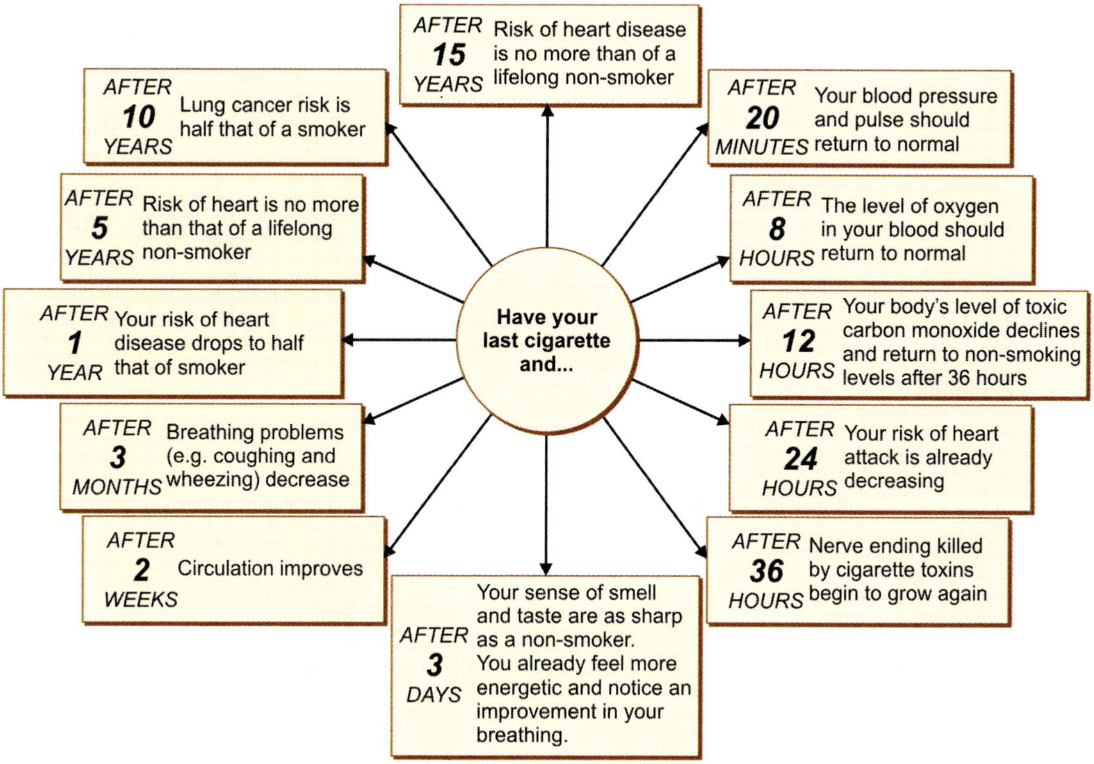

AFTER **15** YEARS Risk of heart disease is no more than of a lifelong non-smoker

AFTER **10** YEARS Lung cancer risk is half that of a smoker

AFTER **5** YEARS Risk of heart is no more than that of a lifelong non-smoker

AFTER **1** YEAR Your risk of heart disease drops to half that of smoker

AFTER **3** MONTHS Breathing problems (e.g. coughing and wheezing) decrease

AFTER **2** WEEKS Circulation improves

Have your last cigarette and...

AFTER **20** MINUTES Your blood pressure and pulse should return to normal

AFTER **8** HOURS The level of oxygen in your blood should return to normal

AFTER **12** HOURS Your body's level of toxic carbon monoxide declines and return to non-smoking levels after 36 hours

AFTER **24** HOURS Your risk of heart attack is already decreasing

AFTER **36** HOURS Nerve ending killed by cigarette toxins begin to grow again

AFTER **3** DAYS Your sense of smell and taste are as sharp as a non-smoker. You already feel more energetic and notice an improvement in your breathing.

Fig 13.2: Benefits of quitting smoking

Non-pharmacological

i. Initial approach towards smoking cessation (Fig. 13.3).[11]

- Ask—every patient, at every visit, about their tobacco usage status
- Advise—the smoking patient to quit
- Assess—the willingness to quit
- Assist—help them in quitting
- Arrange—for a follow-up

ii. If the patient is not willing to quit, "5 Rs" approach can be used to enhance motivation in your discussion:[11]

- Relevance—personal relevance of quitting
- Risks—ask for negative consequences of smoking
- Rewards—tell about rewards after quitting

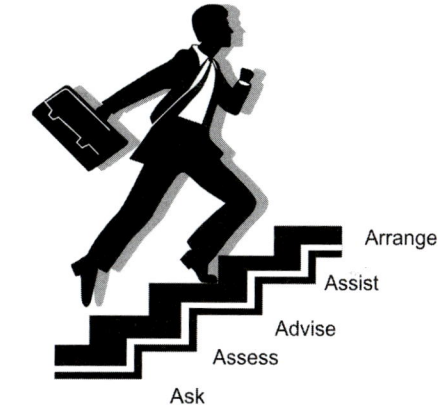

Arrange
Assist
Advise
Assess
Ask

Fig. 13.3: Approach towards smoking cessation

- Roadblocks or barriers toward quitting
- Repeat—Repeat the above process if patient is still unwilling to quit

iii. For those who are willing to quit, the 'STAR' approach (Fig. 13.4).

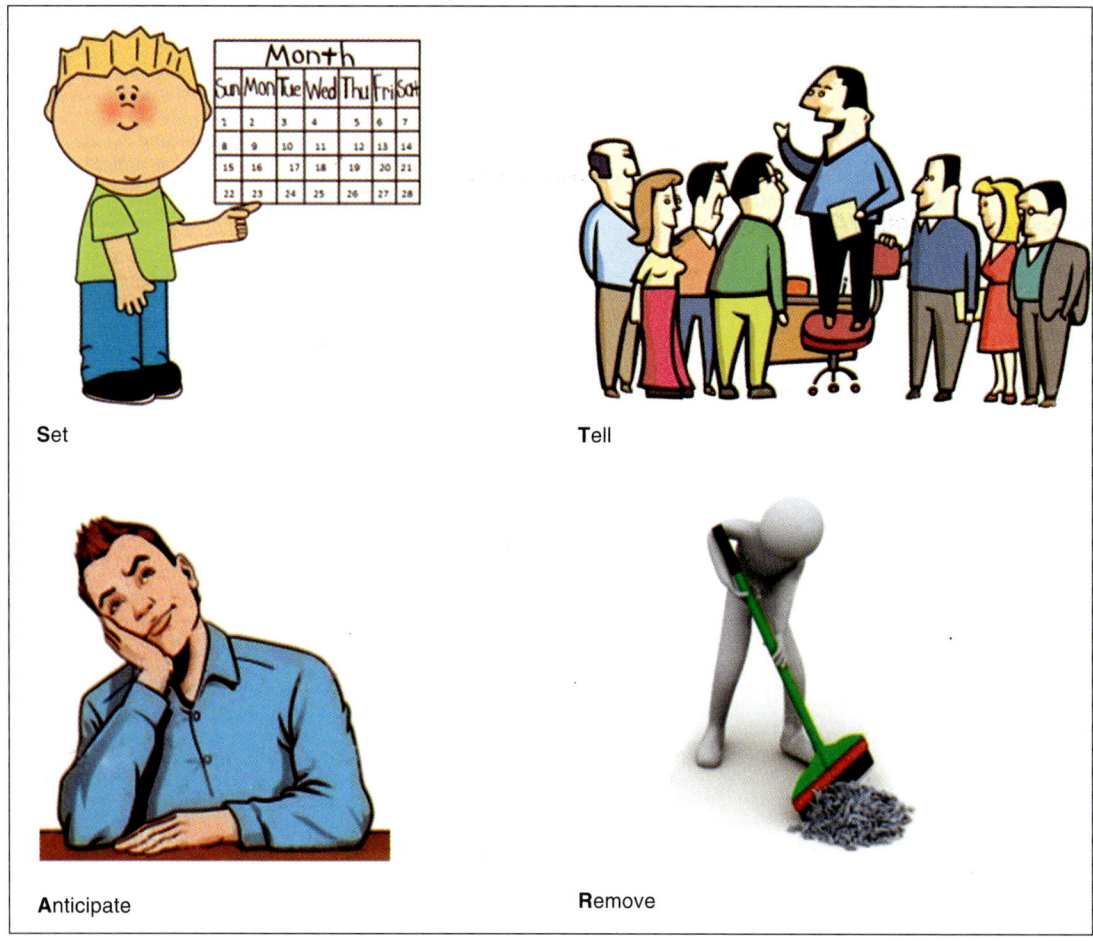

Set

Tell

Anticipate

Remove

Fig 13.4: STAR approach

- **S**et—a quit date
- **T**ell—tell the caregivers, family, friends and co-workers about quitting and request understanding and support and motivation.
- **A**nticipate—anticipate challenges to deal in future
- **R**emove—remove tobacco products from proximity

Pharmacological Therapy

i. **Nicotine replacement therapy (NRT):** The goal of NRT is to provide nicotine to a smoker without using tobacco, thereby relieving nicotine withdrawal symptoms as the smoker breaks the behaviour of cigarette smoking. Differences in the bioavailability of nicotine replacement products provide a rationale for combining NRT products to increase efficacy.[12] The long-acting, slow-onset nicotine patch (Fig. 13.5) is the primary NRT which helps to control baseline withdrawal symptoms.[13] Adding a short-acting form of NRT like lozenge, gum, inhaler or nasal spray helps to control cravings and withdrawal symptoms as and when needed and also enhances quit rates. Trials of NRT have reported to increase the chances of stopping smoking by 50% to 70% (Table 13.1).

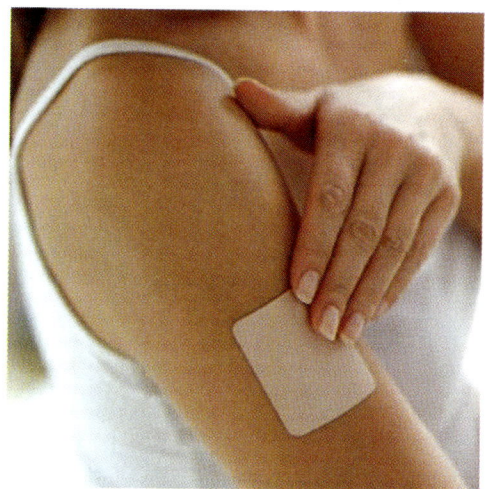

Fig. 13.5: Nicotine patch

ii. **Bupropion,** which was originally developed as an antidepressant, acts through blockade of neuronal reuptake of dopamine and norepinephrine and blockade of nicotinic acetylcholinergic receptors.[15, 16] It was the first non-nicotine medication found to be effective for smoking cessation.

- Bupropion is available as a starter pack of 30 tablets and a continuation pack of 90 tablets.
- The dose of bupropion is 150 mg once per day for the first 3 days
- And then increased to 150 mg twice per day.
- The patient should stop smoking in the second week of treatment.[17]

iii. **Varenicline,** is a non-nicotine medication that was approved by the FDA for the treatment of tobacco dependence. Its proposed mechanism of action is through a partial agonist action on $\alpha_4\beta_2$ nicotinic acetylcholine receptor in the nucleus accumbens of the brain and an antagonist to nicotine by preventing it from binding. Varenicline appeared to decrease the urge to smoke, withdrawal symptom.[18]

Dosage and Administration[17]

- Begin Chantix (varenicine) dosing one week before the date set by the patient to stop smoking or the patient can begin Chantix dosing and then quit smoking between days 8 and 35 of treatment.
- Starting week: 0.5 mg once daily on days 1–3 and 0.5 mg twice daily on days 4–7.
- Continuing weeks: 1 mg twice daily for a total of 12 weeks.
- An additional 12 weeks of treatment is recommended for successful quitters to increase likelihood of long-term abstinence.
- Renal impairment: Reduce the dose in patients with severe renal impairment according to estimated creatinine clearance.

Prevention of Indoor air Pollution and Biomass Burning

Biomass fuels are used for cooking and for other purposes in countries like ours and have adverse effects on health. Biomass burning forms the major source of indoor air pollution and byproducts which are produced by their burning leads to many respiratory complaints and increasing COPD burden in the world. Deaths are reported in women due to COPD.[18] Biomass burning used for the cooking and heating purposes attributes to major cause of COPD in population which is non-smoker. Especially in women, studies have found that association of exposure to solid fuel smoke with chronic bronchitis.[20] Duration of use of these fuels for the cooking purposes is directly proportional to the severity, intensity of symptoms and early progression in deterioration in lung functions. The use of biomass fuels, mainly wood, impairs pulmonary function.

Minimization of biomass fuel exposure can be optimised by:

Table 13.1: Nicotine replacement therapy initial dosing guidelines[13]

	Patient group	Dose	Duration **(weeks)	Contraindications (*adapted from MIMS online May 2014)
Patch	>10 cigarettes per day and weight >45 kg	21 mg/24 hr or 25 mg/16 hr	>8	(Unscheduled) non-smokers; children under 12 years; hypersensitivity to nicotine or any component of the patch; diseases of the skin that may complicate patch therapy
	<10 cigarettes per day or weight <45 kg or cardiovascular disease	14 mg/24 hr or 10 mg/16 hr	>8	
Gum	First cigarette >30 minutes after waking	2 mg 8–12 per day	>8	(Unscheduled) non-tobacco users; known hypersensitivity to nicotine or any component of the gum; children (<12 years)
	First cigarette <30 minutes after waking	4 mg 6–10 per day	>8	
Inhaler	>10 cigarettes per day	6–12 cartridges per day	>8	(S2) Non-tobacco users; hypersensitivity to nicotine or menthol; children (<12 years)
Inhalator	Assessed as tobacco dependent	3–6 cartridges per day	>8	(S2) Non-tobacco users; hypersensitivity to menthol; children (<12 years)
Lozenge	First cigarette >30 minutes after waking	1.5 mg or 2 mg 1 lozenge every 1–2 hr	>8	(Unscheduled) non-smokers; hypersensitivity to nicotine or any component of the lozenge; children (<12 years); phenylketonuria
	First cigarette <30 minutes after waking	4 mg 1 lozenge every 1–2 hr	>8	
Nicotine oral spray	Assessed as tobacco-dependent	Up to 4 sprays per hour	>8	(Unscheduled) non-tobacco users; children (<12 years)
Nicotine oral strips	First cigarette >30 minutes after waking	2.5 mg 1 oral strip every 1–2 hr, use at least 9 strips per day	>8	(Unscheduled) non-tobacco users; children (<18 years)

Source: *Adapted from Smoking cessation guidelines for Australian general practice. Canberra, 2004*

**Use NRT for at least 8–12 weeks for the best chance of stopping smoking in the long term.

I. Education and behaviour changes: Education should be aimed to bring the behaviour changes in cooking, heating, changes in the fuel and stove used. Some habits like being close to the fire while cooking increases the exposure and should be changed. Women should be encouraged to keep their children away from the fire.

II. Improvement in indoor ventilation: Indoor air quality can be improved by good indoor ventilation.[21] Ventilation controls indoor humidity and reduces the level of contaminants and improves indoor air quality. Also it helps to control indoor temperatures and helps in reducing indoor airborne pollutants coming from various sources. The introduction of outdoor air is one important factor in promoting good indoor air quality.

Air ventilation happens in the following ways:

- Through natural ventilation, such as windows and doors—if used properly natural ventilation can at times help moderate the indoor air temperature, without requirement of air-conditioning systems

- Through mechanical means, such as through outdoor air intakes associated with the heating, ventilation and air conditioning (HVAC) system

- Through infiltration, a process by which outdoor air flows into the house through openings, joints and cracks in walls, floors and ceilings, and around windows and doors. Infiltration occurs in all homes to some extent.

There should be a separate cooking area. Chimneys and exhaust fans should be used.

III. Air cleaners: Air cleaners are highly effective at airborne particulate matter removal. In market they are available in different types and sizes ranging from relatively inexpensive table-top models to sophisticated and expensive whole-house systems. Air purifiers are appliances that help in removing pollutants from air and very helpful devices for people who suffer from asthma or allergies. Air purifiers help in getting rid off second hand smoke. Air purifiers serve residential as well as commercial needs. Commercially air purifiers serve various industrial, medical and commercial industries. Air purifiers have HEPA (high efficiency particulate air) filters that aid in cleaning the air around that is circulated. They help get rid off contaminants and impurities from the air. It is possible for the HEPA filter to remove about 99.9% of dust particles bigger than 0.3 microns (the standard measure for microns). HEPA filters can clear the air of dust, pollen, pet dander, smoke and almost all pollutants present in the air.

Air cleaners are tested and rated by the Association of Home Appliance Manufacturers (AHAM), which assigns a number from 0 to 450 known as the Clean Air Delivery Rate (CADR) to indicate how quickly a cleaner filters dust, tobacco smoke, and pollen out of the air. The AHAM also suggests the size of the room (in square feet) for which a particular model is best suited.

When shopping for an air cleaner, compare these four key numbers by looking for the AHAM seal, which the association requires manufacturers to display on their packaging. *Consumer Reports* recommend that you purchase a model with more square-footage capacity than you need, so that you can run the machine effectively on its (quieter) "low" setting.[22]

IV. Use of better stoves: More complete combustion of fuels, increasing the generated heat and decreasing the harmful by-products are the advantages of the improved stoves (high-efficiency/low-emission stoves). Reduction in particulate matter and carbon monoxide concentrations have been described using improved stoves.[23]

V. Use of cleaner fuels: Replacement of wood or other biomass fuels used for cooking or heating with cleaner fuels, like petroleum-derived fuels like LPG and kerosene, industrially processed biomass, and alternative source of energy like thermoelectric energy, electricity, and nuclear energy. Electricity and solar energy (solar cookers) are the alternatives but costly. There is 50 to 90% reduction of particulate indoor air pollution using LPG.[24] As a part of national initiative **Pradhan Mantri Ujjwala Yojana**[25] has been launched by honourable Prime Minister of India Narendra Modi in 2016. The stated objective of the program is providing 50,000,000 LPG connections to women from families below the poverty line.

Target beneficiaries: Woman belonging to BPL group. Selection of beneficiary is further based on economic condition among BPL group too. SC/ST is the given first priority and for rest division of LPG cylinder depends on existing state and existing LPG distribution density.

Eligibility criteria: Age limit for eligibility of woman is 18 plus, applicant should be a woman belonging to BPL group, woman applicant to have an account in any nationalised bank of the country and no other household members must not be an existing LPG subscriber.

How to apply: Form for applying scheme is available with all the LPG distributors all over country free of cost. Basic details, contact and bank account details to be filled. Mandatory documents required are panchayat or municipal issued BPL certificate, BPL ration card, a Photo ID: Aadhar card/Voter ID and passport size photograph.

EXPECTED BENEFITS

- Providing LPG connections to BPL households will ensure universal coverage of cooking gas in the country.
- This measure will empower women and protect their health.
- It will reduce efforts and the time spent on cooking.
- It will also provide employment for rural youth in the supply chain of cooking gas.
- It will possibly reduce incidence of COPD and other smoke-related diseases in women and other family where earlier biomass fuel was used as cooking mode.

Occupational Exposure Related COPD and Prevention

In the current age, occupational respiratory diseases are contributing to the many respiratory diseases ranging from COPD to interstitial lung diseases. In 2003 American Thoracic Society conducted a systematic review which estimated a 15% population attributable risk for COPD related to work burden.[26] Also the occupational exposure leads to the worsening and more frequent exacerbations in COPD patients. In nineteenth century it was found that those working in industries associated with heavy organic dust exposure (e.g. coffee workers, malt workers, flaxseed workers, rag paper makers, and grain millers) had higher incidence of chronic bronchitis. When lung are examined pathologically, they found to have fibrosis and pneumoconiosis, term coined to describe the fibrotic interstitial diseases. According to the recent data, there could be association between work related exposures and chronic bronchitis and emphysema but they do not meet the criteria for COPD. For example, occupational exposure to organic dusts has been associated with variable airflow limitation and acute (as opposed to chronic) bronchitis,[27] nonetheless, these can lead to a stage of disease more akin to COPD than asthma. It is proven fact various studies that the occupational exposure to the dust, gases, fumes leads to development and progression of COPD which is marked by decline in FEV_1 and appearance and worsening of symptoms leading to cough, dyspnoea and increased sputum production. Prevention strategies include risk avoidance, exposure prevention strategies which involve the cooperation between employers, workers, and regulators, and healthcare provider.

Preventive measures are generally classified as below:

I. Strategies are aimed at reducing exposures. These strategies include:
   - Elimination (e.g. substitute alternate materials),
   - Engineering controls (e.g. exhaust ventilation or process enclosure),
   - Administrative controls (e.g. transfer to another job or change in work practices) and
   - Personal protective equipment (e.g. masks or respirators). They have the important role in preventing and reducing the degree and severity of exposures.

II. Medical surveillance programs for early detection and timely intervention. Strategies involve the administration of the short symptom questionnaires before employment and on annual basis thereafter. This will help in medical screening and exposure monitoring.

Spirometry done at annual basis can also help in determining any decline in respiratory function.

III. Institution of appropriate health care and an effort to prevent further progression to end stage disease by early removal from, or reduction of, exposure. Early recognition of the disease and early removal from, or reduction of, exposure, makes it more likely that the patient will have a slower progression of COPD.

Outdoor Air Pollution Minimisation and COPD

Main sources of the air pollution include combustion of the fossil fuels, industrial process, agricultural processes, waste incineration and natural processes like thunderstorms and volcanoes. Outdoor air quality is affected by industrial and agricultural activities, treatment of industrial effluents and domestic residues, traffic, solid waste management, cottage industries and chemical incidents and spills. Outdoor pollution primarily due to release of carbon monoxide, sulphur dioxide, particulate matter, nitrogen oxides, hydrocarbons and other pollutants. Outdoor air pollution (such as ambient air pollution or traffic-related air pollution) is a significant environmental trigger for acute exacerbation of COPD, leading to increasing symptoms, emergency department visits, hospital admissions and mortality. Strategies aimed at improving ambient air pollution are effective measures that may substantially improve the health of the general public. Lung function and exacerbations of chronic obstructive pulmonary disease (COPD) have been associated with short-term exposure to air pollution. However, the effect of long-term exposure to particulate matter from industry and traffic on COPD as defined by lung function has not been evaluated so far.

Chronic exposure to gaseous and particulate matter and living near a major road might increase the risk of developing COPD and can have a detrimental effect on lung function.

A 7 µg/m³ increase in five years means of PM10 (interquartile range) was associated with a 5.1% decrease in FEV_1, a 3.7% decrease in FVC and an odd ratio (OR) of 1.33 for COPD. Women living less than 100 m from a busy road also had a significantly decreased lung function and COPD were 1.79 times more likely than for those living farther away.[27]

Preventive strategies emphasise on public health policy for outdoor air quality as per WHO recommendation. Reducing the public health impacts of outdoor air pollution requires addressing the main sources of outdoor pollution, including inefficient fossil fuel combustion from motor vehicle transport, power generation and improving energy efficiency in buildings and manufacturing. Reducing the health effects from urban outdoor air pollution is largely beyond the control of individuals and requires action by public authorities at the national, regional and even international levels. The public health sector can play a leading role in instigating a multisectoral approach to prevention of exposure to outdoor air pollution, by engaging with and supporting the work of other sectors (i.e. transport, housing, energy, industry) to develop and implement long-term policies and programs aimed to reduce air pollution and improve health. Transport is responsible for around 25 to 70% of urban outdoor air pollution, depending on the city, but there are many other sources that should also be tackled. Action in the energy, industry, and building sectors together with the transport sector holds the greatest potential for reducing the disease burden from urban outdoor air pollution. Although newer motor vehicles have more efficient engines and are using cleaner fuels, the absolute number of vehicles and the power of each engine are still increasing and consequently so are the levels of outdoor air pollution in cities. For example, in parts of Europe where stricter standards and regulations for vehicles have been enforced, outdoor air pollution levels are stable or continue to rise due to the absolute increase in the number of vehicles on the road and in engine sizes. Substituting car trips by public transport, or by walking and cycling, would reduce the number of cars in circulation and help clean the air we all breathe, as well as minimize the health burden from urban outdoor air pollution.

The National Green Tribunal (Fig. 13.6) has been established in India on 18.10.2010 under the National Green Tribunal Act 2010 for effective and expeditious disposal of cases relating to environmental protection and conservation of forests and other natural resources including enforcement of any legal right relating to environment and giving relief and compensation for damages to persons and property and for matters connected therewith or incidental thereto. It is a specialized body equipped with the necessary expertise to handle environmental disputes involving multi-disciplinary issues. The Tribunal shall not be bound by the procedure laid down under the Code of Civil Procedure, 1908, but shall be guided by

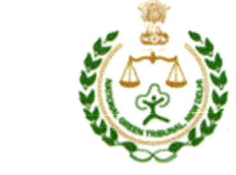

National Green Tribunal

Fig 13.6: The National Green Tribunal

principles of natural justice.[29] The Chairperson of the NGT is a retired Judge of the Supreme Court, headquarter in Delhi. The NGT has the power to hear all civil cases relating to environmental issues and questions that are linked to the implementation of laws listed in Schedule I of the NGT Act. These include the following:

1. The Water (Prevention and Control of Pollution) Act, 1974;

2. The Water (Prevention and Control of Pollution) Cess Act, 1977;

3. The Forest (Conservation) Act, 1980;

4. The Air (Prevention and Control of Pollution) Act, 1981;

5. The Environment (Protection) Act, 1986;

6. The Public Liability Insurance Act, 1991;

7. The Biological Diversity Act, 2002.

E. COPD and Exacerbations Prevention

Chronic obstructive pulmonary disease (COPD) is associated with episodes of acute deterioration in respiratory symptoms and signs are termed "exacerbations." Exacerbations are characterized by a worsening from the usual stable state, especially dyspnoea, increased sputum volume, and purulence. When diagnosing COPD exacerbations, clinicians must also exclude other causes for respiratory deterioration, such as pneumothoraces, pulmonary emboli, and pneumonia, using clinical examination and appropriate investigations if required. Exacerbations are among the most common causes of emergency medical hospital admission and the rate at which they occur seems to reflect an independent individual susceptibility pattern. Exacerbations are important events in the natural history of COPD that help drive lung function decline, increase the risk of cardiovascular events, and are responsible for much of the morbidity and mortality.

GOLD (global initiative in chronic obstructive lung diseases) defined acute exacerbation as the acute event characterized by worsening of the patient respiratory symptoms that is beyond normal day-to-day variations and leads to a change in medications.

Prevention of acute exacerbation is of utmost importance as it causes deterioration in pulmonary reserve, frequent COPD episodes lead to decrease in quality of life, severe exacerbations increase rehospitalization, frequent relapses lead to disability and also increases the risk of mortality, severity of exacerbation is directly proportional to days of hospital stay and also it has a high health care cost.

Early recognition of the acute exacerbation is important. Patient may not recognise the symptoms and delay in presentation to hospital. The early pointers to acute exacerbations include cough which has increased for past more than 2 days, change in colour viscosity and amount of mucus, increase in respiratory distress and dyspnoea causing limitations in activity of daily living. Acute exacerbation can be recognised early by the use of the domiciliary pulse oximetry. It has been seen that there is earlier risk following 8 weeks post-acute exacerbation when recent event of acute exacerbation will recur. A patient reported diary has been found useful in assessing timing and frequency of exacerbation (Fig. 13.7).

Pharmacological and non-pharmacological therapies (Fig. 13.8) on the basis of disease severity are aimed to decrease the preventing and decreasing exacerbations, control the symptoms, improving quality of life. Management of exacerbations in COPD is usually done as per recommended guidelines. Pharmacotherapy is generally added in a stepwise fashion. However, for patients who present with severe disease, a

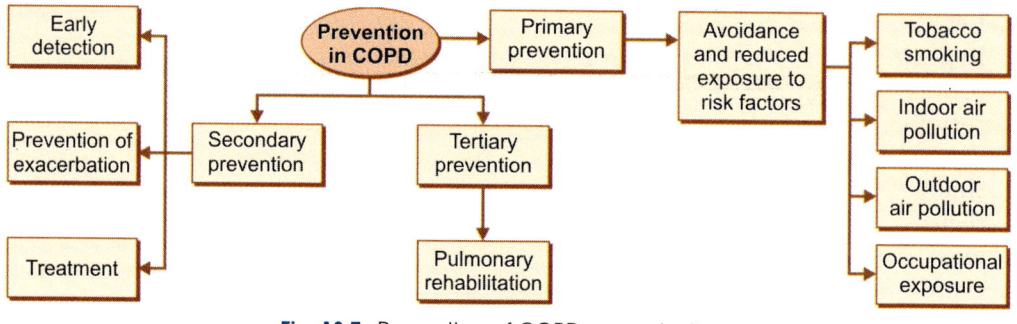

Fig. 13.7: Prevention of COPD exacerbations

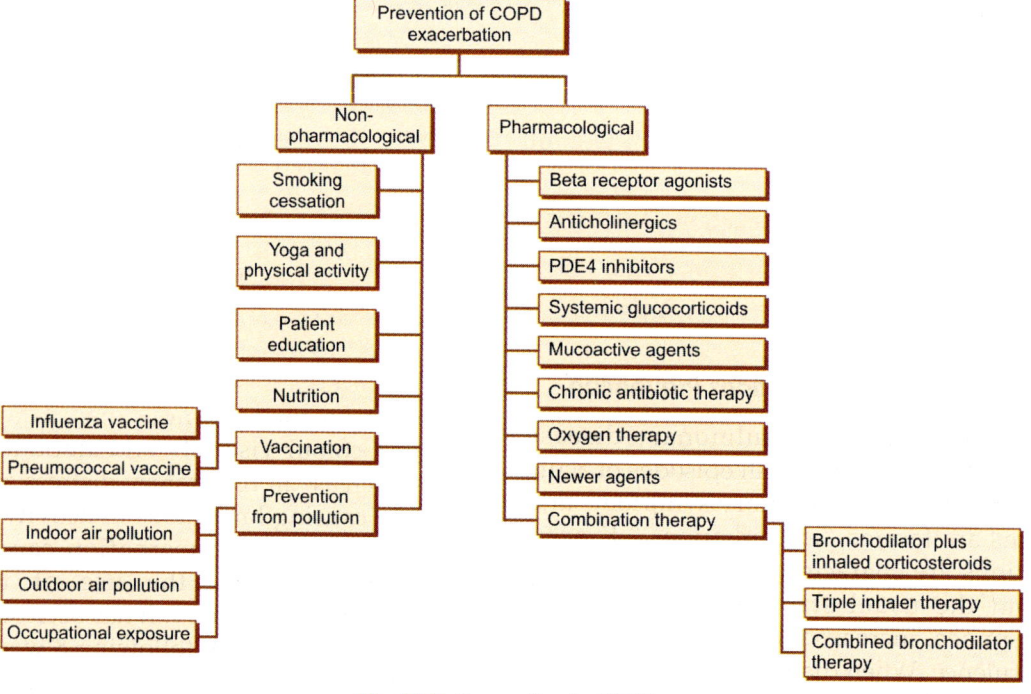

Fig. 13.8: Prevention in COPD

stepwise approach may not always be the best choice, as it may be necessary to initiate several medications at once to achieve symptom control.

Preventive Pharmacological Interventions for Exacerbation

i. **Beta agonists:** The long-acting selective beta 2 agonists (LABAs) have shown promise in TORCH trial, salmeterol significantly decreased rates of exacerbation, improved lung function, and improved health-related quality of life when compared to placebo.[30] Although, LABA were found to be associated with increased risk of arrhythmia. Indacaterol is a once-daily LABA known to decrease in the exacerbation rate that is approved for the treatment of COPD. Olodaterol and vilanterol are newer agents.

ii. **Anticholinergics:** The long-acting anticholinergic medications, also known as long-acting muscarinic agents (LAMAs), include tiotropium, aclidinium, umeclidinium, and glycopyrronium. Tiotropium improves lung function and decreases hyperinflation (an effect also seen with other medications), while also relieving dyspnoea and reducing exacerbations.[32] Tiotropium may slow the rate of decline in FEV_1 and recurrent exacerbations. Tiotropium was more effective at reducing exacerbations.[32] Tiotropium increased the time to the first exacerbation of COPD and reduced the risk of developing an exacerbation by 17 percent. Umeclidinium is a once-daily LAMA with characteristics similar to tiotropium that has been developed for use in a combination inhaler with the long-acting LABA vilanterol.

iii. **Combined bronchodilator therapy:** Some beneficial role of adding a second long-acting bronchodilator from the alternate bronchodilator class (e.g. a long-acting muscarinic antagonist [LAMA] or a long-acting beta-agonist [LABA] bronchodilator) in patients with GOLD stage II–IV COPD whose symptoms are not well-controlled with a single long-acting bronchodilator. Various new combinations include tiotropium-olodaterol, umeclidinium-vilanterol, glycopyrronium-indacaterol, glycopyrrolate-formoterol and aclidinium-formoterol. Aclidinium-formoterol has shown to improve airflows and dyspnoea and decreased the rate of moderate to severe exacerbations compared with either of the individual agents alone or placebo. The combination also decreased the rate of moderate/severe exacerbations relative to placebo.[33]

iv. **Bronchodilators plus inhaled corticosteroids:** Inhaled glucocorticoids are typically used in combination with a long-acting bronchodilator for patients with significant symptoms or repeated exacerbations, despite being on optimal bronchodilator regimen. In the TORCH trial, salmeterol plus fluticasone significantly improved lung function, health status, and exacerbations rate compared to placebo, salmeterol alone, or fluticasone alone.[30] And also decreased mortality compared to placebo. In INSPIRE trial, no difference in the frequency of exacerbations, although salmeterol plus fluticasone improved including mortality and health status. The combination of a long-acting anticholinergic plus an inhaled glucocorticoid has not been compared to a long-acting anticholinergic alone.

v. **Role of triple inhaler therapy:** Triple inhaler therapy with a long-acting beta agonist plus an inhaled glucocorticoid plus a long-acting anticholinergic is often used in patients with COPD patients with severe and persistent symptoms. The benefits of triple therapy are suggested by the UPLIFT trial.[34] In UPLIFT trial, addition of tiotropium to those patients receiving a LABA and an ICS significantly improved airflows, reduced exacerbations, and improved health related quality of life. When tiotropium plus ICS plus LABA were compared to 996 taking ICS plus LABA, the group taking triple therapy had a lower mortality as well as fewer hospital admissions. Other studies have shown a benefit to triple therapy compared with single agent therapy in moderate to severe COPD.[35] In a double-blind trial, 449 patients with moderate or severe COPD were randomly assigned to one of three treatment groups: Tiotropium plus placebo, tiotropium plus salmeterol, or tiotropium plus both salmeterol and fluticasone for one year; the latter two groups were compared with tiotropium alone.[36] Triple therapy, when compared to tiotropium alone, was associated with significant improvements in lung function and disease-specific quality of life and a reduction in all—cause hospitalizations, but not a reduction in overall exacerbation rate.With the use of inhaled budesonide plus formoterol plus tiotropium or to inhaled tiotropium alone,[35] as seen in a study, the number of severe exacerbations was significantly lower in the triple therapy group.

vi. **PDE-4 inhibitors:** Theophylline, roflumilast and cilomilast are three available phosphodiesterase inhibitors.

Roflumilast and cilomilast being a selective PDE4 inhibitor have advantage over theophylline which is a nonselective one in terms of higher potency with an improved therapeutic index. Selective PDE4 inhibitors are more efficacious in improving lung functions, decreasing acute exacerbations. Also selective inhibitors have less toxic effects, whereas theophylline requires a plasma drug monitoring and drug adjustments because of cardiovascular and CNS adverse effects and drug interactions.[36]

Phosphodiesterase-4 (PDE-4) inhibition decreases inflammation and also shown to promote smooth muscle relaxation of airways. Roflumilast is a selective PDE-4 inhibitor, has the proven role and has already been approved to reduce the risk of COPD exacerbations in patients with a history of frequent episode (e.g. at least two per year or one requiring hospitalization), inform if individual therapy or as an adjunct to other agents.[38] In a multicentre trial in

patients with COPD, moderate-to-severe COPD exacerbations were 14 percent lower among those who took roflumilast when compared with those taking placebo. Severe exacerbations requiring hospital admission were decreased by 24 percent. When roflumilast was used in combination with salmeterol, the results were similar.[39]

vii. **Systemic glucocorticoids:** Long-term systemic glucocorticoid therapy is not recommended, even for severe COPD, because of the significant side effects and evidence of increased morbidity and mortality with this therapy.[40]

viii. **Mucoactive agents:** However, it is not certain if these treatments provide additional benefit to patients already being treated with LABA or ICS. Thick sputum can be a major problem in patients with COPD. Thiol derivatives such as N-acetylcysteine (NAC), erdosteine and carbocysteine, are mucolytic agents acting on disulfide bonds of mucoproteins and DNA, leads to reduced mucus viscosity. NAC have antioxidant effects. Evidence for recommending NAC in COPD still lacking.[41] PANTHEON trial in patients with moderate to severe COPD has shown that NAC may reduce the risk of exacerbations.[42] Inhaled NAC has been found to produce bronchoconstriction, hence not recommended in COPD patients. Use of oral expectorants like bromhexine is not recommended has shown limited benefits in COPD and adverse effects. Nebulized water or hypertonic saline is without documented benefit in COPD and may irritate the airways and induce bronchospasm.

ix. **Chronic antibiotic therapy:** Chronic antibiotic therapy is not indicated for the majority of patients but can be used in patients having frequent exacerbation. Macrolides like azithromycin are suggested for the antibiotic prophylaxis due to their anti-inflammatory in addition to antibiotic effect. Chronic antibiotic therapy has a role in COPD patients with bronchiectasis. Antiviral therapy to non-immunized patients with COPD who are at high risk for influenza infection.

x. **Oxygen therapy:** Those with chronic hypoxemia long-term oxygen therapy improves survival and quality of life in hypoxemic patients with COPD.[43] Reduced dyspnoea during exercise leads to improved quality of life which improves performance of activities of daily living. Long-term oxygen therapy (LTOT) should be prescribed for all stable patients with COPD who have chronic, severe hypoxemia at rest (PaO_2 ≤55 mmHg or SpO_2 ≤88 percent).[44] For patients with COPD and moderate hypoxemia at rest or with exertion, a clear benefit of LTOT has not been demonstrated.

xi. **Future therapies:** COPD is an inflammatory condition associated with relative steroid resistance and approaches to restore steroid sensitivity may lead to novel future therapies.[45–47] These include use of low dose daily theophylline which increases histone deacetylase activity, phosphoinositide-3-kinase inhibitors and selective p38 (p38 mitogen-activated protein kinase) inhibitors.

Non-pharmacological Interventions

Apart from smoking cessation and prevention from the indoor and outdoor pollution, several non-pharmacological methods are available towards COPD prevention.

i. **Role of vaccination:** Infection is a common cause of COPD exacerbation. Vaccinations can prevent some infections and should be offered to patients with stable COPD (Fig. 13.9).

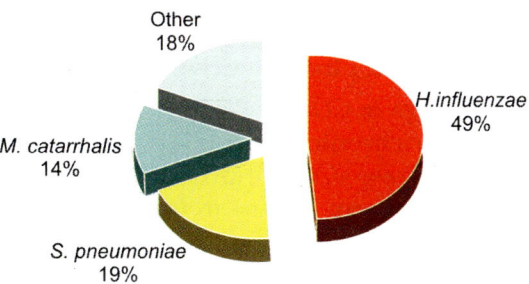

Fig. 13.9: Vaccination in COPD

a. *Influenza vaccination:* In a study on influenza vaccination, it has been found that administration of the vaccine is associated with a 27% reduction in the risk of hospitalization for pneumonia or influenza and a 48% reduction in the risk of death.[48] Also a randomised control trial showed, vaccine effectiveness of 76% in reducing acute respiratory infections in COPD patients.[49] An annual influenza vaccine should be given to all patients, particularly those with COPD.

b. *Pneumococcal vaccination:* Pneumococcal vaccination was associated with reduced risks of hospitalization for pneumonia and mortality in patients with COPD. Though it decreases incidence of community acquired pneumonia in elderly but has no mortality benefit. Significant decrease in rates of community acquired pneumonia is not shown after a trial of pneumococcal polysaccharide vaccine in patients with COPD.[50] Pneumococcal polysaccharide vaccination ($PPSV_{23}$) is advised for patients under age 65 years and $PPSV_{23}$ and pneumococcal conjugate vaccine (PCV_{13}) are advised for patients age 65 years and older.

c. **Combined vaccination:** Combined influenza and pneumococcal vaccination are recommended to all patients with COPD.

ii. **Yoga and physical activity:**

a. **Yoga in COPD:** Existing medications for chronic obstructive pulmonary disease (COPD) do not modify the long-term decline in lung functions. The increasing prevalence of COPD requires the development of interventions beyond the usual medical treatment, with a specific focus on rehabilitation. Yoga is a holistic approach which includes meditation, relaxation, body postures, breath control, and concentration. It invokes endogenous melatonin secretion brings a sense of well being.[51] Controlled breathing (pranayam) is a specific set of respiratory exercises within yoga that has been shown to improvement in lung functions measured as resting respiratory rate, vital capacity, maximum voluntary ventilation, breath-holding time, and maximal inspiratory and expiratory pressures.[52] Pranayam is a useful additional intervention and can be effective in rehabilitation program for individuals with COPD.

The role of yoga in treatment of chronic obstructive pulmonary disease (COPD) is still not defined, and inference is drawn mostly from asthmatic patients or from improve-ment in well-being of healthy people. According to a study, there has been seen the symptomatic and objective improvement in the maximum work performed in COPD patients.[53] Pranayama, asanas, kapalbhati, sithali exercises and meditation, demonstrated to have quality of life and spirometric measures. Improvement in dyspnoea measured by the visual analog scale and improvement in vital capacity, forced expiratory volume in one second (FEV_1), and peak expiratory flow rate, in chronic bronchitis patients.[54] In a study, during the YBT session on room air alone (without the use of supplemental oxygen) in COPD patient, blood oxygen saturation increased from 92% to 94% within 20 minutes of the session.[55] The patient also felt subjectively better and relaxed. As a conclusion short term breathing exercises, pranayam and yoga are recommended. Various proposed mechanisms are discussed in Fig. 13.10.

b. **Physical activity:**[57, 58] Decreased parenchymal elasticity and persistent and progressive airflow limitation is characteristic of COPD which leads to prolonged contracted state of respiratory muscles increasing loads on respiratory muscles and increased ventilatory flow demands. Reduced contractility in these patients leads to stimulation of mechanoreceptors which triggers respiratory centres increasing ventilation eventually

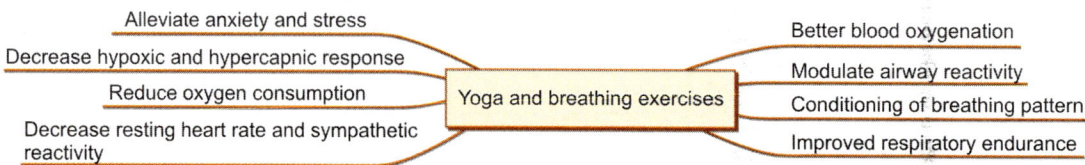

Fig. 13.10: Mechanisms involved in yoga and breathing exercises in COPD prevention

aggravating dyspnoea. Dyspnoea and the shortening of respiratory muscles hamper the performance of activities that require more effort. Aerobic training which aids in capacity building and which eventually reduces dyspnoea should be encouraged as it could be an important intervention in patients with COPD. GOLD guidelines recommends exercise training ranges in frequency from daily to weekly, in duration from 10 minutes to 45 minutes per session, and in intensity from 50% peak oxygen consumption (VO$_2$ max) to maximum tolerated. Also use of a simple wheeled walking aid seems to improve walking distance and reduces breathlessness in severely disabled COPD patients.[59]

iii. **Patient education:** Patient education is an important part of managing patients with COPD and is a routine component of pulmonary rehabilitation. Topics about which patients should be informed include reducing risk factors, appropriate administration and use of medications, recognizing and treating exacerbations, minimizing dyspnoea, recognizing and treating complications, using long-term supplemental oxygen, and making end-of-life decisions.

iv. **Nutrition:** Severe COPD known to have protein-calorie malnutrition. This is associated with increased mortality, impaired respiratory muscle function, and diminished immune competence. High caloric dietary supplements and megestrol acetate (an appetite stimulant) and antioxidants may have beneficial role. Evidence supported by long term studies is scarce.

v. **Patient adherence:** Missing medication is the one the frequent causes of occurrence of exacerbation of symptoms in patient of COPD. Patient adherence serves the important role in prevention in COPD patients, like in many other chronic illness.

Newer drugs added to prescription and drugs for coexisting comorbidities increases the length of the prescription drugs and all intake of these drugs become the major challenge for the patients. This tends to failure to maintain compliance to the maintenance treatment and symptom tends to relapse. Maintenance of patient adherence remains the major challenge for the clinicians for developed and developing countries alike.

Failure to maintain adherence not has poor health outcome but also increase the yearly expenditures which also include increased hospitalisation cost as reported in many studies. Compliance and adherence are terms which are used interchangeably. Adherence has been defined as the ability and willingness to abide by a prescribed therapeutic regimen.[59]

Factors affecting the treatment adherence can be divided into patient related, therapy related, healthcare related, social and economic related and related to disease per se.[60]

Patient related and therapy related factors predominate in COPD patients as seen in daily practice. Patient related factors include knowledge, attitude, behaviour of the patients, forgetfulness and literacy. Therapy related factors include treatment complexities and medication side effects. In developing countries like ours lack of accessibility and difficulty in getting prescriptions filled are also the important factors.

Accurate assessment forms the first step towards improvement of the treatment adherence. It requires the better relationship between treating doctors and patient.[61] A talk with patients can help to assess the factor which leading to non-adherence and proper intervention can be made. Interventions improving the adherence involve the shared role of patients, physicians and caregivers. Use of technology in current era can also improve adherence. Patient counselling has the strategic role in improving drug compliance. Other strategies include keeping drugs at one place, self monitoring of symptoms and medications. Assisted by various mobile applications available which helps the patients to act as alarm and remind them when they miss their medications. Healthcare providers and caregivers can assist and motivate the patients and also ensure that they abide to therapeutic regimen.

COPD and Comorbidities[62]

Comorbidities seem to be present in the majority of COPD patients. Comorbidities associated with poor quality of life in early-stage patients, increases mortality in end-stage patients. It also leads to increased burden of healthcare costs.

COPD and comorbidities coexists. Age and smoking are the major risk factors for a number of illnesses, hence COPD patients demonstrate multiple coexisting comorbidities. Similarities in risk factors and pathophysiology lead to a dilemma that whether COPD increases the susceptibility to other comorbidities or vice versa.

According to GOLD guidelines,[63] the severity of comorbid conditions and their impact on a patient's health status will vary between patients and in the same patient over time. Comorbidities can be categorized in various ways to aid in the better understanding of their impact on the patient, and their impact on disease management.[64] Common pathway comorbidities are the diseases with a common pathophysiology as in the case of COPD, other smoking-related diseases such as ischaemic heart disease and lung cancer. Complicating comorbidities arise as a complication of a specific pre-existing disease as in case of COPD,

pulmonary hypertension and consequent heart failure. Early intervention is directed at preventing complications and the effectiveness of these early interventions should be monitored. Co-incidental comorbidities have unrelated pathogenesis which includes bowel or prostate cancer, depression, diabetes mellitus, Parkinson's disease, dementia, and arthritis. Such conditions may make COPD management more difficult. Inter-current comorbidities are acute illnesses like upper respiratory tract infections which are the most frequent health problem in all age groups, but have a more severe impact and require different treatment in patients with COPD. Some diseases like osteoporosis can arise as a consequence of chronic illness itself or as a side effect of the long steroid treatment in patient with severe COPD. Presence of comorbidities makes the therapeutic decision making difficult.

KEYPOINTS

1. Smoking cessation prevents the COPD exacerbations and reduces further decline in lung functions. Involves the pharmacological and nonpharmacological techniques
2. Use of cleaner fuel, better stoves reduce indoor pollution.
3. Proper screening at workplaces and use of personal protective equipment like mask can reduce occupational exposure.
4. Better policy making is required to reduce air pollution.
5. Early detection and treatment of COPD exacerbation helps to decelerate lung functions and improve the quality of life.
6. Yoga and physical exercises found to be beneficial in improving lung function, preventing exacerbations and pulmonary rehabilitation.
7. Important role of ensuring patient adherence to treatment.
8. COPD and comorbidities coexist, holistic approach to treatment decreases mortality.

SUMMARY

Chronic obstructive pulmonary diseases are responsible for the major disease burden worldwide. Prevention also plays an important role in decreasing morbidity and mortality in COPD, as is true for other diseases also. Smoking is strongly associated with COPD and smoking cessation has shown to improve the lung functions and decrease in burden of diseases. Increasing air pollution and occupational related exposure which is a by-product of increasing vehicles and industrialization has also increased the magnitude of COPD burden. Biomass burning is also a major contributor to indoor pollution. Preventive strategies include risk avoidance, exposure prevention by use of better stoves, cleaner fuels, use of personal protective equipment and laws to regulate air quality.

Pharmacological and non-pharmacological therapies are aimed at decreasing and preventing COPD exacerbations. Role of yoga, breathing exercises and physical exercises have shown some benefit but their role in prevention is being studied.

REFERENCES

1. Global Strategy for the Diagnosis, Management and Prevention of COPD, Global Initiative for Chronic Obstructive Lung Disease (GOLD) 2016. www.goldcopd.org
2. World Health Organization. Burden of COPD. Available from:http: //www.who.int/ respiratory/copd/burden/en/
3. ICMR-MRC Workshop. Building Indo-UK Collaboration in chronic diseases; 2009. p. 16.
4. Reddy KS, Shah B, Varghese C, Ramadoss A. Responding to the threat of chronic diseases in India. Lancet 2005; 366: 1746–51.
5. Lopez AD, Shibuya K, Rao C, Mathers CD, Hansell AL, Held LS, *et al.* Chronic obstructive airway disease: Current burden and future projections. Eur Resp J 2006; 27: 397–412.
6. Petty T. COPD in Perspective. Chest. 2002; 121(5): 116S–120S.
7. Burchfiel CM, Marcus EB, Curb JD, et al. Effects of smoking and smoking cessation.
8. Anthonisen NR, Connett JE, Kiley JP, et al. Effects of smoking intervention and the use of an inhaled anticholinergic bronchodilator on the rate of decline of FEV_1. The Lung Health Study. JAMA. 1994; 272(19): 1497–505.
9. Longitudinal decline in pulmonary function. Am J Respir Crit Care Med 1995; 151: 1778e85.
10. Fletcher C, Peto R. The natural history of chronic airflow obstruction. *BMJ* 1977; i: 1645–8.
11. Tobacco Use and Dependence Guideline Panel. Treating Tobacco Use and Dependence: 2008 Update. Rockville (MD): US Department of Health and Human Services; 2008 May.
12. Rigotti N. Treatment of Tobacco Use and Dependence. New England Journal of Medicine. 2002; 346(7): 506–12.
13. Hartmann-Boyce J Aveyard P. Drugs for smoking cessation. BMJ. 2016; i571.
14. Zwar N, Richmond R, Borland R, Stillman S, Cunningham M, Litt J. Smoking cessation guidelines for Australian general practice. Aust Fam Physician 2005; 34(6): 461–6.
15. Hurt R, Sachs D, Glover E, Offord K, Johnston J, Dale L et al. A Comparison of Sustained Release Bupropion and Placebo for Smoking Cessation. New England Journal of Medicine. 1997; 337(17): 1195–202.
16. Holm K, Spencer C. Bupropion. Drugs. 2000; 59(4): 1007–24.
17. Ebbert JO, Sood A, Hays JT, Dale LC, Hurt RD. Treating tobacco dependence: review of the best and latest treatment options. J Thorac Oncol 2007; 2(3): 249–56.
18. Keating G, Siddiqui M. Varenicline. CNS Drugs. 2006; 20(11): 945–60.
19. Ezzati M, Kammen DM. The health impacts of exposure to indoor air pollution from solid fuels in developing countries: knowledge, gaps, and data needs. Environ Health Perspect 2002; 110: 1057–68.
20. Dennis RJ, Maldonado D, Norman S, Baena E, Martinez G. Wood smoke exposure and risk for obstructive airways disease among women. Chest 1996; 109: 115–9.
21. Dasgupta S, Huq M, Khaliquzzaman M, Pandey K, Wheeler D. Indoor air quality for poor families: new evidence from Bangladesh. Indoor Air 2006; 16: 426–44.

22. Air purifier buying guide. Available from: http://www.consumerreports.org/cro/air-purifiers/buying-guide. Accessed on 24th March 2017.

23. Ezzati M, Mbinda BM, Kammen DM. Comparison of emissions and residential exposure from traditional and improved cookstoves in Kenya. Environ Sci Technol 2000; 34: 578–83.

24. Albalak R, Bruce N, McCracken JP, Smith KR, De Gallardo T. Indoor respirable particulate matter concentrations from an open fire, improved cookstove, and LPG/open fire combination in a rural Guatemalan community. Environ Sci Technol.2001; 35: 2650–55.

25. Pradhan Mantri Ujjwala Yojana (PMUY). Available at http://www.pmujjwalayojana.com/.Accessed on 19th March 2017.

26. Balmes J, Becklake M, Blanc P, et al. American Thoracic Society Statement: occupational contribution to the burden of airway disease. Am J Respir Crit Care Med. 2003; 167(5): 787–97.

27. Eisner MD, Anthonisen N, Coultas D, et al. An official American Thoracic Society public policy.

28. Schikowski T, Sugiri D, Ranft U, Gehring U, Heinrich J, Wichmann H, et al. Long-term air pollution exposure and living close to busy roads are associated with COPD in women. Respiratory Research. 2005; 6(1).

29. The Ministry of Environment, Forests and Climate Change, Government of India. National Green Tribunal (NGT). Available from: http://envfor.nic.in/rules-regulations/national-green-tribunal-ngt. Accessed on 22nd March 2017.

30. Schunemann H. Salmeterol and fluticasone propionate did not reduce mortality in chronic obstructive pulmonary disease. Evidence-Based Medicine. 2007; 12(4): 114–114.

31. O'Donnell DE, Flüge T, Gerken F, Hamilton A, Webb K, Aguilaniu B, Make B, Magnussen H. Effects of tiotropium on lung hyperinflation, dyspnoea and exercise tolerance in COPD. Eur Respir J. 2004; 23(6): 832–40.

32. Vogelmeier C, Hederer B, Glaab T, et al. Tiotropium versus salmeterol for the prevention of exacerbations of COPD. N Engl J Med. 2011; 364(12): 1093–1103.

33. Bateman ED, Chapman KR, Singh D, et al. Aclidinium bromide and formoterol fumarate as a fixed-dose combination in COPD: pooled analysis of symptoms and exacerbations from two six-month, multicentre, randomised studies (ACLIFORM and AUGMENT). Respir Res. 2015; 16: 92.

34. Tashkin DP, Celli B, Senn S, Burkhart D, Kesten S, Menjoge S, Decramer M; UPLIFT Study Investigators. A 4-year trial of tiotropium in chronic obstructive pulmonary disease. N Engl J Med. 2008; 359(15): 1543–54.

35. Welte T, Miravitlles M, Hernandez P, et al. Efficacy and tolerability of budesonide/formoterol added to tiotropium in patients with chronic obstructive pulmonary disease. Am J Respir Crit Care Med. 2009; 180(8): 741–50.

36. Aaron SD, Vandemheen KL, Fergusson, D, et al. 2007. Tiotropium in combination with placebo, salmeterol, or fluticasone-salmeterol for treatment of chronic obstructive pulmonary disease: a randomized trial. Ann Intern Med 146: 545–55.

37. Gruffydd-Jones K, Jones MM. NICE guidelines for chronic obstructive pulmonary disease: implications for primary care. *The British Journal of General Practice*. 2011; 61(583): 91–92.

38. Giembycz MA. Cilomilast: a second generation phosphodiesterase 4 inhibitor for asthma and chronic obstructive pulmonary disease. Expert OpinInvestig Drugs. 2001; 10: 1361–79.

39. Fabbri LM, Calverley PM, Izquierdo-Alonso JL, et al. Roflumilast in moderate-to-severe chronic obstructive pulmonary disease treated with long acting bronchodilators: two randomised clinical trials. Lancet. 2009; 374(9691): 695–703.

40. Horita N, Miyazawa N, Morita S, et al. Evidence suggesting that oral corticosteroids increase mortality in stable chronic obstructive pulmonary disease. *Respiratory Research*. 2014; 15(1): 37. doi: 10.1186/1465–9921–15–37.

41. Poole P, Chong J, Cates CJ. Mucolytic agents versus placebo for chronic bronchitis or chronic obstructive pulmonary disease. Cochrane Database Syst Rev. 2015; (7): CD001287.

42. Zheng JP, Wen FQ, Bai CX, et al.Twice daily N-acetylcysteine 600 mg for exacerbations of chronic obstructive pulmonary disease (PANTHEON): a randomised, double-blind placebo-controlled trial. Lancet Respir Med. 2014; 2(3): 187–94.

43. Long term domiciliary oxygen therapy in chronic hypoxic corpulmonale complicating

chronic bronchitis and emphysema. Report of the Medical Research Council Working Party. Lancet. 1981 Mar 28; 1(8222): 681–6.

44. Qaseem A, Wilt TJ, Weinberger SE. & et al. Diagnosis and management of stable chronic obstructive pulmonary disease: A clinical practice guideline update from the American college of physicians, American college of chest physicians, American thoracic society, and European respiratory society. Annals of Internal Medicine. 2011; 155: 179–91.

45. Ito K, Lim S, Caramori G, Cosio B, Chung KF, Adcock IM, Barnes PJ. A molecular mechanism of action of theophylline: Induction of histone deacetylase activity to decrease inflammatory gene expression. Proc Natl Acad Sci USA. 2002; 99(13): 8921–6.

46. Marwick JA, Caramori G, Stevenson CS, et al. Inhibition of PI3K delta restores glucocorticoid function in smoking-induced airway inflammation in mice. Am J Respir Crit Care Med. 2009; 179(7): 542–8.

47. Renda T, Baraldo S, Pelaia G, et al. Increased activation of p38 MAPK in COPD. Eur Respir J. 2008; 31(1): 62–9.

48. Nichol KL, Nordin JD, Nelson DB, et al. Effectiveness of influenza vaccine in the community-dwelling elderly. N Engl J Med. 2007; 357(14): 1373–81.

49. Wongsurakiat P, Maranetra KN, Wasi C, et al. Acute respiratory illness in patients with COPD and the effectiveness of influenza vaccination: a randomized controlled study. Chest. 2004; 125(6): 2011–20.

50. Alfageme I, Vazquez R, Reyes N, et al. Clinical efficacy of anti-pneumococcal vaccination in patients with COPD. Thorax 2006; 61(3): 189–95.

51. Harinath K, Malhotra AS, Pal K, et al. Effects of Hatha yoga and Omkar meditation on cardiorespiratory performance, psychologic profile, and melatonin secretion. J Altern Compl Med. 2004; 10: 261–68.

52. Cooper S, Oborne J, Newton S, et al. Effect of two breathing exercises (Buteyko and pranayama) in asthma: a randomised controlled trial. Thorax. 2003; 58: 674–79.

53. Tandon MK. Adjunct treatment with yoga in chronic severe airways obstruction. Thorax. 1978; 33: 514–17.

54. Behera D. Yoga therapy in chronic bronchitis. J Assoc Phys India. 1998; 46: 207–8.

55. Vedanthan P. Yoga Breathing Techniques (YBT) in Chronic Obstructive Pulmonary Disease (COPD): A Preliminary Study. International Journal of Yoga Therapy.2003; 13: 51–4.

56. Paulin E, Brunetto AF, Carvalho CRF. Effects of a physical exercises program designed to increase thoracic mobility in patients with chronic obstructive pulmonary disease. J Pneumol. 2003; 29(5): 287–95.

57. Spruit MA, Singh SJ, Garvey C, et al. ATS/ERS Task Force on Pulmonary Rehabilitation An official American thoracic society/European respiratory society statement: key concepts and advances in pulmonary rehabilitation. Am J Respir Crit Care Med. 2013; 188(8): 13–64.

58. Yohannes AM, Connolly MJ. Early mobilization with walking aids following hospital admission with acute exacerbation of chronic obstructive pulmonary disease. Clin Rehabil. 2003; 17(5): 465–71.

59. Inkster ME, Donnan PT, MacDonald TM, Sullivan FM, Fahey T. Adherence to antihypertensive medication and association with patient and practice factors. J Hum Hypertens. 2006; 20(4): 295–7.

60. Jin J, Sklar GE, Min Sen Oh V, Chuen Li S. Factors affecting therapeutic compliance: A review from the patient's perspective. Therapeutics and Clinical Risk Management. 2008; 4(1): 269–86.

61. Martin LR, Williams SL, Haskard KB, DiMatteo MR. The challenge of patient adherence. Therapeutics and Clinical Risk Management. 2005; 1(3): 189–99

62. [Internet]. 2017 [cited 5 February 2017]. Available from: http://www.who.int/respiratory/copd/GOLD_WR_06.pdf

63. Schellevis FG, Van de Lisdonk EH, Van der Velden J, et al. Consultation rates and incidence of intercurrent morbidity among patients with chronic disease in general practice. Br J Gen Pract. 1994; 44(383): 259–62.

64. Available at http://envfor.nic.in/rules-regulations/national-green-tribunal-ngt (Last visited on June 4, 2015)

Recent Advances and Future

Hemant Kumar Aggarwal, Amit Kumar Verma

INTRODUCTION

Globally, obstructive airway diseases including chronic obstructive pulmonary disease (COPD) are one of the leading causes of morbidity and mortality. The available treatment options control airway inflammation to an extent, however, with the advent of better technology and more effective medical and surgical treatment strategies are being developed. Newer bronchodilators with longer duration of action and lesser side effects along with more combination therapies are being developed. Bronchoscopic procedures are coming up as noninvasive techniques for treatment of COPD. In this chapter we will also discuss about the asthma–COPD overlap syndrome which is a diagnostic challenge, unless a proper approach be used to diagnose this entity.

MEDICAL THERAPY

Newer Bronchodilator

The mainstay of medical management is in the form of inhaled bronchodilators. It provides symptomatic relief and improves the quality of life significantly, primarily by emptying the trapped air by dilating the small airways.

Long-acting β_2 Agonist (LABA)

Initially LABA was administered twice a day, however, the newer drugs available aim at increasing compliance to therapy and are available in easy once a day dosing schedule. The newer LABA, available are indacaterol, vilanterol, olodaterol (Table 14.1).

Indacaterol is an ultra long-acting inhaled β_2 agonist used for the treatment of COPD. Clinical studies have proven its long duration of action (hence, once a day convenient dose), fast onset of action, and improved cardiovascular safety profile.[1] Its onset of action is 5 minutes, that peaks after 2–3 hours and is maintained for 24 hours after dosing with all doses evaluated.[2] It is available as dry powder inhaler.

The INLIGHT 1 study assessed the 12-week efficacy and safety of indacaterol

Table 14.1: Long-acting β_2 agonist (LABA)

Long-acting bronchodilators	Onset of action	Duration of action	Half life	Dose (μg)
Indacaterol	5 minutes	24 hours	40–56 hours	150–300
Vilanterol	3 minutes	24 hours	21.3 hours	25
Olodaterol	5 minutes	24 hours	7.5 hours	5–10

150 µg od in patients with moderate-to-severe COPD.[1] It confirmed the 24-hour sustained bronchodilation produced by indacaterol with a significantly reduced rescue medication use when compared with placebo.[1] Indacaterol is now known to be more effective than salmeterol or formoterol. Once-daily treatment with 150 µg indacaterol had a clinically relevant bronchodilator effect over 24-hour post-dose and improved health status and dyspnoea to a greater extent than twice-daily 50 µg salmeterol as seen in the INLIGHT 2 study.[3] It was shown in the INVOLVE study that 300 µg indacaterol increased 24-hour post-dose FEV_1 after 12 weeks by 170 ml (both doses) versus placebo and by 100 ml versus formoterol. These significant differences were maintained at 52 weeks. Indacaterol was well tolerated and had a good overall safety profile, including minimal impact on QTc interval and systemic β_2-mediated events.[4] In the study there was more common occurrence of post-inhalation cough but it was not reported as troublesome.[3] Doses of 150 µg and 300 µg have been studied to determine which dose is more apt for use and investigations have shown that doses of 150–300 µg once daily are equally effective.[5] In the INHANCE study, patients with moderate-to-severe COPD were randomized to double-blind indacaterol 150 or 300 µg or placebo, or open-label tiotropium 18 µg, all once daily, for 26 weeks. The incidence of adverse events, low serum potassium, high blood glucose, and prolonged QTc interval was similar across treatments. Indacaterol was an effective once-daily bronchodilator and was at least as effective as tiotropium in improving clinical outcomes for patients with COPD.[6] The magnitude of the bronchodilator effect achieved with indacaterol compares favourably with that reported in other studies for salmeterol, formoterol and tiotropium.[3] It is available in stand-alone form or with glycopyrronium.

Vilanteroltrifenatate (formerly named compound 13f.triphenylacetate or GSK-642444) is an ultra LABA. It is a highly lipophilic molecule. Its affinity for the β_2 receptor is higher than formoterol, indacaterol, and olodaterol but comparable with that of salmeterol in a dose-dependent rapid bronchodilation in healthy subjects and in patients with stable COPD and is maintained over 24 hours. In India it is available in combination with fluticasone furoate and umeclidium.[7]

Olodaterol (BI 1744 CL) is a novel once-daily LABA designed with the aim of improving β_2-adrenoreceptor (AR) selectivity and intrinsic activity. Both 5 and 10 µg dose of olodaterol significantly improved the FEV_1 and these improvements were evident at weeks 24 and 48 also. Interestingly, improvements in FEV_1 with olodaterol were evident from 5 minutes after the first dose. Over 48 weeks, use of rescue medication was also significantly reduced. It is administered as a solution via a Respimat soft mist inhaler.[8] It has been approved to be administered in combination with tiotropium.

Long-acting Muscarinic Antagonist (LAMA)

The LAMAs like tiotropium are selective M3 receptors blocker in the lungs. They have a better and sustained bronchodilator effect. LAMAs reduce rate of progress of disease by reducing COPD exacerbations thus reducing mortality.[9] Newer LAMAs include glycopyrronium, aclidinium, umeclidinium, etc.

Glycopyrronium bromide (NVA237) is a once-daily dry-powder formulation of the LAMA for the treatment of COPD.[10] It blocks muscarinic type 1 (M1) and type 3 (M3) receptors producing bronchodilatation.[11–12] Once-daily dose of glycopyrronium provides sustained 24-hour bronchodilation. It has a rapid onset of action and is safe and well tolerated. Dose of glycopyrronium bromide is 50–100 µg once daily (tolerated up to 200 µg). GLOW1 study showed that glycopyrronium bromide resulted in improvement in trough FEV_1 at 12 weeks, reduced the risk of moderate or severe COPD exacerbations and was associated with reduced rate of exacerbations. It has a safe cardiac profile due to high affinity for M_3 receptors and low affinity for M_2 receptors.[10] It is an inhalation powder available in hard capsules. It is available in stand alone form or in combination with indacaterol.

Aclidinium bromide is a novel inhalational long-acting muscarinic antagonist compound with low systemic activity. The efficacy and safety of aclidinium 200 µg and 400 µg bid versus placebo over 12 weeks (ACCORD) and 24 weeks (ATTAIN) in patients with moderate to severe COPD reported significant improvements in bronchodilation, health status and COPD symptoms. There were no differences between the safety profiles of the two doses.[13]

Umeclidinium bromide (GSK573719) is a new LAMA used in COPD. It acts preferentially on the M3 receptor. Bronchodilation peaks at 3 hours after a dose and is sustained for 24 hrs. A randomized, *double-blind, placebo*-controlled, parallel-group study evaluated three once-daily doses of umeclidinium (125, 250 and 500 µg) for 28 days. It showed significantly increased trough FEV_1 over placebo, reductions in *salbutamol* use and improvements in FVC.[14] It is available as a combination of umeclidinium bromide-vilanterol (62.5 µg/ 25 µg).

Combinations (Table 14.2)

According to GOLD 2016, combination therapy is the first line treatment for patients in group C and group D COPD. Combi-

Table 14.2: Various combinations therapies available for COPD medical management

S.No.	Drug	Inhaler (µg)	Duration of action	Trial
1.	Formoterol/aclidinium	12/340 (DPI)	12 hours	Augment COPD study[15] Acliform-COPD study[16]
2.	Indacaterol/ glycopyrronium	85/43 (DPI)	24 hours	Van, et al[17] Enlighten study[18] Shine study[19] Illuminate study[20] Spark study[21] Beacon study[22] Glow6 study[23] Flight 1 and flight 2 study[24] Lantern study[25] Flame study[26] etcc
3.	Olodaterol/tiotropium	5/5 (SMI)	24 hours	Maltais, et al[27] Aalbers, et al[28] Energito study[29]
4.	Vilanterol/umeclidinium	25/62.5 (DPI)	24 hours	Feldman, et al[30]
5.	Vilanterol/Fluticasone furoate	25/100 (DPI)	24 hours	Summit study[31] Martinez, et al[32] Kerwin, et al[33]

nation therapy presently available and in the pipeline include inhaled corticosteroid and LABA in a single inhaler, LABA and LAMA in a single inhaler and triple therapy including inhaled corticosteroid, LAMA and LABA. Table 14.2 lists the newer combination therapies available around the world and their status in India.

Drugs In The Pipeline

A number of other newer drugs are being developed and are in different phases of trials (Table 14.3). These include newer bron-

chodilators, combination therapy, MABA (muscarinic-antagonist β_2-agonist), anti-oxidants, anti-inflammatory, statins, regenerative therapies and anti-ageing therapy. Table 14.3 enlists these newer drugs.[9]

Antibiotics

In recent years a number of studies have been done on the role of macrolide-azithromycin in COPD. Macrolide antibiotics have immunomodulatory, anti-inflammatory, and antibacterial effects. It has been concluded that in patients with chronic

Table 14.3: Newer drugs in the pipeline for COPD

S.No.	Drug Category	Drugs
1.	Bronchodilators a. Ultra long-acting β_2 agonists b. Ultra long-acting anti-muscarinic agents	Carmoterol, milveterol hydrochloride, GSK-642444, BI-1744-CL, saligenin or indole containing β_2 agonists, UK-503590 etc. TD-4208, QAT-370, CHF 5407, darotropium bromide, dexpirronium
2.	Combinations a. MABA (Muscarinic-antagonist-β_2-agonist) b. LABA and ICS c. LABA, LAMA and ICS	 GSK-91081, Bicyclohept-7-ylamine derivatives Carmoterol and budesonide, formoterol and mometasone (MFF258), formoterol and ciclesonide, indacaterol and mometasone (QMF-149), indacaterol and QAE-397 (a novel corticosteroid), fluticasone furoate and GSK-642444. Tiotropium and salmeterol and fluticasone/ciclesonide, indacaterol and glycopyrronium and mometasone, milveterol hydrochloride and darotropium and fluticasone furoate, GSK-642444 and dartropium and fluticasone furoate.
3.	PDE4 Inhibitors	Cilomilast
4.	Anti-inflammatory drugs	Cytokine inhibitors, chemokine antagonists, TGF-β inhibitors, antiproteases, nuclear factor-κB inhibitors, 7. p38 MAP kinase inhibitors, PI3k inhibitors, PAR agonists
5.	Anti-oxidants	N-acetyl cysteine (NAC) derivatives, NRF-2 activators
6.	Statins	Simvastatin, Atorvastatin, Pravastatin
7.	Regenerative therapies	Retinoic acid
8.	Anti-ageing therapy	SIRT1 activators

obstructive pulmonary disease at increased risk for exacerbations, once-daily azithromycin for 1 year reduced frequency of exacerbations and improved quality of life but increased hearing loss and increased incidence of bacterial resistance.[34]

Gold 2017 suggests, azithromycin (250 mg/day or 500 mg three times per week) or erythromycin (500 mg two times per day) for one year in patients prone to exacerbations reduced the risk of exacerbations compared to standard treatment.[35]

Previously pulse therapy with moxifloxacin (400 mg/day for 5 days every 8 weeks) was also studied in chronic bronchitis patient with frequent exacerbations, however, it had no overall beneficial effect.[35]

Role of Vitamin D

Studies suggest that Vitamin D may be involved in the pathogenesis of COPD, it may reduce the frequency of respiratory infections, impairing response to pathogens, and inhibiting the proliferation of airway smooth muscle. There are contradictory studies on the role of vitamin D deficiency in development of COPD. A meta-analysis suggested that the low serum level of 25(OH)D was not associated with COPD susceptibility, but the high rate of 25(OH)D deficiency was associated with COPD severity. It also suggests that vitamin D supplementation can inhibit COPD exacerbation.[36]

BRONCHOSCOPIC MANAGEMENT OF COPD (LUNG VOLUME REDUCTION PROCEDURES)

In emphysema there is alveolar destruction causing hyperinflation. Severe emphysema reduces diaphragmatic contraction and hence reduces capacity of lung. Hypoxia due to severe emphysema causes pulmonary arterial hypertension by hypoxia induced pulmonary vasoconstriction. In such situations most of medical treatment like bronchodilators, do not relieve symptoms. In such cases treatment modalities which reduce hyperinflation will help in the management of severe emphysema. Figure 14.1 depicts the various bronchoscopic methods for treatment of COPD.

Surgical management of COPD via bullectomy, lung volume reduction surgery and lung Transplant are known treatment for COPD. Nowadays various bronchoscopic methods are under trial for non-invasive or minimal invasive management of emphysema.

In selected patients of COPD, with heterogeneous or homogeneous emphysema and significant hyperinflation, refractory to optimized medical care, bronchoscopic

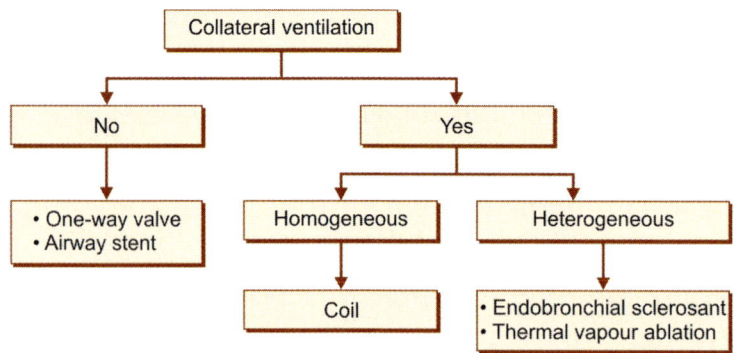

Fig 14.1: Suggesting assessment of the patient for bronchoscopic treatment of COPD

modes of lung volume reduction may be considered according to GOLD 2017.[35]

It depends on a number of factors including the extent and pattern of emphysema on HRCT, the presence of interlobar collateral ventilation measured by fissure integrity on HRCT, or physiological assessment, and patient and provider preferences.[35]

Criteria of endoscopic LVR[37] are as follows:

1. (a) Severe air trapping (RV>225%, IC/TLC<25%), (b) hyperinflation of chest (TLC>150%), (c) severe functional impairment (FEV$_1$ and DLco> 20%)
2. Careful chest CT scan and endobronchial balloon occluding system should be used to see collateral ventilation and distal flow.

Treatment Modalities

1. **Endobronchial valves** (Fig. 14.2): These are umbrella or fish mouth appearing endobronchial valve. These are one-way valve which are deployed in bronchus of maximum emphysema without significant collateral ventilation (less than 10% collateral ventilation). These valves allow air to come out during expiration but prevent air to go in while inspiration so causes atelectasis of that lobe.[38] Best

results are seen in patients with heterogeneous emphysema. Most studies show increase in mean FEV$_1$ (~7%) compared to standard medical care in patients with severe to very severe COPD and improvement in chronic dyspnoea. These changes were statistically significant.[39, 40] Its adverse events include nonmassive hemoptysis, pneumothorax and pneumonia.

2. **Endobronchial coil implants** (Fig. 14.3): These are wire-like structure which modifies its shape according to airway anatomy (memory shape coil). It can be used in homogeneous emphysema as it is collateral independent. It acts by causing compression of adjacent lung tissue and has tethering effect on small bronchi which helps in keeping open airways while expiration to empty the lung. Small studies show improvement in FEV$_1$.[41] Its side effects include pneumonia and COPD exacerbation.

3. **Endobronchial sclerosant therapy:** Sclerosant materials are usually made up of aminated polyvinyl alcohol and glutaraldehyde, and are injected in distal airway. It reduces emphysema by tissue remodelling rather than atelectasis of lung. Studies show improvement in lung function and quality of life at 6 and 12 months.[42, 43]

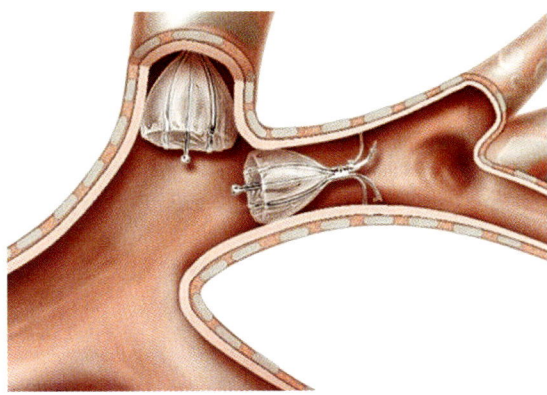

Fig: 14.2: Endobronchial valves

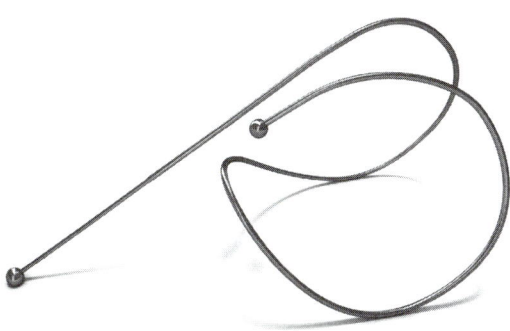

Fig: 14.3: Endobronchial coil implants

4. **Biological LVR:** Biological substances like fibrinogen and thrombin solution are injected into distal airway by bronchoscopy.[37] These substances polymerize and produce local inflammatory reaction, causing tissue remodelling and atelectasis. So there is lung volume reduction in 1–2 months. Another small study was done with autologous blood and thrombin, used as biological sealant.[43] This modality of treatment is collateral independent. Studies show improvement in exercise tolerance and quality of life. There were two mortality in one randomised control trial and number of serious adverse events was higher than that of other modality of LVR.[45]

5. **Endoscopic thermal vapour ablation LVR:** Endoscopic thermal vapour ablation LVR uses heated water to produce thermal injury to distal airway. It is more useful in heterogeneous emphysema and independent of collateral ventilation. Studies show improvement in lung functions, exercise tolerance and quality of life.[46,47] It is reported to cause adverse events like pneumonia, exacerbation of COPD, etc.

6. **Airway bypass stents:** Airway bypass stents create passage between airway and emphysematous lobe by a stent. There should be complete absence of collateral ventilation. To date there is no significant improvement in outcome.[39]

In ELVR, one-way valve is treatment of choice when there is heterogenous emphysema and no colllateral ventilation. In conditions where there is significant collateral ventilation and homogenous emphysema, coil implant is treatment of choice for ELVR.

Table 14.4 summarizes various bronchoscopic methods to treat COPD.

Further studies are required to demonstrate the effect of bronchoscopic lung volume reduction surgery on survival or other long-term outcomes or in comparison to LVRS.

Treatment of Non-emphysematous COPD (Chronic Bronchitis)

For patients who suffer from chronic bronchitis or the non-emphysematous COPD, the upcoming procedures are targeted lung denervation and endobronchial cryospray.

Targeted lung denervation: Lung is innervated by vagus nerve which has parasympathatic action by releasing acetylcholine (Bronchoconstrictor). So, thermal ablation of vagus nerve complex around main bronchi by water-cooled radiofrequency energy prevents broncho-

Table: 14.4: Summary of the various bronchoscopic methods to treat COPD			
Technique	*Collateral ventilation*	*Emphysema*	*Reversibility*
One-way valve	Should be absent	Heterogeneous	Fully reversible
Coil implant	Independent	Heterogeneous or homogeneous	Partially reversible
Endobronchial sclerosant, biological, thermal vapour ablation	Independent	Heterogeneous	Irreversible
Airway stent	Should be absent	Heterogeneous	Partially reversible

constriction. By unknown mechanism, there is increased sensitivity of bronchi with anticholinergic drugs after lung denervation procedure. Pilot study shows improvement in FEV$_1$ and dyspnoea grade.[48]

Endobronchial cryospray: This is bronchoscopic procedure by which bronchial mucosa is exposed to repeated rapid freeze-thaw cycles by cryoprobe. This procedure leads to cell death and regeneration of normal mucosa.[49]

DIAGNOSIS AND NEWER TESTS

Thoracic CT scanning can be used to quantify the extent, type, distribution, and progression of emphysema. However, measurement of airway dimensions is difficult. The presence of emphysema is associated with a more rapid decline in FEV$_1$ and with increased mortality. Studies show relationships between both the extent of emphysema, airway thickening and the frequency of exacerbations. CT chest can help diagnose other lung conditions, such as bronchiectasis, obliterative bronchiolitis, and diffuse panbronchiolitis and to assess comorbidities such as coronary artery disease by measuring coronary artery calcification.[50] However, till date there are no guidelines incorporating the use of CT scan in the diagnosis of COPD.

BIOMARKERS

Classically a biomarker is defined as "a unique marker such as a molecule, cell, tissue or material that indicates the existence of a disease.[51]" However, functional assessment and imaging may also be considered as a marker of the disease occurrence. Biomarkers help in the early diagnosis of a particular disease, aid in the treatment strategy, facilitate monitoring the progression of the disease, foretell response to treatment and also predict mortality in certain cases.[52]

Blood Biomarkers

In COPD patients, biomarkers can be measured in the blood, sputum or breath. The most promising blood biomarker is fibrinogen. It has been associated with the risk of COPD, disease progression and mortality, independent of other established risk factors.[53] Although the data on the role of fibrinogen as a biomarker in disease progression and exacerbation is variable, its role in predicting mortality is promising. Danesh et al have demonstrated that a 1 g/L increase in fibrinogen level is associated with a 3.5 times increase in COPD mortality.[54]

Other blood biomarkers include serum amyloid protein (SAA) and C-reactive protein (CRP). SAA is an excellent biomarker in predicting exacerbation of COPD. SAA levels increase by 6.5 fold in exacerbations as compared with levels observed during periods of clinical stability and there is a 92% decrease in the SAA levels on treatment.[42] CRP is a non-specific acute phase reactant. Although theoretically it is good in predicting exacerbation and mortality[55] in COPD patient, practical use of CRP remains to be seen.

Fibrinogen, SAA, and CRP are regulated by IL-6. Serum IL-6 levels have been assessed as a possible biomarker in COPD. In the ECLIPSE study, serum IL-6 level was significantly related to total mortality.[56] However, one of its major drawbacks is that it is non-repeatable, as levels return to baseline after prolonged periods of time.[56]

Other blood biomarkers are surfactant protein D (SP-D) and Clara cell secretory protein-16 (CCSP-16).[57] They are also called pneumoproteins since they are mostly synthesized in the lungs.

CCSP-16 is produced by club cells and noncilliated bronchiolar cells in the airways and hence plasma levels vary according to the performance of these cells in the lungs.[57] According to ECLIPSE study, CCSP-16 was the best biomarker of disease progression.[58] It showed that one SD increase in serum CCSP-16 level was associated with a 33 ml increase in baseline FEV_1.[59]

SP-D has a weak association with COPD exacerbation and its levels are sensitive to corticosteroid treatment.[59]

Pulmonary and activation-regulated chemokine (PARC/CCL-18) is another lung-predominant inflammatory protein that is found in serum.[57] It has been associated with an increased risk of mortality. However, it has a relatively low repeatability index.[57]

Other upcoming biomarkers are receptor for advanced glycation end products (RAGE) and its ligand, advanced glycation end products (AGE). These glycated lipid or protein molecules bind non-specifically to normal tissue, such as endothelium or epithelium, altering their structure and function.[57] Wu et al have shown that patients with COPD have increased protein expression of AGE and RAGE in the airways.[60]

Sputum Biomarkers (Table 14.5)

COPD is considered a neutrophilic airway inflammatory disease. In the recent years, a number of molecules, released by activated respiratory tract cells have been found in variable amount in COPD lungs. These include cytokines, chemokines, lymphokines, growth factors, molecules related to oxidative stress, proteases and antiproteases etc. However, more studies are needed to clarify their role and utility in diagnosing COPD.[60] Table 1.3 lists the sputum biomarkers currently being studied in COPD patients.[61]

Exhaled Breath Analysis

This is a non-invasive method to analyse the airway inflammation that occurs in COPD patients. Different technologies are used such as gas chromatography-mass spectrometry and the electronic nose.[62]

Exhaled Breath Condensate (EBC)

Collection of cooled exhaled breath as condensate is a non-invasive method of evaluating the airways and epithelial lining fluid that is exposed to the environment. EBC levels are lower in former smokers with GOLD stage III to IV COPD, compared to stage I,[63] suggesting that airway acidification could be a marker of airway inflammation and disease severity in COPD.[63] EBC pH is also reduced during acute exacerbations.[65]

Table: 14.5: Sputum biomarkers in COPD	
Cytokines	TNF-α, IL-1β, and IL-6
Chemokines	CCL2, CXCL1, CXCL8, CXCL9, CXCL10, CXCL11 and CCL5
Growth factor	GM CSF, VEGF
Molecules related to oxidative stress	Myeloperoxidase (MPO), superoxide dismutase (SOD), 8-isoprostane, nitrotyrosine
Proteases and antiproteases	Matrix metalloproteinases (MMPs) MMP8, MMP 9, MMP12 neutrophil elastase (NE), HNP (human neutrophil peptide)
Others	Leukotriene B_4 (LTB$_4$)

Volatile Organic Compounds (VOCs)

The exhaled breath contains some VOCs. Electronic noses are small portable devices that emulate the human nose. They have an ability to detect VOCs by adsorbing them onto sensors to produce a change in conductivity, colour or oscillation of a crystal, leading to readouts that are analysed.[62]

However, before extensive use in the clinical setting, validation is required.

The search for the perfect biomarker in COPD continues. The ease of collecting the sample and reproducibility remains a major concern at present.

ACOS: ASTHMA COPD OVERLAP SYNDROME

Definition and Epidemiology

Asthma COPD overlap syndrome or ACOS, as it is popularly known, is the occurrence of features of both, asthma and COPD simultaneously in an individual. According to a joint document by the global initiative for asthma (GINA) and global initiative for chronic obstructive lung disease (GOLD) 2016, ACOS is a clinical diagnosis, and it is characterized by persistent airflow limitation with several features usually associated with asthma and several features usually associated with COPD.[66]

The Dutch hypothesis[67] states that asthma and COPD are a part of the same spectrum of airway diseases. Why some patient have a benign course with reversible airway obstruction in the beginning which responds to inhaled bronchodilators and while others have a more malignant course in the form of fixed airway obstruction, is a matter of study. However, a few factors have been attributed to the development of ACOS. These include advancing age, smoking, airway inflammation, bronchial hyper-reactivity and airway remodelling.[68]

Studies suggest that in patients younger than 50 years of age the prevalence of ACOS is 10%, whereas the prevalence is up to 50% in age groups more than 80 years.[69]

Since there are no established diagnostic criteria till date for ACOS, the epidemiological data is scarce. Most studies on COPD exclude the history of atopy and reversible airflow obstruction while studies on asthma, exclude smokers. Depending on the population considered, different studies estimate a prevalence of ACOS between 5 and 20%.[70]

Clinical Features

The patients with ACOS present at an earlier age than COPD. The symptoms are same as that of obstructive airway disease including shortness of breath, productive cough, whitish expectoration and wheezing. These patients have more severe exacerbations, both in intensity and frequency. They have more frequent hospital admissions, longer hospital stays and poorer quality of life as compared to patients with either COPD or asthma alone.[71] Patients with ACOS also show poorer lung function tests than patients with COPD alone. It may show a partially reversible airway disease in smokers or irreversible airflow obstruction in patient with history of personal or family atopy, the diffusion capacity may be normal or it could be reduced. Chest radiography is usually normal or suggestive of features of hyperinflation.[72] CT scan of the thorax shows greater airway wall thickness and more air trapping as compared to COPD.[72]

Guidelines

There are no universal guidelines in existence for ACOS, making the diagnosis a difficult task for a primary care and respiratory physician. There is a need for an diagnostic criteria which can ascertain standardized treatment to all patients falling into this phenotype of obstructive airway disease. There are a few criteria proposed to diagnose a patient with ACOS in patients who have been previously diagnosed with chronic obstructive airway disease, listed in Table 14.6. However, they are neither sensitive nor specific.

GINA and GOLD joint document 2016,[66] suggests a 5-step syndromic approach to chronic obstructive airway diseases. The first step is ascertaining if an airway disease is present. This is done by detailed history taking and examination along with radiological tests. Next it is assessed whether the symptoms are more in favour of COPD,

Table 14.6: Various criteria are proposed by different studies for diagnosing ACOS in a patient, with pre-existing chronic obstructive airway disease

Study	*Criteria proposed*	
Spanish consensus guideline[73]	Major criteria: 1. Positive bronchodilator response (increase in FEV_1 ≥15% and 400 ml) 2. Sputum eosinophilia 3. Personal history of asthma **Minor criteria:** 1. Increased total serum IgE 2. Previous history of atopy 3. Positive bronchodilator test (>200 ml and >12% in FEV_1) on at least two occasions	Two major or one major and two minor criteria
Zeki et al[74]	1. Asthma with partially reversible airflow obstruction, with or without emphysema or DLCO<80% 2. COPD with emphysema accompanied by reversible or partially reversible airflow obstruction, with or without environmental allergies or reduced DLCO	Presence of one of the two clinical phenotypes
Louie et al[75]	**Major criteria:** 1. A physician diagnosis of asthma and COPD in the same patient. 2. History or evidence of atopy, e.g. hay fever, elevated IgE 3. Age> 40 years 4. Smoking > 10 pack years 5. Post-bronchodilator FEV_1<80% and FEV_1/FVC <70 **Minor criteria:** 1. >15% increase in FEV_1 or 12% and 200 ml increase in post-bronchodilator treatment with albetrol.	
Hardin et al[76] and Miravitlles, et al[77]	Previous diagnosis of asthma before the age of 40	

asthma or there are equal features of both, suggesting ACOS. This is followed by spirometry and initial treatment in the form of inhaled therapy. If however, the patient does not respond to the initial therapy, further tests are warranted and require a specialist's attention.

Diagnosis and Algorithm

Diagnosing ACOS is a challenging task. To avoid confusion we ought to follow a systematic stepwise approach. Figure 14.5 is a flowchart aiding in the diagnosis of ACOS.

Abbreviations: OAD: Obstructive airway disease, COPD: Chronic obstructive airway disease, BA: Bronchial asthma, ACOS:

Asthma COPD overlap syndrome, hx: History, CXR: Chest X-ray, DLCO: Diffusion capacity.

Treatment

There are a few evidence-based studies on the treatment strategies of ACOS. Most of current knowledge is extrapolated from the research done in either asthma or COPD.[78] Like all obstructive airway diseases, the treatment is divided into two parts: Supportive measures and the main therapy. Supportive therapy includes smoking cessation, avoiding exposure to allergens and biomass fuel, vaccination against influenza and pneumococcus, pulmonary

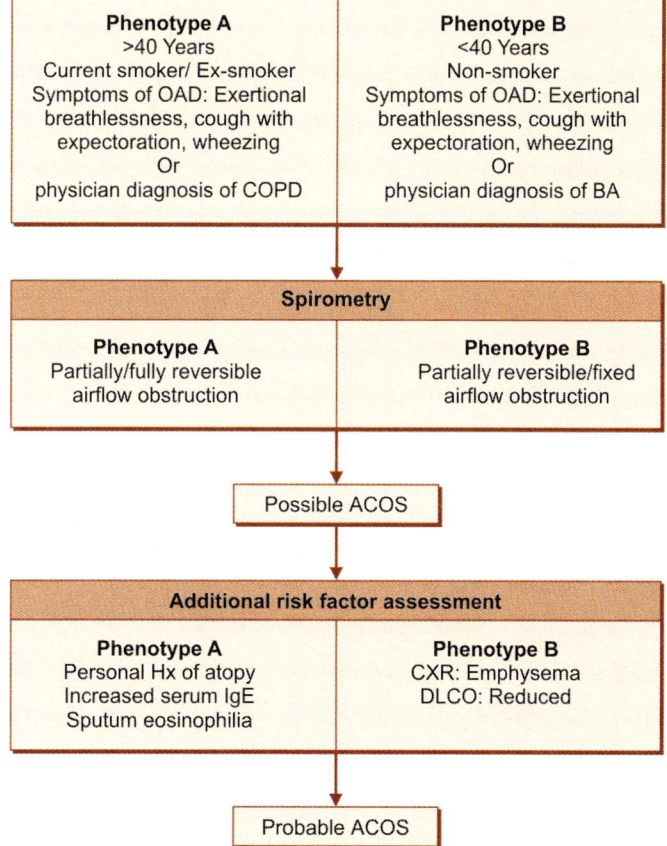

Fig. 14.5: Proposed stepwise approaches for patients with overlapping features of COPD and asthma

rehabilitation, oxygen therapy and non-invasive ventilation in the more advanced stages.

Inhaled corticosteroids form the core of treatment. As compared to COPD, ACOS warrants early use of inhaled steroids to suppress the eosinophilic airway inflammation that is associated with it.[70] Inhaled bronchodilators (LAMA OR LABA) are used along with inhaled steroids.[70] Whether ICS/LABA/LAMA combination is preferred to ICS/LABA, remains to be studied.[78] The dose of inhaled corticosteroids must be adjusted as per the severity of the disease. The role of theophyllines, anti-leukotrienes, phospho-diesterase inhibitors, macrolides and n-acetyl cysteine in the treatment of ACOS is not known. Table 14.7 illustrates the treatment strategies for ACOS.

ACOS is a difficult to treat airway disease (Table 14.7). Before switching to additional therapy, the physician must ensure compliance to the medication. The inhaler technique must be cross-checked and if found to be incorrect, taught to the patient. Besides treating ACOS, it is imperative to treat the comorbidities which may be associated with rhinosinusitis, obstructive sleep apnoea, gastro-esophageal reflux disease and psychiatric illnesses such as depression and anxiety disorders.

Table 14.7: Criteria proposed for diagnosing ACOS in a patient, with pre-existing chronic obstructive airway disease

POSSIBLE/PROBABLE ACOS

Supportive therapy
- Smoking cessation
- Avoiding exposure to allergens and biomass fuel
- Vaccination against influenza and pneumococcus
- Pulmonary rehabilitation
- Nutrition
- Oxygen therapy
- Non-invasive ventilation

Main therapy

Inhaled CS + LABA

Other options: Inhaled CS + LABA + LAMA

Additional therapy

Theophylline

Leukotriene receptor antagonist

Phosphodiesterase 4 inhibitors: Roflumilast

Treatment of comorbidities

GERD

Obesity and obstructive sleep apnoea

ARS

Depression

Anxiety

Refer to specialist for special investigations if no improvement

Acute exacerbations of ACOS are common and more frequent than COPD. There are no clear treatment guidelines for the same. In our experience, acute exacerbation of ACOS requires a much more aggressive approach. Oxygen therapy, injectable corticosteroid, and nebulized short-acting bronchodilators are the mainstay of treating the exacerbation. Frequent ABG (arterial blood gas) analysis must be done to look for early signs of hypoxia and hypercapnia. Non-invasive ventilation may eliminate the need for mechanical ventilation. These patients may require longer ICU and hospital stay as compared to COPD patients.

There is very limited literature on ACOS as of today. More studies are required to give us an exact picture of the patho-physiology of this complex disease entity. A better understanding of its cause will help formulate guidelines to diagnose the disease, thus standardizing the management and making decisions easier for the physician and the patient. Till then one can contemplate and make use of the current consensus based guidelines available.

Abbreviation: CS: Corticosteroid, LABA: Long-acting β_2 agonist, LAMA: Long-acting anti-muscarinic agents, GERD: Gastro-esophageal reflux disease, ARS: Allergic rhinosinusitis

SUMMARY

The available treatment options control airway inflammation to an extent, however, with the advent of better technology and more effective medical and surgical treatment strategies are being developed. Ultra long-acting β_2 agonists like indacatrol, vilantrol have made possible once day dosing. Their onset of action is 5 mins or less and is maintained for 24 hrs. The LAMAs like tiotropium (M3 receptors blocker), glycopyrronium bromide (M1, M3 receptor blockers) are also prescribed in once a day dose.

A number of other newer drugs are being developed, which includes newer bronchodilators, combination therapy, MABA (Muscarinic antagonist-β_2 agonist), anti-oxidants, anti-inflammatory, statins, regenerative therapies and anti-ageing therapy, etc.

Bronchoscopic procedures like one-way valves, coil implants, endobronchial sclerosant, biological, thermal vapour ablation, airway stent, are coming up as non- invasive techniques for treatment of COPD.

In diagnostic aspect many blood and sputum markers are being evolved.

REFERENCES

1. G. Feldman, T. Siler, N. Prasad, D. Jack, S. Piggott, R. Owen, *et al.* Efficacy and safety of indacaterol 150 microg once-daily in COPD: a double-blind, randomised, 12-week study. BMC Pulm Med, 10 (2010), p. 11.
2. A dose-ranging study of indacaterol in obstructive airways disease, with a tiotropium comparison. Respir Med. 2008 Jul; 102(7): 1033–44.
3. O. Kornmann, R. Dahl, S. Centanni, A. Dogra, R. Owen, C. Lassen, B. Kramer. Once-daily indacaterol vs. twice-daily salmeterol for COPD: a placebo-controlled comparison. EurRespir J, 37 (2) (2011), pp. 273–9.
4. R. Dahl, K.F. Chung, R. Buhl, H. Magnussen, V. Nonikov, D. Jack, *et al.*Efficacy of a new once-daily long-acting inhaled β_2-agonist indacaterol versus twice-daily formoterol in COPD Thorax, 65 (6) (2010), pp. 473–9.
5. Barnes PJ, Pocock SJ, Magnussen H, et al. Integrating indacaterol dose selection in a clinical study in COPD using an adaptive seamless design. Pulm Pharmacol Ther 2010; 23: 165e71.
6. J.F. Donohue, C. Fogarty, J. Lotvall, D.A. Mahler, H. Worth, A. Yorgancioglu, *et al.* Once-daily bronchodilators for chronic obstructive pulmonary disease: indacaterol versus tiotropium. Am J Respir Crit Care Med, 182 (2) (2010), pp. 155–162.

7. Caramori G, Chung KF, Adcock M. Profile of fluticasone furoate/vilanterol dry powder inhaler combination therapy as a potential treatment for COPD. Int J Chron Obstruct Pulmon Dis. 2014 Feb 24; 9: 249–56.

8. Matera MG, Ora J, Cazzola M. Differential pharmacology and clinical utility of long-acting bronchodilators in COPD - focus on olodaterol. Ther Clin Risk Manag. 2015 Dec 4; 11: 1805–11.

9. Rahul Kodgule, AbhijitVaidya, Sundeep Salvi. Newer Therapies for Chronic Obstructive Pulmonary Disease. Supplement to JAPI, February 2012, Vol. 60.

10. D'Urzo A, Ferguson GT, van Noord JA, et al. Efficacy and safety of once-daily NVA237 in patients with moderate-to-severe COPD: the GLOW1 trial. Respir Res 2011; 12: 156.

11. Fogarty C, Hattersley H, Di SL, Drollmann A: Bronchodilatory effects of NVA237, a once daily long-acting muscarinic antagonist, in COPD patients. Respir Med 2011, 105: 337–342.

12. Verkindre C, Fukuchi Y, Flemale A, Takeda A, Overend T, Prasad N, Dolker M: Sustained 24-h efficacy of NVA237, a once-daily long-acting muscarinic antagonist, in COPD patients. Respir Med 2010, 104: 1482–89.

13. Fuhr R, Magnussen H, Sarem K, et al. Efficacy of aclidinium bromide 400 μg twice daily compared with placebo and tiotropium in patients with moderate to severe COPD. Chest 2012; 141: 745.

14. Decramer M, Maltais F, Feldman G, Brooks J, Harris S, Mehta R, Crater G. Bronchodilation of umeclidinium, a new long-acting muscarinic antagonist, in COPD patients. Respir Physiol Neurobiol. 2013 Jan; 185(2): 393–9.

15. D'Urzo AD, Rennard SI, Kerwin EM, Mergel V, Leselbaum AR, Caracta CF, AUGMENT COPD Study Investigators Efficacy and safety of fixed-dose combinations of aclidinium bromide/formoterolfumarate: the 24-week, randomized, placebo-controlled augment COPD study. Respir Res. 2014; 15(1): 123.

16. Singh D, Jones PW, Bateman ED, et al. Efficacy and safety of aclidinium bromide/form oterol-fumarate fixed-dose combinations compared with individual components and placebo in patients with COPD (ACLIFORM-COPD): a multicentre, randomised study. BMC Pulm Med. 2014; 14: 178.

17. vanNoord JA, Buhl R, LaForce C, et al. QVA149 demonstrates superior bronchodilation compared with indacaterol or placebo in patients with chronic obstructive pulmonary disease. Thorax. 2010; 65: 1086–91.

18. Dahl R, Chapman K, Rudolf M, et al. QVA149 administered once daily provides significant improvements in lung function over 1 year in patients with COPD: the ENLIGHTEN study [abstract]. EurRespir J. 2012; 40 (Suppl 56): P2896.

19. Bateman ED, Ferguson GT, Barnes N, et al. Dual bronchodilation with QVA149 versus single bronchodilator therapy: the SHINE study. Eur Respir J. 2013; 42: 1484–94.

20. Vogelmeier CF, Bateman ED, Pallante J, et al. Efficacy and safety of once-daily QVA149 compared with twice-daily salmeterol-fluticasone in patients with chronic obstructive pulmonary disease (ILLUMINATE): a randomised, double-blind, parallel group study. Lancet Respir Med. 2013; 1: 51–60.

21. Wedzicha JA, Decramer M, Ficker JH, Niewoehner DE, Sandström T, Taylor AF, D'Andrea P, Arrasate C, Chen H, Banerji D. Analysis of chronic obstructive pulmonary disease exacerbations with the dual bronchodilator QVA149 compared with glycopyrronium and tiotropium (SPARK): a randomised, double-blind, parallel-group study. Lancet Respir Med. 2013 May; 1(3): 199–209.

22. Dahl R, Jadayel D, Alagappan VK, Chen H, Banerji D. Efficacy and safety of QVA149 compared to the concurrent administration of its monocomponents indacaterol and glycopyrronium: the BEACON study.Int J Chron Obstruct Pulmon Dis. 2013; 8: 501–8. doi: 10.2147/COPD.S49615. Erratum in: Int J Chron Obstruct Pulmon Dis. 2014; 9: 85.

23. Vincken W, Aumann J, Chen H, Henley M, McBryan D, Goyal P. Efficacy and safety of coadministration of once-daily indacaterol and glycopyrronium versus indacaterolalone in COPD patients: the GLOW6 study. Int J Chron Obstruct Pulmon Dis. 2014 Feb 24; 9: 215–28.

24. Donald A. Mahler, Edward Kerwin, Tim Ayers, Angel FowlerTaylor, Samopriyo Maitra, ChauThach, Mark Lloyd, Francesco Patalano, and Donald Banerji. FLIGHT1 and FLIGHT2: Efficacy and Safety of QVA149 (Indacaterol/Glycopyrrolate) versus Its Monocomponents

and Placebo in Patients with Chronic Obstructive Pulmonary Disease. Am J Respir Crit Care Med. 2015 Nov 1; 192(9): 1068–79.

25. Zhong N, Wang C, Zhou X, Zhang N, Humphries M, Wang L, Thach C, Patalano F, Banerji D.LANTERN: a randomized study of QVA149 versus salmeterol/fluticasone combination in patients with COPD.Int J Chron Obstruct Pulmon Dis. 2015 Jun 5; 10: 1015–26.

26. Wedzicha JA, Banerji D, Chapman KR, Vestbo J, Roche N, Ayers RT, Thach C, Fogel R, Patalano F, Vogelmeier CF. Indacaterol-Glycopyrronium versus Salmeterol-Fluticasone for COPD. N Engl J Med. 2016 Jun 9; 374(23): 2222–34.

27. Maltais F, Beck E, Webster D, et al. Four weeks once daily treatment with tiotropium + olodaterol (BI 1744) fixed dose combination compared with tiotropium in COPD patients [abstract]. Eur Respir J. 2010; 36 (Suppl 54): 1014s.

28. Aalbers R, Maleki-Yazdi MR, Hamilton A, et al. Dose-finding study for tiotropium and olodaterol when administered in combination via the Respimat® inhaler in patients with COPD. Eur Respir J. 2012; 40 (Suppl 56): 525s.

29. Beeh KM, Derom E, Echave-Sustaeta J, Grönke L, Hamilton A, Zhai D, Bjermer L.The lung function profile of once-daily tiotropium and olodaterol via Respimat(®) is superior to that of twice-daily salmeterol and fluticasone propionate via Accuhaler(®) (ENERGITO(®) study). Int J Chron Obstruct Pulmon Dis. 2016 Feb 4; 11: 193–205.

30. Feldman G, Walker RR, Brooks J, Mehta R, Crater G. Safety and tolerability of the GSK573719/vilanterol combination in patients with COPD [abstract]. Am J Respir Crit Care Med. 2012; 185: A2938.

31. Vestbo J, Anderson JA, Brook RD, Calverley PM, Celli BR, Crim C, Martinez F, Yates J, Newby DE.Fluticasone furoate and vilanterol and survival in chronic obstructive pulmonary disease with heightened cardiovascular risk (SUMMIT): a double-blind randomised controlled trial. Lancet. 2016 Apr 30; 387 (10030): 1817–26.

32. Martinez FJ, Boscia J, Feldman G, Scott-Wilson C, Kilbride S, Fabbri L, Crim C, Calverley PM.Fluticasone furoate/vilanterol (100/25; 200/25 µg) improves lung function in COPD: a randomised trial. Respir Med. 2013 Apr; 107(4): 550–9.

33. Kerwin EM, Scott-Wilson C, Sanford L, Rennard S, Agusti A, Barnes N, Crim C. A randomised trial of fluticasone furoate/vilanterol (50/25 µg; 100/25 µg) on lung function in COPD. Respir Med. 2013 Apr; 107(4): 560–9.

34. Albert RK, Connett J, Bailey WC, et al; COPD Clinical Research Network. Azithromycin for prevention of exacerbations of COPD. N Engl J Med. 2011; 365: 689–98.

35. Biyuan Zhu1, Biqing Zhu2, Chaolie Xiao, Zhiwen Zheng. Vitamin D deficiency is associated with the severity of COPD: a systematic review and meta-analysis. International Journal of COPD 2015: 10 1907–16.

36. Global initiative for chronic obstructive lung disease. Global statergy for the diagnosis, management and prevention of chronic obstructive pulmonary disease. 2017. Available from: www.goldcopd.org.

37. Update on Nonsurgical Lung Volume Reduction Procedures J. Alberto Neder and Denis E. O'Donnell Canadian Respiratory JournalVolume 2016, Article ID 6462352, 6 pages http://dx.doi.org/10.1155/2016/6462352.

38. D. Gompelmann, R. Eberhardt, and F. Herth, "Endoscopic volume reduction in COPD-a critical review," *Deutsches ¨ Arzteblatt International*, vol. 111, no. 49, pp. 827–33, 2014.

39. H. Iftikhar, F. R. Mguire, and A. I. Musani, "Efficacy of bronchoscopic lung volume reduction: a meta-analysis,"*International Journal of Chronic Obstructive Pulmonary Disease*, vol. 9, pp. 481–91, 2014.

40. M. Choi, W. S. Lee, M. Lee et al., "Effectiveness of bronchoscopic lung volume reduction using unilateral endobronchial valve: a systematic review and meta-analysis," *International Journal of Chronic Obstructive Pulmonary Disease*, vol. 10, pp. 703–10, 2015.

41. Z. Zoumot, S. V. Kemp, S. Singh et al., "Endobronchial coils for severe emphysema are effective up to 12 months following treatment: medium term and cross-over results from a randomised controlled trial," *PLoS ONE*, vol. 10, no. 4, Article IDe0122656, 2015.

42. Herth FJ, Gompelmann D, Stanzel F, et al. Treatment of advanced emphysema with emphysematous lung sealant (AeriSeal1). Respiration 2011; 82: 36–45.

43. Kramer MR, Refaely Y, Maimon N, et al. Bilateral endoscopic sealant lung volume reduction therapy for advanced emphysema. Chest 2012; 142: 1111–7.

44. Y.Mizumori, Y.Mochiduki, Y. Nakahara et al., "Effects of bronchoscopic lung volume reduction using transbronchial infusion of autologous blood and thrombin in patients with severe chronic obstructive pulmonary disease," *Journal of Thoracic Disease*, vol. 7, no. 3, pp. 413–21, 2015.

45. C. E. Come, M. R. Kramer, M. T. Dransfield et al., "A randomised trial of lung sealant versus medical therapy for advanced emphysema," *European Respiratory Society*, Vol. 16, no. 3, pp. 651–62, 2015.

46. G. Snell, F. J. F.Herth, P.Hopkins et al., "Bronchoscopic thermal vapour ablation therapy in the management of heterogeneous emphysema," *European Respiratory Journal*, Vol. 39, no. 6, pp. 1326–33, 2012.

47. Herth FJ, Valipour A, Shah PL, et al. Segmental volume reduction using Thermal vapour ablation in patients with severe emphysema: six month randomized controlled trial (STEP-UP) results. Lancet Respir Med 2016.

48. Slebos DJ, Klooster K, Koegelenberg CF, et al. Targeted lung denervation for moderate to severe COPD: a pilot study. Thorax 2015; 70: 411–9. Initial clinical trial with first in human data of targeted vagal nerve ablation in a cohort of COPD patients.

49. Finley DJ, Dycoco J, Sarkar S, et al. Airway spray cryotherapy: initial outcomes from a multiinstitutional registry. Ann Thorac Surg 2012; 94: 199–203.

50. Peter Lange, David M Halpin, Denis E O'Donnell, William MacNee.Diagnosis, assessment, and phenotyping of COPD: beyond FEV$_1$. International Journal of COPD 2016: 11.

51. Cazzola M, MacNee W, Martinez FJ, et al. Outcomes for COPD pharmacological trials: from lung function to biomarkers. Eur Respir J 2008; 31: 416–69.

52. Morrow DA, de Lemos JA. Benchmarks for the assessment of novel cardiovascular biomarkers. Circulation 2007; 115: 949–52.

53. Duvoix A, Dickens J, Haq I, et al. Blood fibrinogen as a biomarker of chronic obstructive pulmonary disease. Thorax 2013; 68: 670–6.

54. Danesh J, Lewington S, Thompson SG, et al. Plasma fibrinogen level and the risk of major cardiovascular diseases and nonvascular mortality: an individual participant meta-analysis. JAMA 2005; 294: 1799–809.

55. Bozinovski S, Hutchinson A, Thompson M, et al. Serum amyloid as a biomarker of acute exacerbations of chronic obstructive pulmonary disease. Am J Respir Crit Care Med 2008; 177: 269–78.

56. Dickens JA, Miller BE, Edwards LD, et al. COPD association and repeatability of blood biomarkers in the ECLIPSE cohort. Respir Res 2011; 12: 146.

57. Agusti A, Sin DD. Biomarkers in COPD. Clin Chest Med. 2014 Mar; 35(1): 131–41.

58. Vestbo J, Edwards LD, Scanlon PD, et al. Changes in forced expiratory volume in 1 second over time in COPD. N Engl J Med 2011; 365: 1184–92.

59. Faner R et al. Lessons from ECLIPSE: a review of COPD biomarkers. Thorax. 2014 Jul; 69(7): 666–72.

60. Wu L, Ma L, Nicholson LF, et al. Advanced glycation end products and its receptor (RAGE) are increased in patients with COPD. Respir Med 2011; 105: 329–36.

61. Paone G et al. Blood and sputum biomarkers in COPD and asthma: a review.Eur Rev Med Pharmacol Sci. 2016; 20(4): 698–708.

62. Shaw JG, Vaughan A, Dent AG et al. Biomarkers of progression of chronic obstructive pulmonary disease (COPD). *J Thorac Dis* 2014; 6(11): 1532–47.

63. Papaioannou AI, Loukides S, Minas M, et al. Exhaled breath condensate pH as a biomarker of COPD severity in ex-smokers. Respir Res 2011; 12: 67.

64. MacNee W, Rennard SI, Hunt JF, et al. Evaluation of exhaled breath condensate pH as a biomarker for COPD. Respir Med 2011; 105: 1037–45.

65. Warwick G, Thomas PS, Yates DH. Non-invasive biomarkers in exacerbations of obstructive lung disease. Respirology 2013; 18: 874–84.

66. Global Initiative for Asthma. Global Stratergy for Asthma Management and Prevention, 2016. Available from: www.ginasthma.org.

67. Orie NGM, Sluiter HJ, eds. Bronchitis. Assen, the Netherlands: Royal van Gorcum,1962.

68. Papaiwannou A et al. Asthma-chronic obstructive pulmonary disease overlap syndrome (ACOS): current literature review *J Thorac Dis 2014; 6(S1): S146–S151.*

69. Soriano JB, Davis KJ, Coleman B, et al. The proportional Venn diagram ofobstructive lung disease: two approximations from the United States and the United Kingdom. Chest 2003; 124: 474–81.

70. Barrecheguren M, Esquinas C, and Miravitlles M. The asthma–chronic obstructive pulmonary disease overlap syndrome (ACOS): opportunities and challenges. Curr Opin Pulm Med 2015, 21: 74–79.

71. Menezes AM, Montes de Oca M, Pérez-Padilla R, et al. Increased risk of exacerbation and hospitalization in subjects with an overlap phenotype: COPD-asthma. *Chest.* 2014; 145(2): 297–304.

72. Hardin M, Cho M, McDonald ML, et al. The clinical and genetic features of COPD-asthma overlap syndrome. *Eur Respir J.* 2014; 44(2): 341–50.

73. Soler-Cataluna JJ, Cosio B, Izquierdo JL, et al. Consensus document on the overlap pheno-type COPD-asthma in COPD. Arch Bronconeumol 2012; 48: 331–7.

74. Zeki AA, Schivo M, Chan A, et al. The Asthma-COPD Overlap Syndrome: A Common Clinical Problem in the Elderly. J Allergy (Cairo) 2011; 2011: 861926.

75. Louie S, Zeki AA, Schivo M, et al. The asthma-chronic obstructive pulmonary disease overlap syndrome: pharmacotherapeutic considerations. Expert Rev Clin Pharmacol 2013; 6: 197–219.

76. Hardin M, Silverman EK, Barr RG, et al. The clinical features of overlap between COPD and asthma. Respir Res 2011; 12: 127.

77. Miravitlles M, Soriano JB, Ancochea J, et al. Characterisation of the overlap COPD-asthma phenotype. Focus on physical activity and health status. Respir Med 2013; 107: 1053–60.

78. Kostikas K, Clemens A, Patalano F. the asthma–COPD overlap syndrome: do we really need another syndrome in the already complex matrix of airway disease? International Journal of COPD 2016; 11: 1297–306.

Index

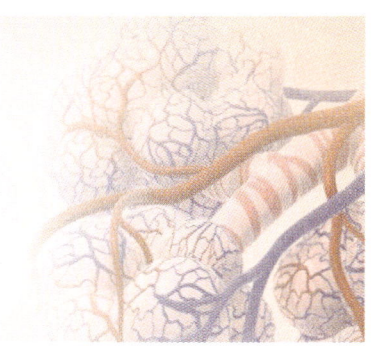

A

6MWT 142
ACCORD study 200
ACE inhibitors 119
Acebrophylline 86, 93
Acetylcholine 17
Aclidinium 188, 199
ACOS 207
Acute angle closure glaucoma 84
Acute rejection 101
Adhesion molecule 33
Administrative control 185
Adrenaline 16
Advice 94, 179
Aerobic
   exercises 168
   training 193
AGE biomarker 206
AHAM seal 183
Air purifiers 183
Airway bypass stent 204
Airway clearance techniques 172
Albuterol 82
Alpha-1 antitrypsin 34
   deficiency 19, 63, 93
Alpha-2 microglobulin 34
Ambroxol 91
Aminophyllin 93
Anaemia 68, 128
Angina 21, 69
Anthonisen criteria 106
Antibiotics 107
Anticipate 180
Anticoagulants 143
Antidepressant 181
Antioxidants 150
Anuvittasana 173

Anxiety 102
ARB 119
Arrange 94, 179
Arrhythmia 68, 84, 108
Arterial blood gas (ABG) 109, 115, 126
Ask 94, 179
Assess 94, 179
Assist 94, 179
ATTAIN study 200
Auscultation 52
AVAPS 115
Awareness 7
Azithromycin 191

B

Barrier filter 25
Bellows or diaphragm type spirometer 22
β_2 adrenergic receptors 82
Biceps curl 168
Bidi 6, 150
Bioelectrical impedence analysis 97
Biological LVR 204
Biomass fuel 7, 14, 49, 99, 181
BiPAP 113, 149
Bisoprolol 120
Bloating 156
Blocking 13
Blue bloaters 43
BMI 157
BODE index 65, 101
BOLD 133
Breathing training 165
Bronchial dehiscence 101
Bronchial stent 101
Bronchiectasis 53
Bronchiolitis obliterance 101
Bronchodilators 107

Bronchospasm 115
Bulla 61
Bullectomy 101, 201
Bupropion 94, 96, 181

C

C-reactive protein 107
Cachexia 21, 128
CADR 183
Calcium channel blocker 119, 143
Calf stretch 170
Carbocysteine 91, 190
Carboxyhemoglobin 63
Cardinal symptoms 106
CAT score 60
CAT 79, 135
CCR-2 38
CCSP-16 205
Centriacinar emphysema 43
CFTR gene 38
Chakrasana 173
Chantix 181
Cheese 160
Chillum 6, 150
Chimneys 183
Chronic bronchitis 13, 79
Chronic persistent asthma 53
Chronic renal failure 68
Ciliary dysfunction 19
Cilomilast 190
Claustrophobia 112
Compensatory emphysema 44
Confusion 102
Congestive heart failure 129
COPD diagnostic questionnaire 60
Cor pulmonale 51, 128, 143
CPAP 113, 149
C-reactive protein 205
Crop residue 97
CRQ 80, 134
Custard 160
Cyclic AMP 82

D

Dal 156
DALY 4
Depression 21, 68, 71, 97, 121, 129, 152, 194
Diabetes mellitus 68, 119, 121, 129, 194
Diaphragmatic 166, 167
   dysfunction 129
Dietary counseling 154

Distal acinar emphysema 43
Dizziness 69
Domiciliary oxygen 116
Dopamine 181
Doxofyllin/doxophyllin 85
DPI 126
Drug compliance 116
Dry mouth 84
Dutch hypothesis 207
DXA 144
Dynamic hyperinflation 89

E

ECLIPSE study 67, 205
Eggs 160
Elastic recoil 20, 81
Elimination 185
Emphysema 13, 79
Endobronchial
   coil 203
   cryospray 205
   sclerosant therapy 203
   unidirectional valve 101
   valves 203
Endoscopic thermal vapour ablation LVR 204
Endotracheal intubation 111
Engineering control 185
Environmental tobacco smoke 16, 97
Eosinophilia 91, 107, 190
Erythropoietin 72
Essential hypertension 119
Exaggerated somatic tremor 84
Exercise training 165
Exhaust fans 183

F

Facial puffiness 51
Fasting plasma sugar 121
Fat free mass index 97
FEF 25
FEV_1 25
FEV_6 25
Fibrinogen 205
Fibrosis 13
Folic acid 152
Fish 156
Flavonoids 151
Flexibility exercises 170
Flow time display 55
Formoterol 82, 93, 199
FVC 25

G

GARD 8
GERD 68, 120
Glucocorticoids 190
Glutamate 17
Glycopyrronium 189, 199
Goblet cell 20
Grand mal seizures 85

H

H. influenzae 109, 110
Haemodynamic stability 126
Haemoptysis 129
Head tilt 170
Heart failure 108
Hemoptysis 24
HEPA filters 183
Hepatojugular reflex 52
Histone deacetylase (HDAC) 87
   activity 84
Home walking program 168
Hookah 6, 150
Huffing 172
Hypercapnia 22, 108
Hypertension 24, 68, 144
Hypokalemia 84
Hypotension 108
Hypoxemia 108

I

ICMR 5
ICS 93, 125
IFN-γ 38
IL-6 205
IL-8 38
Immunosuppression 147
Indacaterol 82, 92, 93, 198, 211
Indoor air pollution (IAP) 6
Indoor ventilation 183
Industrialization 195
Infiltration 183
Influenza 94, 191
Inhaled corticosteroids 86, 210
Inhaler technique 116
Injectable corticosteroids 211
INLIGHT-1 study 198
INLIGHT-2 study 199
INSEARCH 3, 5
Insomnia 69
Inspection 52
Inspiratory muscle training 171

Intersitital emphysema 44
Intractable cough 102
INVOLVE study 199
Iodinated glycerol 91
Ischaemic heart disease 69

J

JVP 128

K

Kapalbhati 192
Klebsiella pneumonia 110

L

LABA 92, 125, 210
LAMA 92, 125, 210
Lean body mass 97
Leg raise 168
Leptin 148
Lipophilic 82
Liquid diet 160
LTB_4 38
LTOT 113
Lung
   age 178
   cancer 129
   health study 178
   senescence 40
   transplantation 81
   volume reduction coil 101
LVRS 100, 101
Lymphoproliferative disorder 101

M

M. catarrhalis 109, 110
M_2 receptors 200
M_3 receptors 200
Magnesium 151
Malnutrition 147
Matrix metallo-proteineases 34
MCP-1 38
Mechanical ventilation 111
Mediterranean diet 150
Metabolic syndrome 72
Metallic taste 84
Metformin 123
Metoprolol 120
Micronutrients 148
MIP-1α 38
mMRC 79, 128
Montelukast 91

Mosquito coil 7
Mouthpiece 25
Mucolytic agent 89
Mucus hypersecretion 19
Muscle deconditioning 125
Muscle wasting 128
MVV 26
Myeloperoxidase 38, 187
Myocardial
  infract 24
  perfusion 120
Myopathy 87, 91
Myosin light chain kinase 82

N

N-acetylcysteine 91, 93, 190
Nabivolol 120
National green tribunal 186
Natural ventilation 183
Nausea 85
Nebulizaton 126
  therapy 88, 108
Neutrophil elastase activity 87
Neutrophilic inflammation 21
Nicotine 16
  chewing gum 94, 95
  inhaler 96
  nasal spray 95
  patch 180
  replacement therapy 180
NIPPV 8
Non-invasive ventilation (NIV) 112
Non-smoker's COPD 3, 7
Nortriptyline 94, 96
Nosocomial pneumonias 125
Noxious particles 3, 132
Nuisance dust 17

O

Obliterative bronchiolitis 53, 79
Obstructive sleep apnoea 68
  syndrome 74
Occupational
  dust 7, 8
  exposure 184
Olodaterol 199
Omega-3 fatty acid 156, 162
Oral candidiasis 74, 123
Organic dust 185
Osteoporosis 21, 128, 129, 144

Oxidative stress 32
Oxygen therapy 211

P

Pack year 15
PAL 9
Palliative care 102
Palpation 52
Panacinar emphysema 43
Paneer 156
PANTHEON trial 190
Paracicatricial emphysema 44
Parkinson's disease 194
Paroxysmal noctournal dyspnoea 69
Paschimottanasana 173
Pedal oedema 51
PEF 25
Percussion 52
Peripheral oedema 22
Personal protective equipment 185
Perspiration 69
Phosphodiesterase inhibitors 84
Phosphorus 150
PHQ-2 71
PHQ-9 71
Physiotherapy 165
Pink puffers 45
Pleurocentesis 123
Pleurodesis 123
pMDI 126
PMUY 10
Pneumococcal 191
  vaccination 94
Pneumonia 68, 130
Pneumotachograph 22
Pneumothorax 68, 107
Pores of Kohn 44
Post-parendial plasma sugar 123
Post-TB COPD 7
Potassium 156
Poultry 156
PPSV 23 191
Pranayam 192
Prednisone 109
Primary prevention 177
Pseudomonas aeruginosa 109, 110
Pseudostratified columnar epithelium 42
Pulmonary artery hypertension 97, 143
Pulmonary artery pressure 69
Pulmonary hypertension 143
Pulmonary rehabilitation 97
Pursed lip 166

Q

QTc 84
Quadriceps stretch 170
Quarts 17
Quitters 178

R

RAGE biomarker 206
Reactive nitrogen species 32
Reactive oxygen species 32
Recovery 107
Reflux 70
Refractory dyspnoea 102
Rehabilitation 99, 127, 130, 135
Rehospitalization 187
Reid index 42
Relaxation techniques 99
Relevance 179
Reliever 116
Remove 180
Repeat 179
Resistance 166
Respiratory acidosis 64, 116
Resting energy expenditure 148
Restrictive lung pathology 58
Rewards 179
Right sided heart failure 69
Right ventricular failure 143
Risks 179
Roadblocks 179
Roflumilast 87, 93, 190
Rolling seal type spirometer 22, 23
RSSDI 123

S

S. pneumonia 109, 110
SABA 92, 125
Salmetrol 82, 93, 199
SAMA 92
Second-hand smoking 6
Secondary hypertension 119
Secondary polycythemia 21, 62
Secondary prevention 177
Selenium 152
Serum amyloid protein 205
Serum iron 121
Set 180
SGRQ 80, 134
Shoulder roll 170
Side lift 168

Silica 17
Sinus tachycardia 84
Sithali exercise 192
Skeletal muscle dysfunction 68, 70, 121
Smoking
  cessation 94, 135, 178
  index 15
Social aspect 126
Soft diet 157
Sphingolipids 36
Spironolactone 120
Split virion 94
SpO$_2$ 128
Sputum biomarkers 206
Squamous metaplasia 20
Star approach 179
Statins 91
Stationary bicycle 168
Steroids 107
Stoves 184
Stretchy resistance bands 168
Sublingual tablet 94
Subunit vaccine 94
Surfactant protein D 205
SVC 25
Systemic hypertension 129

T

Tachyphylaxis 84
Tadasana 172
Targeted lung denervation 204
Targeted thermal vapour ablation 101
Tell 180
Terbutaline 92
Terminal bronchioles 13
Tertiary prevention 177
Theophyllin 190
Thiazide diuretic 119, 120
Tiotropium 84, 188
TNF-α 38, 97, 107
  converting enzyme 38
Tracheostomy 129
Transdermal patch 94, 95
Treadmill 168
Tremors 85
Tricuspid regurgitation 63
Tuberculosis 68
Type-1 muscle fibers 167
Type-2 muscle fibers 167

U

Umeclidinium 188, 199
Underweight 152
UPLIFT trial 189

V

Vaccination, 94, 135, 191
Vanishing lung syndrome 61
Varenicline 94, 96, 181
VGEF 35, 36
Vilanterol 82, 93, 211
Vital capacity 83
Vitamin C 151
Vitamin D 152, 201
Vocal fremitus 74

Volatile organic compounds 207
Volume time curve 26, 55

W

Water seal type spirometer 22
Weaning 114
Welding fumes 17
Wheezes 134
WHO-FCTC 9
Workplace 97

Y

Yoga 172, 192

Z

Zinc 151

Reader's Notes